BIOLOGY AND LANGUAGE

Let us never grow so pedantic that we shall frown on any brother who occasionally goes off the reservation of biological orthodoxy to refresh himself in other fields. He may bring back from his excursion a treasure which those who stay at home can never find.

EDMUND W. SINNOTT, *Science*, 1939, vol. **89**, p. **44**.

BIOLOGY AND LANGUAGE

An Introduction to the
Methodology of the Biological Sciences
including Medicine

BY

J. H. WOODGER, D.Sc.

Professor of Biology in the
University of London

THE TARNER LECTURES
1949–50

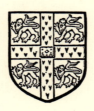

CAMBRIDGE
AT THE UNIVERSITY PRESS
1952

PUBLISHED BY
THE SYNDICS OF THE CAMBRIDGE UNIVERSITY PRESS

London Office: Bentley House, N.W.1
American Branch: New York

Agents for Canada, India, and Pakistan: Macmillan

Printed in Great Britain at the University Press, Cambridge
(Brooke Crutchley, University Printer)

To
ALFRED TARSKI
MY FRIEND AND TEACHER

CONTENTS

PART III. METHODOLOGICAL PROBLEMS IN NEUROLOGY AND RELATED SCIENCES

PREFACE

In these days, when so many books are published, and there is so little time in which to read them, it would seem to be the duty of an author to give some guidance to a possible reader in deciding whether to read his particular book or not. Such guidance is not altogether easy to give because the answer will depend, not only on the quality of the book, for which alone the author is responsible, but also on the interests of the reader. I take it to be the primary business of a book to please and interest the reader; if he also finds it useful in a narrower sense so much the better. This book is addressed chiefly to biologists, and biologists are interested first and foremost in organisms. But here is a difficulty: this book is not primarily about organisms at all, but about *statements* which speak about organisms. Any biologist, therefore, who is not at all interested in statements is strongly recommended to proceed no further. But any biologist whose interest *does* extend to statements about organisms—their laws and the part they play in biology (which are discussed in the first two lectures)—will find that some problems connected therewith have been solved, and some muddles removed, in this book. To learn how this has been done may give the interested reader some intellectual pleasure. But how far he will find such learning useful in the narrower sense it is difficult to say. Whether a book is useful in this sense again depends not only on the author, but on what the reader does with it. If this book provides an incentive, to readers who are prepared to overhaul their linguistic habits, to solve the many problems, and to clarify the many muddles that remain, and if the method of doing so here advocated proves to be helpful for that purpose, then it will be useful. If not, not.

I have already published two books dealing with method, *The Axiomatic Method in Biology* and *The Technique of Theory Construction*. These books were rather technical. The first, especially, was committed to a close adherence to the methods and notation of Whitehead and Russell's *Principia Mathematica*. Since writing those books I have had an opportunity of learning more about these matters and of thinking independently about them. This has enabled me to simplify and clarify the procedure to a very great extent, and I hope the present book will have a wider appeal and be of greater and more direct help in improving the language of biology. It also deals with an aspect of the growth and development of science with which those former books did not deal; namely, with the way in which theoretical statements come to be constructed on the basis provided by observations and experiments. It is hoped that biologists who are interested in such questions, and in the difficult problems connected with the relation between theory and observation, will find here some suggestions to stimulate, and possibly to guide, their own thinking about them.

A few words should perhaps be added in explanation of the occurrence of the words 'including medicine' in my sub-title. The general principles of scientific methodology are the same for all the sciences, and in so far as medicine is a practical application of the biological sciences the methodological principles which especially concern the latter will also apply to the former. To illustrate these principles I have chosen examples from genetics, neurology and medical psychology. I therefore include the word 'medicine' in my sub-title in order to catch the eye of the occasional medical man who is interested in these topics but who would not otherwise suppose that this book was addressed to him.

In parts of this book, especially Part II, symbols and formulas are used. This will be a stumbling block to some. There was opposition at first to the use of formulas in chemistry. Whewell quotes some remarks of the chemist Berzelius on this question:

The use of Formulae has always, for a person who has not accustomed himself to them, something repulsive; but this is easy to overcome. I agree with my opponent, who says that nothing can be understood in a Formula which cannot be expressed in words; and that if the words express it as easily as the Formula, the use of the latter would be a folly. But there are cases in which this is not so; in which the Formula says in a glance what it would take many lines to express in words; and in which the expression of the Formula is clearer and more easily apprehended by the reader than the longer description in words.*

Berzelius then gives an example of a chemical formula which occupies less than half a line of print but which requires eleven lines when expanded into words. As far as chemistry is concerned the verdict of history has been on the side of Berzelius, not on that of his opponent. But abbreviation is not the only or even the primary aim in the introduction of formulas into scientific discourse. Their more important merits (which were not understood at the time at which Berzelius wrote) can only be explained at some length and after the general principles of scientific linguistics have been understood. It is the primary purpose of this book to explain these general principles. Any reader with an inflexible objection to symbols and formulas is recommended to proceed no further. But a reader who is prepared to make an effort to overcome such a dislike will find that no symbols are used here quite arbitrarily but always with reference to a well-established plan and with full explanations, and that all he needs for the operation, if he has the will, are provided within the covers of this one book.

It is also my hope that readers interested in scientific methodology rather than in biology will find something to appeal to them in this book, and that they may feel urged to improve upon what I have done. In this connexion I would draw attention to Part II, and especially to the D-operator, the combined algebra, the composition functor, the method of defining maximized and mutually relativized sets and the theory of the joining of sets by one-one relations (p. 223). In order to avoid going too deeply into technicalities, which would be out of place in this book, I have not attempted a very full working out of these procedures. I hope the explanations given will

---

* W. Whewell, *Novum Organon Renovatum* (1858), p. 360.

suffice to make clear to the non-biological reader what is required. One of the future tasks for biological methodology is the discovery of the kind of mathematics that is required for biology. Considerable use has already been made of some existing branches of mathematics, but these branches have been developed, to a very large extent, to meet the special demands of physics. It will be interesting to discover what new mathematical topics will arise in relation to the needs of biology. Important contributions to the theory of statistics have already been made from this standpoint. I hope the present book may contain some hints which will suggest new mathematical topics arising out of biological problems.

Because scientific statements constitute the subject-matter of methodology it is often necessary to quote examples from well-known authors as specimens for examination. But I am told that in doing this one runs a risk of being rude and of hurting people's feelings. As I do not wish to be rude, and as no useful purpose can be served by hurting people's feelings, I have taken the precaution, in all instances where there seems to be any risk of the results of methodological discussions of this kind giving offence, of omitting the name of the author and the bibliographic reference of the specimen quoted. I can assure the reader that all my specimens are selected from reliable and eminent sources. Given that assurance I do not think anything important is lost if the precise reference is withheld. We *all* make mistakes. If we can learn enough from them to enable us to avoid repeating them in the future, the purely personal question of who made them is of no scientific importance.

The lectures, with the exception of those in Part II, which required much rewriting, have been published almost exactly as they were delivered. But it has been necessary, for reasons given in Lecture I, to supplement them with notes at the end of each Part which qualify or amplify what is stated in the lectures. These notes are to be regarded as an essential part of the book. I have also added, in an Appendix to each Part, other methodological studies which were not used in the lectures.

By the very terms of his appointment a Tarner Lecturer is compelled to deal with some topics in which he cannot possibly be an expert. To all the experts upon whose fields I have trodden with amateurish feet, especially in connexion with Appendix C, I offer my humblest apologies.

I wish to express my thanks and appreciation to the Council of Trinity College, Cambridge, for the honour they have done me in inviting me to become Tarner Lecturer, and for their generous hospitality during my tenure of the lectureship. These lectures were delivered exactly thirty years after the first series was given by A. N. Whitehead, and it is indeed an honour to be a successor of Whitehead in this office, from whom, as well as from many other of my predecessors, I have learnt so much.

Throughout the preparation of these lectures I have been very greatly helped by my son, Michael Woodger, and I am also indebted to the following for reading them in whole or in part and helping me with their criticism: Professors A. J. Ayer, R. Martin, K. Mather, W. V. Quine and A. Tarski; Doctors H. Daitz and W. H. Thorpe; and Messrs B. Dunham and R. Withers. I am further obliged to Mr M. Woodger and to Dr E. Hutten for help in proof reading. For permission to quote a passage from O. Jespersen's *Language, Its Nature, Development and Origin* I am indebted to Messrs George Allen and Unwin Ltd.; and for permission to quote from his translation of Harvey's *De motu cordis* I am obliged to Dr C. D. Leake and the publisher, Charles C. Thomas of Springfield, Illinois, U.S.A. Finally this book and its author owe a great deal to the skill, care and patience that have been devoted to it by all members of the staff of the Cambridge University Press who have been concerned in the production of the book.

J. H. WOODGER

MIDDLESEX HOSPITAL
MEDICAL SCHOOL
LONDON, W.I
July 1951

PART I

GENERAL METHODOLOGY

It will be proved to thy face, that thou hast men about thee, that usually talk of a noun, and a verb, and such abominable words, as no Christian ear can endure to hear.

King Henry VI, Part 2, iv, vii.

LECTURE I

§ 1. BIOLOGY AND THE BOOLE-FREGE MOVEMENT

It is the duty of Tarner lecturers to discuss the Philosophy of the Sciences and the relations or want of relations between the different departments of knowledge. I propose to deal with the relations, and more especially with the want of relations, between the biological sciences and a department of knowledge which, if we date it from Boole's first work (1847) is a little more than, and if we date it from Frege's first work (1879) is considerably less than, one hundred years old.* This is a department of knowledge which is still actively developing, is still so young that it has not yet acquired a very suitable name, and is but little understood except among a comparatively small band of specialists—mostly philosophers and mathematicians —who pursue it for its own sake. Its bearing upon natural science has hardly been considered at all. This seems, therefore, to be an instance of want of relations between the departments of knowledge which should provide a suitable topic for a course of Tarner lectures.

One of the two departments of knowledge whose relations we are to consider being thus relatively unfamiliar, I can best introduce my plan from the standpoint of the other, namely, biology. When we reflect upon what biologists do we find that their most conspicuous activity is the making and recording of observations, which may or may not involve experimentation. But they also do other and less obvious things which, being less obvious, may be overlooked. The making of observations does not take place in an intellectual vacuum, but is preceded and followed by the invention of hypotheses which are tested by recourse to further observations. At very rare intervals these hypotheses have a tremendous effect: they open up entirely new lines of research—creating new branches of science as well

* See Note 1, p. 60.

as affecting older existing branches. Familiar examples are the hypotheses introduced into biology by William Harvey, Charles Darwin, Gregor Mendel and Louis Pasteur. The part played by hypotheses in the work of these celebrated men is obscured by the way in which, in histories of science, they are represented not so much as inventors of hypotheses but as discoverers. Thus Harvey is commonly referred to as the discoverer of the circulation of the blood. But what he actually did was something much more important. He invented a *hypothesis* concerning the action of the heart which had many revolutionary *consequences* for physiology, that there was a circulation of the blood being but *one*.* In this way the distinction between the making of observations and the invention of hypotheses tends to be blurred, and it is even possible to find biologists who deny that hypotheses play any part in their science whatever. They are unaware that they are living on the intellectual capital bequeathed to them by the inventors of hypotheses which they could not have invented themselves and without which their own work would be impossible.†

Some new hypotheses also lead to the invention of new apparatus for observation, and the new observations so made possible suggest further hypotheses, and so on. This process is better illustrated by physics than by biology.

Now in addition to making and recording observations and in addition to inventing hypotheses, there is yet a third and still more obscure activity for biologists. From time to time such questions as the following may arise: Is this biological hypothesis compatible with that one? Does this new hypothesis contradict existing hypotheses? What modification must be made to this theory in view of that recent observation? And so on.

Let us for the present call this third activity *criticism*. Then it is at once obvious that criticism, although it is connected with biological problems, and is part of the activity of biologists, nevertheless deals with the subject-matter of biology only

* See Appendix A, p. 75.   † See Note 2, p. 60.

indirectly—so to speak at second hand. For hypotheses and theories are not organisms, but statements and systems of statements related in some characteristic way. When therefore we turn to criticism, we at the same time change our subject-matter; we are no longer speaking about organisms but about statements. It is important to be clear about this change of subject-matter. Talking biology and talking *about* biology (as we do when we venture upon criticism) are quite different things, although current terminology does not distinguish between them.

It is clear that what I have called criticism can be considered from two points of view. We can regard it, as I have suggested, as an activity intimately connected with the pursuit of biology —one that is rendered necessary by the fact that biology is a growing subject, and its growth is not a simple matter of accretion, but involves frequent readjustment between theory and observation. But we can also regard it as an application to biology of a distinct branch of science which is itself much more general. For it is clear that questions about particular biological hypotheses and theories raise, or are themselves instances of, much wider questions, such as: What sort of object is a hypothesis? Exactly what part do hypotheses play in natural science and how do they play it? What happens when a scientific hypothesis is tested? What constitutes a scientific explanation? How do we decide whether one hypothesis is compatible with another? And so on. The investigation of these wider questions is the task of a distinct science which I will call general scientific methodology. What I have called criticism in biology can be viewed as an application of this science to biology and can be called biological methodology. Its subject-matter, I have said, consists of biological statements.

Now statements are the units of language, and language is just as indispensable a tool for the pursuit of biology as microscopes, kymographs and other instruments. If observations are impossible without the one, their recording and the construction of hypotheses are no less impossible without the other.

This being so, a knowledge of how this tool works in the service of science would seem to be as necessary as it is in the case of other tools used in biology. An understanding of the pitfalls to which a too naïve use of language exposes us is as necessary as some understanding of the artifacts which accompany the use of microscopical techniques. But at present biologists in general receive no instruction in such matters in university courses which otherwise provide for subjects which are considered to be essential in a biological training, and biological criticism is therefore conducted on a purely intuitive basis.*

The reason for this is not far to seek. For one thing no such instruction is believed to be necessary. It is considered sufficient if every biologist is able to speak and write his native language in accordance with the rules of grammar and current usage. I hope to convince you that this belief is quite without foundation.

But even if the necessity or desirability of some such instruction is admitted, it might be argued that no scientific basis for it exists. But this is not true. There *is* available a body of such knowledge, and this brings me back to the second member of the pair of departments of knowledge whose lack of relations we are to investigate. I said at the beginning that the movement which began with Boole and Frege has not yet acquired a very suitable name. I had in mind the fact that this movement is commonly associated with the name 'symbolic' or 'mathematical' logic. But what this movement has in fact provided us with is a general methodology, a new science of scientific languages, and this is not at all suggested by the title 'logic'. It is true that one outcome of this movement has been a great extension of logic beyond the bounds set to it by the Greek and medieval logicians. But what can strictly be called logic forms but a part of what has already been achieved by the Boole-Frege movement.

Nor are the adjectives 'symbolic' and 'mathematical' especi-

* See Note 3, p. 61.

ally illuminating. The use of symbols in this connexion is important and in practice almost indispensable, but it is by no means indispensable in principle. The word 'mathematical' owes its presence here, historically speaking, to the fact that most of the creators of this new discipline were mathematicians, because the motive for its creation sprang from the need to clarify mathematical statements and to investigate the foundations of mathematics.

Boole called his great work *An Investigation of the Laws of Thought*, but what he was in fact investigating were the laws of scientific language. For science can only deal with shared thoughts, and thoughts can only be shared effectively by the use of language.* When I speak of biology I shall mean the system of accepted written or printed biological statements. For whilst it is true that at every moment biology is actively growing in the thoughts of biologists in laboratories all over the world, these thoughts cannot be the subject of scientific study until they have been communicated by the help of marks on paper. This, then, is the other member of the pair of topics whose relations or want of relations we are to consider: the laws governing the use of language in the service of science.

Let me give some of the reasons why methodological considerations are sooner or later forced upon us. First, because biology, considered as a system of statements, is distributed among a number of natural languages, English, French, Russian, etc., and these European languages have been greatly influenced in their development by Greek logic and Greek metaphysics as well as by the naïve realism of everyday life. In so far, therefore, as it may become necessary to consider the significance of such influences for science, it will also be necessary to bear in mind these peculiarities of the languages which are the vehicles of science.

Again, English is not only used for purposes of communication in the scientific sense. It is also used for the writing of poetry, for religious devotion, for political controversy and for

* See Note 4, p. 62.

persuading people to buy some of the products of industrial activity which they would not otherwise want. But these pursuits make demands upon language which are very different from those made by science. The requirements of science prove on investigation to be quite surprisingly meagre, and the excessive riches of a natural language like English are a source of embarrassment. They tempt us to employ linguistic devices borrowed from extra-scientific usages which can have unfortunate consequences. Metaphors, for example, with which some branches of biology abound, are often suggestive and may be harmless enough if they are recognized for what they are. But at best they are makeshifts and substitutes for genuine biological statements, and the fact that recourse is had to them is surely a sign of immaturity. Science demands great linguistic austerity and discipline, and the canons of good style in scientific writing are different from those in other kinds of literature.

Yet again, biology, like other sciences, begins with observations on the familiar things of everyday life, and its results are at first adequately expressed in the language of everyday life. But as it advances it widens the scope of its observations. The invention of successful hypotheses brings with it the invention of new apparatus for observation. The records of observations made with such apparatus are meaningless apart from the theory of the apparatus—the hypotheses which have led to its invention. Is it not to be expected then that sooner or later the linguistic habits of everyday life will cease to do justice to this increasing complexity and novelty of observation and hypothesis? If we consider the kind of activities in which English-speaking people have been engaged, during the long period in which the language has been developing, it will not surprise us to find that this language cannot, without some modification, cope with the problems with which embryology and genetics now have to deal. This seems to be one reason why recourse is so often had to metaphors in these sciences.

Then there is another important point. Language resembles dress in this respect, that what is suitable to one occasion of its use may be quite unsuitable to another. Moreover, in both cases people may differ very much regarding what is suitable. Suppose we could arrange linguistic expressions in a scale of increasing precision, and suppose we could arrange the occasions of their use in a similar scale of increasing requirement of precision, then we could see that there are two ways in which the two scales could be out of correlation. We may be using a language which is more precise than the occasion demands, or we may be using one which is not precise enough. In the first case we have a name in common use for the situation: we say we are being pedantic. But in the second case there does not seem to be a corresponding word—a derogatory word—in common use. And yet, this is just the situation which is likely to arise with the development of science. I am assuming that as a science develops and gets further and further away from everyday observations, its language will lag behind its needs, unless especial care is taken from time to time to see that the necessary readjustments are made.

It must also be understood that language in science is not only used for the purpose of communication, for recording of observations and for formulating hypotheses. It is also used for calculation. That is to say, it should be such as to facilitate the working out of the consequences of our hypotheses so that we may test them. But so long as we confine ourselves to a natural language like English, such calculation becomes exceedingly difficult and tedious as soon as the statements become long and complicated. We are then forced to construct languages which are at least in part symbolic or we must make use of one which has already been constructed. Surely it is no accident that the two sciences which are most highly developed are also the two which most use symbolic languages. I refer of course to physics and chemistry. It seems reasonable to suppose that the invention of chemical equations has played an important part in the development of chemistry. And these equations, unlike those of physics, are not mathematical equations, because they contain symbols which do not belong to the vocabulary of mathematics. In a later lecture I shall submit to you some biological equations which, for the same reason, are also not mathematical equations. Among the things which the results of the Boole-Frege movement can do for us is the provision of guidance for the construction of such scientific languages.

I have already emphasized the distinction between talking biology and talking *about* biology, and I have called the science which talks about biology biological methodology. But there is another more general pair of terms which is often convenient and, although it will be my aim to restrict technical terminology as far as possible, I think the following pair of terms is sufficiently general and useful to warrant introduction here. The language *in which* we speak may be called the *object* language, and the language we use when we speak *about* the object language is then called its *metalanguage*. Similarly, we may speak of a theory and its metatheory. Thus biology will be our theory and the methodology of biology will be our metatheory.*

Within any given metalanguage there is a further subdivision which is of the greatest importance. Every language has at least two aspects. It consists of words or other signs which, when combined in appropriate ways, yield statements. This is the structural or syntactical aspect. But these words or other signs (or some of them) have reference to something which is not part of the language but which constitutes its subject-matter. They are said to 'have meaning', and the statements constructed from them are said to be true or false. This aspect is therefore called the semantical aspect. In consequence of this, every metalanguage will have two branches: a syntactical branch which enumerates the signs of the object language, and enunciates the rules of their meaningful combinations and their truth-preserving transformations, and a semantical branch which deals with the connexion between the object language and its subject-matter, the questions of denotation and truth.

I must hasten to add that these distinctions are of little importance in connexion with natural languages. From both

* See Note 5, p. 62.

the syntactical and the semantical points of view natural languages are incredibly complicated and unruly. The rules of ordinary grammar are quite insufficient from the standpoint of the requirements of science, and the problems connected with meaning and truth in relation to natural languages are enormously complicated and perhaps insoluble. If therefore we require a precise object language for some scientific purpose we are driven to construct one deliberately, using English as metalanguage. The syntactical statements will tell us what is in it, and the semantical ones will tell us under what conditions some of its statements are true. In this way a small area of the wilderness is walled off and tamed and so made manageable.

These lectures will fall into three parts. In Part I, I shall explain the structure and classification of biological statements and the way in which they are related to one another in theories. In Part II the results of Part I will be applied to certain methodological problems of genetics. It will be shown how a workable, partly symbolic, language can be constructed for genetics, and how this can be used to clarify certain obscurities which have been a source of controversy in that science. In Part III some methodological problems connected with neurology and related sciences will be discussed.

I should explain that these topics do not lend themselves very readily to exposition by lecture. They are better studied in books. All that can be attempted in a lecture is the stimulation of interest and the explanation of the bare outline of the scheme proposed. But to do no more than this would be to create a false impression of the procedure. The results of applying general methodology will only be impressive and useful if they are carried out in complete and convincing detail in relation to particular topics. The reason why these topics are not suitable for exposition by lecture is not at all on account of the difficulty of the subjects treated but simply because they are complicated and take time to explain. To give lists of definitions and strings of formulas in a lecture would be tedious and useless, because no audience would be expected to absorb them in the time allotted to a few lectures. But it is the custom to publish these lectures in book form. I shall therefore attempt a compromise: with the help of lantern slides I shall show you in outline what I have done and leave the details to be expounded in the book.

Finally, I feel that I ought to make it quite clear that I cannot claim to be an expert on the Boole-Frege movement and its results. Neither can I claim to be an expert on any branch of biology. But I have devoted a great deal of time to the study of possible ways in which one can help the other, and I hope I have learnt at least enough of both to enable me to make a beginning in working out some of these possibilities. On this I therefore feel that I can speak with some authority, although I am very far from supposing that I shall not make mistakes. One thing I beg of you: that you will not attribute to the Boole-Frege movement any blame for my errors of execution, for the seeming triviality of my examples or for the shortcomings of my exposition.

§ 2. THE CLASSIFICATION OF BIOLOGICAL STATEMENTS

I propose to divide biological statements in the first instance into two mutually exclusive groups: (1) observation records and (2) theoretical statements. Observation records are statements of the kind we usually find in the field or laboratory note-books of biologists. They rarely find their way into general treatises or even into the papers published in the learned journals. But by no means all statements found in laboratory note-books are observation records. A botanist, for example, might record in his note-book that from a certain plant a certain quantity of carbon dioxide had been evolved during a certain night. But this would not be an example of what I mean by an observation record. For the botanist would not in fact have observed the evolution of so many grammes of carbon dioxide. He would have observed, perhaps, the formation of a precipitate in a glass vessel, and the number of weights required to balance it after it had been collected and dried. It is convenient to record the final result as so many grammes of carbon dioxide, but it is only possible to do so with the help of a considerable amount of chemical theory. By observation records I shall mean, therefore, statements which record observations with the help of no more theory than is inevitably involved in common-sense language. It seems clear that all scientific observation records, however recondite they may be and however elaborate the apparatus involved in making the observations, must be translatable into common-sense statements about objects which we can look at or touch.

Let us first examine some observation records from the structural or syntactical point of view. Suppose a geneticist is using rats in an experiment and has labelled his animals 'a', 'b', 'c', ..., etc. Then he might write down in his note-book such statements as:

(1) a is black,
(2) a weighs 6 ounces,
(3) a is female parent of b,
(4) b was mated to c on 1 May 1947.

From the syntactical point of view it is customary to recognize *two* kinds of linguistic elements in these statements. First there are the rat labels 'a', 'b', 'c' and the date label '1 May 1947', and then, coupled with these, are such phrases as 'is black', 'weighs 6 ounces', 'is female parent of' etc. Let us call the rat labels and the date label *individual names*, and let us call all the other phrases *functors*. Then we can say that (1) and (2) both consist of one individual name coupled with a functor, (3) consists of two individual names coupled with a functor, and (4) is constructed by means of a functor associated with three individual names. Clearly these form the first few terms of a sequence which could be continued.

The number of occurrences of individual names which must be coupled with a functor to yield a complete statement is called the *degree* of the functor. Thus 'is black' is of degree one; 'is female parent of' is of degree two, and so on. I shall assume that every observation record of the simplest type (i.e. one which does not contain a proper part which is a statement) consists of a functor of some finite degree n coupled with n individual names.

By way of illustration of the fact that English frequently does not reveal the form of statements we may consider the following examples:

> (5) Tom loves Mary,
> (6) Tom loves dogs,
> (7) Tom loves justice,

and

> (8) Tom is going to Oxford,
> (9) Tom is going to sleep.

At first sight it might appear that all these statements contain one functor of degree two; and this does seem to be the case in (5) and (8); but since 'dogs' and 'justice' can hardly be regarded as individual names—and the same applies to 'sleep' —the remaining statements must have a more complicated, but concealed, structure than (5) and (8).

The consideration of these examples involves reference to the semantical aspect of these statements. The individual names 'a', 'b', etc., seem at first sight to present no great difficulty. Each labels a particular rat which is assumed to persist in its cage throughout the experiment and to be easily recognizable from one day to the next. We can think of the letter as being punched on a metal disk and fastened round the neck of the rat. In war-time even Tom and Mary may have their identity disks, and a date can be labelled by means of a calendar hanging on the wall, which is changed every twenty-four hours. But in the case of 'is black', 'is female parent of', 'loves', 'dogs' and 'justice' this will not do. They do not seem to label anything which can have an identity disk and yet they are said to 'have meaning', otherwise the statements in which they occur would not convey any information, as they evidently do.

There are two traditional ways of dealing with this problem which may be called the intensional and the extensional methods. According to the first, functors name *properties* or attributes, and a statement, formed by coupling the appropriate number of individual names with the functor, asserts that the individual objects named *have* the property, or attribute. According to the second or extensional method, functors name *sets* or *classes*, and a statement formed with a functor asserts that the individual objects named are *members* of the set or class named by the functor.

There are objections to both of these methods. For one thing they both appear to commit us to the recognition of abstract entities in addition to individual particular objects. The first alternative raises such questions as: How does a property differ from an individual object, and what precisely is meant by saying that one 'has' the other? The extensional method leaves us with the problem: What do we mean by a set or class?

If we had to choose between these two alternatives I have no doubt that, for the purpose of natural science, the extensional procedure is the better one. But I should like to offer a third possibility which avoids the objectional features of both of the foregoing. Let me introduce what I have to say on this subject by means of a fictitious story of my own invention. I call it the story of Naamba:

Once upon a time, long long ago, there dwelt in a village which later was called Naamba (the precise geographical location of which need not detain us) a people endowed with the power of recognition and speech but, to begin with, a very limited vocabulary. They had demonstrative pronouns and made great use of gestures, but they had no proper names, nouns or adjectives.

The results of acts of recognition in space they expressed in the form:

'here is another of those';

and the results of acts of recognition in time they expressed in the form:

'here is another of those' *or* 'here is that again'.

Finding this highly inconvenient one of these people—a man of great originality—invented proper names. This man, whenever he recognized his pet dog, said:

'here is Fido again',

and whenever he recognized another object which was more like Fido than anything else, but at the same time obviously *not* Fido again, he said:

'here is *another* Fido'.

But this also proved to be inconvenient and insufficient, because another inhabitant, copying the first, had decided to call his dog 'Dido'. So instead of one saying 'here is another Fido' and the other saying 'here is another Dido' they agreed each to keep his own name for his own pet, but both to say:

'here is another bobo',

when they recognized Fido-like *or* Dido-like objects.

Along these lines the inhabitants of Naamba gradually began to enlarge their language. They also devised ways of speaking about objects when they were not actually present.

One day, many years later, the same two men, being of a philosophical turn of mind, fell into a dispute about the difference between 'Fido', which one of them applied to his pet, and 'bobo', which each used for either pet and for any animal like them. One of these men maintained that, whilst 'Fido' was a label for one individual object, namely, his pet dog, 'bobo' was not a name for a concrete object at all, but for something abstract and intangible of which, as he expressed it, all Fido-like objects partake. The other man maintained that 'bobo' was a name for the class or set of all Fido-like objects, which must be carefully distinguished, not only from each particular one, but even from the physical collection of all such objects then living, because it included all the dead ones and all those not yet born.

At this stage in the discussion, after the same arguments had been repeatedly advanced on both sides, a third philosopher, the oldest man in the village, tottered up to the pair. He had at first been opposed to the introduction of names. Leaning heavily on his stick, be began:

'What's this I hear? Abstract, intangible entities? Sets and classes? Stuff and nonsense! The situation is really quite simple, but you create all sorts of difficulties with your fine talk. Let me explain.

'When we decided to use names we applied them, in the first instance, to objects of an enduring kind in our immediate day-to-day experience which we could recognize as being the same objects from one day to another. You called one of these objects Fido, you chose Dido for yours. I call mine Carno. Now there is no reason why they should not have *other names* as well. So we have called them, in effect, bobo Fido, bobo Dido and bobo Carno. If another object like these strays into the village we are able to call it bobo also, and to say: Here is another bobo; although we may not know, until its owner turns up, what other names it may have. So there is the answer to your problem. It is not two kinds of *objects* that you have to distinguish, but two kinds of *names*, namely, *shared names* and *unshared names*. And that is all there is to it, so don't let me hear any more of this nonsense. Why, bless my soul, haven't you both decided to call yourselves 'Jumbo' because you both live in the same hut—you being Fumbo Jumbo and you Dumbo Jumbo? There the situation is exactly the same.'*

So ends the story of Naamba. It will be seen that the old philosopher was advocating the type of nominalistic attitude towards the problems I mentioned at the beginning which has been characteristic of the English empiricists from Hobbes onwards. We must now see whether the hints he offered can be worked out in more detail.

What I wish to suggest is that 'Fido is a dog' and 'Fido has the properties of a dog' and 'Fido is a member of the set of dogs' are all different ways of saying that, in English-speaking communities, the object to which the name 'Fido' has been

* See Note 6, p. 62.

assigned by its owner is also named by the shared name 'dog'. Against this it may be objected that this merely tells us something extrinsic and accidental about Fido, namely, how certain people apply names to him, and that 'Fido is a dog' expresses a fact of natural history which would still be the case even if no one existed to name Fido at all. But in discussing the statement 'Fido is a dog' we are not speaking about natural history but about a linguistic unit and the parts of such units called names. Shared names are not assigned to objects quite arbitrarily, otherwise the purposes of communication would not be realized. Fido is named by 'dog' because of his resemblance, his recognizable likeness, to other objects to which that name is applied—because of the shapes and colours we see when we look at him, because of the sounds we hear when he barks, and the smells we smell when he is to windward of us. Moreover, Fido eats meat, not hay. All this and much more is asserted when we say that 'dog' names Fido. *Which* name is assigned in the first instance in a given community is of course arbitrary, but when once a name has been assigned its further application is *not* arbitrary if communication is to be achieved.

A certain element of arbitrariness does, however, enter the situation owing to the fact that dog-like animals shade off into other animals such as foxes, wolves, etc. This must be allowed for and our interpretation must be amended to read:

'Fido is *sufficiently like* other objects named by "dog" to be also named by "dog".'

Moreover, there is yet a further complication. Not only is Fido named by 'dog' but also by 'Dog' and by 'DOG' and by '*dog*'. This is because we regard all these marks as being *sufficiently like* one another to be all instances of what we call 'the same name'. Accordingly we must expand 'Fido is a dog' into:

'Fido is sufficiently like other objects that are named by "dog" to be also named by any written or printed mark which is sufficiently like "dog".'

The phrase 'Fido is sufficiently like other objects' thus involves a tacit reference to some *community of persons* within which there is agreement regarding the degree to which two objects may differ and still both be named by 'dog', and also regarding the degree to which two marks may differ and still both be regarded as instances of the same name. In ordinary language such degrees of allowable diversity are rarely expressed verbally, and even scientific classification, which attempts to formulate them, is frequently confronted with difficulties which can only be resolved by establishing arbitrary barriers to the assignment of names. These difficulties are well exemplified by the disputes among biologists regarding species, some (the splitters) being inclined to accept distinctions which others (the lumpers) are prepared to disregard. Their disputes are therefore about where the process of subdivision should stop.

I believe it should be possible to express all that can be expressed in the class theory with the help of the notion of naming and by the division of names into (i) unshared names, i.e. names which name exactly one object, and (ii) shared names, or names which name *more* than one object.

Let us suppose that we have a language in which names are divided in this way, small letters being used for unshared and capital letters for shared names, and let us further suppose that statements of the simplest form are constructed in this language simply by the *juxtaposition* of two names. We also lay down the very simple semantical rule that such a simple statement is to be accepted if and only if everything named by the first (or left-hand) name is also named by the second (or right-hand) name. Then there are three and only three possibilities for accepted statements constructed in this way:

(1) both names are unshared: e.g. 'xy';

(2) the first is unshared, the second shared: e.g. 'yX';

(3) both names are shared: e.g. 'XY'.

In a language in which shared names are regarded as names of classes we should have, corresponding to (1): '$x = y$'; and corresponding to (2) we should have statements of the form 'y is a member of the set X'; and finally, corresponding to (3), we should have statements of the form 'the set X is included in the set Y'.

This very simple language would thus be able to cover a great deal of the ground covered by traditional set theory without using the notion of set. But now the question arises what shall we do about sets of sets? In the language of *Principia Mathematica*, for example, '9' is defined as the set of all sets which have exactly nine members, so that to say that the set of planets is a member of this set is to say that there are exactly nine planets. This problem could be solved, I believe, by introducing a new linguistic entity which is not a name at all but is called an *abbreviator*. When juxtaposed with a shared name to the right of it we obtain a statement which is an abbreviation for a longer statement which contains the shared name but not the abbreviator. But an example of this device cannot be given until the structure of theoretical statements has been explained in the next lecture.

I offer this as a possible answer to the question: What is a class or set? It answers by refusing to recognize such objects as sets. But it does not reject sets in favour of properties as is done in *Principia Mathematica*. It speaks only of concrete objects, of two kinds of names, and of abbreviators. I shall return to this point later. Meanwhile having said this I shall continue to speak of sets because this is more familiar.*

There is, however, one point where the account given by the old philosopher of Naamba requires correction. He fell into the error of supposing that proper names were unshared names. Let us consider some familiar name, such as 'Winston Spencer Churchill'. In 1909 the person named by this name was a member of the Liberal party, and in 1949 the person so named was a member of the Conservative party. But the Liberal party in 1909 and the Conservative party in 1949 have no members in common. Consequently the object named by 'Winston Spencer Churchill' in 1909 is not identical with that so named in 1949. Therefore 'Winston Spencer Churchill' is a shared name.

It is difficult to formulate this argument in ordinary language in a way which is free from objections. To meet such objections

---

* See Note 7, p. 63.

we must proceed more analytically. Let us use 'W' as an abbreviation for the name 'Winston Spencer Churchill', 'L' as an abbreviation for the name 'member of the Liberal party during 1909' and 'C' as an abbreviation for the name 'member of the Conservative party during 1949'. Let us further suppose that the following statements are accepted:

> something is named by both 'W' and 'L';
> something is named by both 'W' and 'C';
> nothing is named by both 'L' and 'C'

(because everything named by 'L' begins and ends in 1909 and everything named by 'C' begins and ends in 1949, and an object x cannot be identical with an object y unless the beginning of x is identical with the beginning of y and the end of x is identical with the end of y, *strict* identity being intended). If all this is granted, then the object named by both 'W' and 'L' must be distinct from the object named by 'W' and 'C'. Hence 'W' names at least two distinct objects and so is not an unshared name.

Nevertheless, there is a very important difference between a shared name of this kind and a shared name like 'man', or 'dog'. It is possible to have two objects, both called or named 'man', which have the same time but different space coordinates, whereas if 'Winston Spencer Churchill' is a genuine proper name any two objects named by it must have different time coordinates. There is, moreover, another difference. Between any two objects named by such a proper name there is, in time, either a continuum of such objects or they overlap in a common part which also shares the name. But nothing of this kind is true of two objects with the same time coordinates named by 'man'. In order to distinguish these two types of shared name let us call those of the 'Winston Churchill' type *proper* names and those of which 'man' is the type common or *general* names.

I have dealt with these points at some length because they are important from the point of view of biological language.

Let me expand these remarks a little further in order to explain the terminology I shall use.

I call any continuous part of the time extent of an organism a *time-stretch* of that organism. I take the word 'stretch' from *Principia Mathematica* (*215).* There the authors say: 'A *stretch* of a series is any piece taken out of it, and not having any gaps; that is, it is a class contained in the series, and containing all the terms which come between any two of its terms.' But an intuitive understanding of a time-stretch is sufficient for our present purposes. I treat time-stretches as individuals, not as classes.

If the beginning of a time-stretch is identical with the beginning of the organism of which it is a time-stretch then I call it a *life*. If the end of the one also coincides with the end of the other, then time-stretch and organism are one and the same thing and I speak of a life which is *complete in time*. If we adopt the usual assumptions regarding the continuity of time there will be an infinity of lives which are parts of any given complete life, all of which are named by the proper name. If we want an unshared name for any one of these lives we use the proper name coupled with a date-name or with a designation of some time-length or age, as we call it, because two distinct lives which are both parts of the same complete life cannot have the same end. For example: a certain short time-stretch of Winston Spencer Churchill will be called 'Winston on his first birthday', another will be called 'Winston at age 4', another will be 'Winston on 1 January 1940', and so on. These of course are not lives but time-stretches with unspecified beginning.†

Among our first examples of observation records we had '*a* is black', where '*a*' was called an individual name of a rat and was supposed to be punched on a metal disk round the neck of the animal. It is clear that '*a*' is what I am now calling a proper name and hence a shared name. In order that the above should be an observation record there must be an unshared name intro-

* A. N. Whitehead and B. A. W. Russell, *Principia Mathematica* (1927), vol. II, p. 665.   † See Note 8, p. 64.

duced, and so there is, but in this case it is only tacit. The observer will no doubt have written the date at the top of the page of his note-book, and it will be rat a on this date which is black.

Let me summarize this somewhat complicated discussion about observation records. An observation record is a statement composed of a functor or shared name of degree n, coupled with n occurrences of individual or unshared names. A functor of degree 1 names single objects, one of degree 2 names ordered couples of objects, and one of degree n names ordered n-tuples of objects. For example: in 'York is north of London' the functor 'north of' names the ordered couple York, London, but not the ordered couple London, York. Incidentally 'York, London' is not an unshared name, so unless a date-name is added 'York is north of London' is not an observation record.

Let me now attempt the somewhat difficult task of explaining further why the extensional point of view is superior in natural science to the intensional.

For one thing, mathematics is purely extensional, and the theory of sets or classes is, in more than one sense of the word, the most elementary part of mathematics. Hence in using set-theory we have already begun to employ mathematical methods. For that reason the distinction between intension and extension seems to me to be basic to the more often discussed, but not always clear, distinction between 'qualitative' and 'quantitative'. Mathematics is always extensional but not necessarily always quantitative.*

But the use of the extensional method in natural science does not enable us to avoid all use of property-words. For in natural science, unlike mathematics, we do not deal with sets in the abstract, but only with certain empirically specified sets. But as a rule we can only specify the sets in which we are interested by the use of some property-word which names all the members of the set. But even here a superiority of the extensional method reveals itself; for if two property-words name exactly the same

* See Note 9, p. 64.

objects they both determine the same set. Thus if it is the case that every rational animal is a featherless biped and every featherless biped is a rational animal, then there is only one set involved whether we specify it as the set of featherless bipeds or as the set of rational animals.

But although we must use property-words in order to specify sets, there is all the difference in the world between using property-words for that purpose and *talking about properties*. I firmly believe that, if biologists could be persuaded to avoid this latter procedure we should witness an enormous improvement in biological writing.* This is well illustrated by genetics. Geneticists speak about properties or characters and also about phenotypes. Now a phenotype is a set of organisms or lives specified by the help of one or more property-words of a certain sort. So long as we speak about phenotypes we are therefore speaking about sets and are being extensional. This has the further advantage of facilitating the linking of genetics with embryology, which deals with lives and their parts but not with characters. But now, if instead of saying

the pea-plant a is tall

we say

tallness characterizes a,

we are tempted to construct such statements as

tallness in peas is a dominant character,

which in itself is harmless enough because it can easily be translated into the extensional statement:

> All the offspring from crossing a homozygous tall pea with a dwarf pea are tall.

But we then easily slip into such statements as

tallness is handed down from parent to offspring,

which is at best an unfortunate metaphor and at worst a most misleading product of the intensional point of view which has generated enormous confusion during the short history of genetics.

* See Note 10, p. 65.

Now let me give an example of an analogous procedure from embryology.

It is found that certain embryonic parts will pass through a developmental process of a certain kind provided they are in a certain spatial relation to certain other parts, and provided they are not too young and not too old. Within this prescribed temporal stretch the embryonic parts in question are said to be *competent* with respect to the type of developmental process concerned. Thus we can construct statements of the form

the part a is competent with respect to process P.

So far so good. But now the abstract noun *competence* is introduced and used in such contexts as the following:

it is clear that several competences may exist side by side in the same cell-region.

Now when we say

a and b exist side by side in the same cell-region

'a' and 'b' will denote cells or cell-parts and so competences will be cells or cell-parts. But in that case the statement quoted will simply state that several cells or cell-parts may exist side by side in the same cell-region. And this cannot be what is intended. What presumably is intended is simply that one and the same cell-region can be competent with respect to two or more distinct kinds of developmental process. But, if this *is* what is meant, nothing seems to be gained by the introduction of the word 'competence'. It does not denote a set of individual objects, and consequently when we speak of competences existing side by side we are being highly metaphorical and only creating obstacles to further progress and better understanding. Finally, when we encounter such statements as

it must be the gene which determines the properties of the competence,

we have a further step in the piling up of abstract entities. For we now not only have such monstrosities as competences to contend with but also *their properties*! Nothing is easier than to slip into the habit of using elliptical expressions of this kind without being able to say precisely what they assert, and hence without properly knowing what we are saying. This illustrates what I mean when I say that more is involved in scientific writing than conformity with English grammar and English usage. At the same time this habit is not difficult to avoid. It is a good practical maxim, when we are confronted with a word, about the scientific respectability of which we are in doubt, to ask: What is its extension? What is its degree? If a clear answer is not forthcoming the word should be regarded with suspicion and used with caution. A number of words in common use in embryology and genetics do not emerge very well from this test.*

There is another difficulty about properties which must be dealt with at this stage. I must explain what I mean by *sensible objects*. Suppose you are taken blindfold to a stable where horses are kept. Sooner or later you are likely to become aware of a characteristic odour and you may give utterance to the statement:

I smell a horse,

or that is a smell of a horse,

and you will agree, I hope, that what you are referring to by 'that' is the smell, not the horse, and that 'I smell a horse' is an abbreviated way of saying

I smell a smell which is *of* a horse.

If you prolong your stay a little you may hear a characteristic sound and you may say

that is a sound of a horse.

Next you may come to closer quarters, and by extending your hand you may experience a characteristic warm silky feel and say

that is a feel of a horse.

These smells, sounds and feels are examples of what I mean by *sensible objects*, and they are all clearly distinct from the horse or the parts of the horse.

* See p. 180.

But now the bandage is removed from your eyes and behold, you proclaim:

I see a horse.

But do you? Is not this (as was the case with the smell) an abbreviated way of saying

I see a look or view which is *of* a horse?

It is true that in everyday life we do not usually distinguish between a look and the object *of which* it is a look (and this is a good example of the way in which a false theory can nevertheless be successful); it is also true that some philosophers have maintained that a look is actually part of the surface of that of which it is a look, but I must confess I can see no justification for making such a fundamental distinction between visual sensible objects and others.* Looks behave in quite a different manner from the way the objects of which they are looks are believed to behave. We all believe that railway lines are parallel, but if we stand in the middle of the track and look along the lines the looks are not parallel. Moreover, in dreams we may become aware of looks and other sensible objects which are not *of* anything, certainly not *of* horses. We do not stable horses in our bedrooms.

I do not wish to discuss sensible objects any further at this stage. I should say, however, that I am not assuming that they are in any way discrete entities, in spite of the fact that we can discriminate them from the continuum in which they are embedded. Neither do I wish to call them sense *data* because that might seem to suggest that I am assuming more about them than in fact I am assuming.

I am chiefly interested in the relation denoted by the little word 'of' in the contexts in which I have been using it. Let us consider this relation a little further, and in order to emphasize it let us promote its designation to capital letters and write it **OF**. In order to have a non-committal terminology I should like to borrow a couple of technical terms from the relation theory

* See, for example, *The Philosophy of G. E. Moore* (1942), p. 646.

of *Principia Mathematica*.* There the set of all objects which stand in a given relation R *to* something is called the *domain* of that relation. In the case of the relation **OF** the domain will consist exclusively of sensible objects, although not *all* sensible objects belong to it. Now the set of all objects *to which* something stands in a given relation R is called the *converse domain* of R. In the case of **OF** the converse domain will therefore be the set of all objects to which sensible objects stand in this relation. Some people might say that the converse domain of **OF** is identical with the set of all physical objects. But there are objects spoken of in science and called physical to which nothing stands in **OF**, and I shall maintain later that there are objects belonging to the converse domain of **OF** which are not physical objects, and in any case, in pursuit of my aim to use a non-committal terminology I shall simply call this set the converse domain of **OF**.†

Now throughout its history there has been a more or less deliberate striving to restrict the vocabulary of natural science to the names of objects belonging to the converse domain of **OF**. For example:

rat a now is female parent of rat b now

makes no explicit reference to sensible objects. It asserts that, at some time prior to now, rat a gave birth to rat b. It thus asserts that two members of the converse domain of **OF** stand in a certain relation to one another; in other words, that the shared name 'mother of' of degree 2 names the ordered pair a now, b now. There is of course an implicit reference to sensible objects in the sense that unless someone had observed certain sensible objects which are **OF** rats a and b there would be no grounds for asserting that the parental relation holds between them.

On the other hand

rat a now is black

---

* See *Principia Mathematica*, vol. I, p. 247; or my *Axiomatic Method in Biology* (1937), p. 32.

† More is said about this in Part III, see p. 262.

involves an explicit reference to a sensible object. But I wish
to maintain that this also asserts that a certain relation holds
between two objects—one belonging to the domain, and one
to the converse domain of **OF**. I wish to maintain that the
above statement asserts that a sensible object named 'black' in
English stands in **OF** to the object named 'rat a now'. No
doubt anyone who wrote such a statement in his note-book
would *intend* much more than that. He would no doubt believe,
and perhaps intend to say, that, since as a rule when once a
rat is black it stays black, rat a will continue to look black.
But such considerations take us out of the set of observation
records, and at the moment we are only considering observation
records, and the above was offered as an example of one. If
we write down

Mr Smith's temperature now is 102° F.

(which is an observation record) we do not intend this to suggest
that we believe that Mr Smith's temperature will be 102° F.
to-morrow.

I hope no one will suppose that I am deliberately making
mountains out of molehills or wilfully displaying unnecessary
subtlety. Nothing of the sort is intended. I am merely trying
to be consistently nominalistic, and to show how we can avoid
the pitfalls which spring from a failure to be nominalistic.

I will conclude these remarks on observation records with
a few explanations regarding notation. When we have to deal
with complicated functors it is often a great help to use single
letters as abbreviations for them. For this purpose I shall use
capital letters such as F, G, H, etc., or letters specially chosen
to aid the memory. As unshared names I shall use small letters
like a, b, c, etc. In order to construct statements with functors
of degree 1, I shall use the usual sign of set-membership 'ϵ'.
Thus '$a \epsilon F$' will be read: a is a member of the set F.* In the
case of functors of degree 2, which are said to denote two-

---

* Where single letters are being used for illustrative purposes I sometimes
write 'Fa' instead of '$a \epsilon F$'.

termed relations, or sets of ordered couples, I shall write statements of the form '*aGb*' which are to be read: *a* stands in relation *G* to *b*. Finally, in the case of functors of degree greater than 2, I shall write first the functor, followed by the appropriate number of unshared names enclosed in brackets and separated by commas.* Thus if '*H*' is of degree 3, '*H(a, b, c)*' will be read: *a*, *b* and *c* stand in the three-termed relation *H* to one another; or the ordered triple *a*, *b*, *c* belongs to the set *H* of triples; or, finally, '*H*' names the triple *a*, *b*, *c*.

---

* Some functors are of no fixed degree but can be used with different numbers of individual designations. Such functors are said to be *multigrade*. The technical terminology in this and the next lecture is very largely borrowed from W. V. Quine's *Mathematical Logic* (1940).

LECTURE II

§ 1. THEORETICAL STATEMENTS

In the last lecture I spoke about observation records. Such statements rarely find their way into print. Our next task is therefore to consider those biological statements which are not observation records. I shall call them *theoretical statements*.* Theoretical statements are distinguished from observation records by the fact that they contain no unshared names; they are general statements, not statements about particular objects. Theoretical statements of the simplest kind are those which I shall call generalizations of observation records. William Harvey found, in the animals on which he experimented, that the spurting of blood from a punctured artery immediately followed the systole of the heart, not the diastole, as his contemporaries believed. From these observations on *particular* vertebrates he passed to the general statement that this was so in *all* vertebrates. Pasteur's observations on the correlation between invasion of the body by micro-organisms and certain diseased conditions led to the generalization that *all* diseased conditions were so correlated with some specific parasitic invasion. This generalization was subsequently falsified by the discovery of the deficiency diseases, although only after prolonged controversy, during which the curious argument was used that 'a *positive* condition of disease could not be caused by a *negative* factor, such as a deficiency in the diet'†—in spite of the fact that mankind had for centuries been only too familiar with the deficiency disease known (at least to the laity) as starvation.

The characteristic feature of this type of theoretical statement

---

* In thus contrasting observation records and theoretical statements I do not *at all* wish to suggest that what I am calling observation records are in *no* sense theoretical, but only that in natural science they are usually adopted as basic statements by which all others are tested. Within natural science their further 'justification' is usually not discussed.

† J. C. Drummond and A. Wilbraham, *The Englishman's Food* (1940), p. 320.

is thus the passage from a finite number of observation records to a statement which appears to be about an inaccessible *all*. 'All rats have two parents' is a generalization (from a multitude of observation records) which we do not know to be true because we cannot examine all rats.

But the set of theoretical statements in biology is by no means exhausted by generalizations of observation records. When in some branch of investigation a number of such generalizations have been established, it may be possible to construct a statement which is such that all these generalizations (and many others) *follow from* it as necessary consequences. I shall call these additional theoretical statements *explanatory hypotheses* of the *first order* or *level*.*

But the process of theory building need not end here. With the still further development of the particular branch of science concerned, a number of such explanatory hypotheses may come to be set up, and then it may be possible—if our inventive powers are equal to the task—to repeat the former process by introducing a new theoretical statement which will have all the first-order hypotheses among its necessary consequences. We thus reach explanatory hypotheses of the *second order* or level. Clearly this process can, in principle, be continued indefinitely.

In this way a pyramid of layers of hypotheses is built up, each member of a given level (except the top level) being a consequence of at least one member of the level immediately above it. We can call the generalizations of observation records hypotheses (but not explanatory hypotheses) of *zero level*. All the statements belonging to the pyramid are hypotheses in the sense that each *says more* than is asserted by the statements which have suggested its introduction.

We can thus far discern three roles which hypotheses play in science: (1) they have a classificatory role, grouping generalizations into larger and larger groups; (2) by virtue of the links thus established between them each generalization receives a much wider support than it does from the observation records upon

* See Note 11, p. 67.

which it directly stands. Thus the generalization, 'All adult mammals have a heart', is a consequence of certain physiological hypotheses which rest on a far wider basis than the observation records which assert that certain mammals have been opened and found to have a heart. We should find it very difficult to-day to take seriously a report that someone had dissected a mammal and found no heart. But in ancient times, when there was no physiological theory, it was not so. Plutarch at least, in his life of Julius Caesar, thought it worth while to record that, shortly before his assassination

Caesar himself also doing sacrifice unto the goddes, found that one of the beastes which was sacrificed had no hart: and that was a straunge thing in nature, how a beast could live without a hart.*

(3) Hypotheses have a directive role: they give both a stimulus to further investigation, since they challenge falsification, and a direction to such effort because their unexpected consequences will suggest new experiments.

I must explain that I am using the words 'hypothesis' and 'theory' in a sense somewhat different from some of their current uses. Very often a hypothesis is only called a hypothesis when it is young and has not been much tested. After a while when it has withstood a good deal of testing it may be called a *theory*. And when it has been accepted for a long time it may finally be called a *fact*. For example, we sometimes hear people speak of the fact of evolution. The evolutionary hypothesis is an interesting example of one which was not accepted until one of higher order, namely, the hypothesis of natural selection, had been introduced. But it is surely clear that a hypothesis does not cease to be a hypothesis simply because it has been tested and is believed by a lot of people. So I say: once a hypothesis always a hypothesis, although I do not deny that some hypotheses have withstood testing much longer than others, and that it may be useful to indicate this by some change of name. By a *theory* I shall mean, not a single hypothesis but a system of hypotheses related by the consequence relation.

* Sir Thomas North's translation.

§ 2. THE CONSEQUENCE RELATION.
OPERATIONS ON STATEMENTS

Before anything can be said about the structure of theoretical statements, or about the relation of *following from* in the pyramid constituting a theory, it is necessary to say something about another topic which concerns both observation records and theoretical statements. So far we have considered statements as units having no parts which are statements. We must now consider how such units can be combined to form *compound statements*. For scientific purposes there are *five* such *operations on statements* in common use. One is an operation on single statements and the remainder couple two statements.

(1) The introduction of 'not' into a statement (in the place prescribed by the syntactical rules of the language we are using) yields a new statement called its negation or *denial*.

(2) The joining of two statements by 'and' yields a new statement called their *conjunction*.

(3) The joining of two statements by 'or' yields a new statement called their *disjunction*.

(4) Filling in the blanks of 'if...then...' by two statements yields a new statement called their *conditional*, and this can be done in two ways, yielding two distinct conditionals, according to which statement occupies the first blank. The first statement is called the *antecedent* and the second the *consequent* of the conditional.

(5) Filling in the blanks of '...if and only if...' yields a new statement called their *biconditional*, the order in this case being indifferent.

These operations can clearly be repeated on their products indefinitely to produce statements of increasing complexity.

I shall make—and in subsequent lectures test—the assumption that the above five are the only modes of statement composition needed for scientific purposes. This is important for the following reason among others. In order to discover whether a statement compounded in this way is true or false, no matter

how complicated it may be, it is sufficient to know, for each of
its constituent unit statements, whether it is true or alternatively false. Thus if I know that a given statement 'A' is true
I also know that its denial is false. If I know that both 'A'
and a second statement 'B' are true I know that both their
conjunction '$A \& B$' and their disjunction 'A or B' are true.*
But if I only know that one of them is true I know that their
disjunction is true but I can say nothing about their conjunction. The interpretation of the conditional is apt to be
puzzling and to give rise to misunderstanding owing to the
almost irresistible impulse to read into it more than is intended.
In its scientific use a conditional is understood to be true under
all conditions except one, namely, when the antecedent is true
and the consequent false. Thus 'if A then B' is true except when
'A' is true and 'B' is false.* A biconditional is true when both
its constituent statements are true and also when both are
false.

The conditions under which compound statements are true
or false can best be displayed by means of tables called *truth
tables*. Tables for the four binary operations are given here:

(1)			(2)			(3)			(4)		
A	and	B	A	or	B	A	$\supset$	B	A	$\equiv$	B
T	T	T	T	T	T	T	T	T	T	T	T
F	F	T	F	T	T	F	T	T	F	F	T
T	F	F	T	T	F	T	F	F	T	F	F
F	F	F	F	F	F	F	T	F	F	T	F

They are constructed as follows: we first write down under the
two statements the four possible combinations of truth (T) and
falsehood (F), and then, in the column under the operation sign,
we indicate whether the compound as a whole is true or false
for each of the four possibilities. I have used the customary
symbols '$\supset$' and '$\equiv$', in place of 'if...then...' and '...if and
only if...' respectively, in order to have a single sign between
the statements and thus to bring them into line with 'and' and

* See Note 12, p. 67.

'or'. These tables thus fix the meaning or use of the words 'and', 'or', 'if...then...' and '...if and only if...' for scientific purposes.

We can use truth tables for determining the truth conditions of *any* compound constructed in the above ways. Let us agree to form the denial of a statement by simply writing 'not' in front of it. Then we can construct the table (5) for '(not A) or B' as follows: The column under 'not A' will have 'F' wherever that under 'A' has 'T', and 'T' wherever the latter has 'F'. The compound as a whole, being a disjunction, will have 'F' only where 'not A' and 'B' both have 'F'. This will occur in the third row from the top. Reference to table (3) shows that 'if A then B' and '(not A) or B' have the same truth conditions.

(5)

(not A)	or	B
F	T	T
T	T	T
F	F	F
T	T	F

Now consider the *biconditional* of '(not A) or B' and 'if A then B'. Table (4) shows that this will have 'T' wherever corresponding rows of the column for '(not A) or B' and 'if A then B' both have a 'T' or both have an 'F'. But since the two columns are identical this must be the case for *every* row. Consequently we shall have a compound statement whose column contains *only* 'T'. In other words, it must be true for *all* possibilities, independently of the truth of 'A' and 'B'. When the biconditional of two statements is true they are said to be *equivalent*. When their biconditional is true independently of the truth of the two statements they are said to be *analytically* equivalent.

When two compounds are analytically equivalent either follows from the other, and either can be substituted for the other without altering the truth value of any compound in which it may occur; that is to say, the latter compound will remain true if it was true before the substitution and will remain false if it formerly was false.

In addition to analytical biconditionals we can also have analytical conditionals which are true independently of the truth of the constituent statements. In this case the consequent follows from the antecedent.

Since two compounds must be analytically equivalent when the columns of their truth conditions are identical, every compound which has no 'F' in its column is analytically equivalent to any disjunction of the form, 'A or (not A)', which itself has no 'F' in its column. Such a disjunction is called a *tautology*, and any statement which is analytically equivalent to it is called a tautology.

The following can easily be shown to be tautologies:

(1) A if and only if not (not (A)).

This is the principle of double denial.

(2)   (If A then B) if and only if (if not (B) then not (A)).

This is the principle of transposition.

(3)   If (if (A & B) then C) then (if A then (if B then C)).

This is the principle of exportation.

(4)   If (if A then (if B then C)) then (if (A & B) then C).

This is the principle of importation.

(5)   If (A & (if A then B)) then B.

On the other hand, we do not find that the following is a tautology: If ((if A then B) & B) then A.

This is shown in the following truth tables:

$(A$ & $(A \supset B))$ $\supset$ B				$((A \supset B)$ & $B)$ $\supset$ A		
T T	*TTT*	*T T*		*TTT*	*T T*	*T T*
F F	*FTT*	*T T*		*FTT*	*T T*	*F F*
T F	*TFF*	*T F*		*TFF*	*F F*	*T T*
F F	*FTF*	*T F*		*FTF*	*F F*	*T F*

Consequently if, in a scientific theory, we have a statement of the form 'if A then B' and we obtain 'B' we cannot infer that

'A' is true.* This is important and deserves to be more widely known than it seems to be among biologists. On the other hand, if we obtain 'not B' we *can* say, by the principle of transposition, that 'A' is false.

(6)   If ((if A then B) & (if B then C)) then (if A then C).
In *Principia Mathematica* this is called the principle of syllogism.

It may be asked: What is the use of tautologies in natural science? The answer is that they can be used in the same way in which mathematical formulas are used. That is to say, we can use them for transforming one statement into another with the assurance that, if the initial statement is true, that obtained by the transformation will also be true. In other words, the latter will follow from, or be a consequence of, the former, so that if we admit the first into our theory we must also admit the second. This is done by substituting actual biological statements for the unspecified 'A' and 'B' of the general formulas. But there is another way in which tautologies may be used. We may use them as a basis for formulating rules in our *metalanguage* which tell us what truth-preserving operations can be performed upon the statements of our object language. I will mention two such rules which will be used in a later example:

(1) *Rule of adjunction.* If 'A' and 'B' are accepted statements in a scientific theory, then 'A & B' is also an accepted statement in that theory.

(2) *Rule of abruption.* If both the antecedent of a conditional and the conditional itself are accepted statements in a scientific theory, then the consequent of that conditional is also an accepted statement of that theory. This is based on the fifth of the above tautologies.†

---

* See the quotation from Lord Russell in Note 17, p. 71.

† 'Abruption' is here used as a translation of the German 'Abtrennung'. It is an English word of respectable antiquity meaning 'a breaking off'. It occurs in *Troilus and Cressida*, III, ii. This rule enables us to break off the consequent from a given conditional if we are also given the antecedent.

It might be thought that nothing of importance could issue from the use of such obvious tautologies and rules. But their obviousness is their principal virtue. It is found that by the repeated use of such principles, and a few others, we can derive the consequences from systems of statements of any degree of complexity, consequences which are often very far from obvious.

Certain additional rules are necessitated by the special peculiarities of general statements which have not yet been described. The discussion of the structure of general statements has been postponed until the five operations on statements had been explained. To this topic we must now return.

§ 3. THE STRUCTURE OF GENERAL STATEMENTS

In English, general statements are commonly expressed in the manner of:

All rats have two parents.

How are we to express such statements in a way which will show the connexion between their structure and that of observation records? This can be done with the help of a very important device which is familiar enough in mathematics but not in natural languages, although the use of pronouns in the latter is closely related to it. This consists in the use of *dummy names* in the place of unshared names, and for this purpose it is customary to use small letters from near the end of the Roman alphabet.* Thus we can replace 'Tom' in the statement

Tom is bald

by 'x' and obtain the expression

x is bald,

which is clearly not a statement, just as

he is bald

is not a statement. But just as a statement can be constructed with the help of 'he is bald' by embedding it in a suitable context, so a statement can be constructed with the help of

* See Note 13, p. 67.

'x is bald' by placing it in the context of a certain prefix. Thus, if I write

$$\text{for every } x, x \text{ is bald,}$$

I obtain a statement which expresses what is commonly expressed by writing:

$$\text{everything is bald,}$$

which is a general statement.

The expression 'x is bald' still retains the form of an observation record constructed with the help of a functor of degree 1. It differs from an observation record only in having a dummy name in the place of a genuine name.

An expression consisting of a suitable functor coupled with at least *one* dummy name, which becomes a statement when all the dummy names are replaced by genuine names, is called a *statement-forming matrix*. Thus: 'Tom loves y', 'x loves y', 'Tom is sitting between Jack and z', 'x is sitting between y and z' are all statement-forming matrices. Such a matrix becomes a statement when, for *each* dummy name in it, we either (1) substitute a genuine name or (2) write in front of it a suitable prefix containing the dummy name in question. Thus 'Tom loves y' becomes a statement when I substitute 'Mary' for 'y' and also when I write 'for every y' in front of it. In the latter case I obtain a general statement which asserts that Tom loves everybody. Such a prefix is called a *quantifier*, and a dummy name which occurs both in a matrix and in a quantifier prefixed to it is said to be *bound*. An unquantified dummy name is said to be *free*.

Now we must turn to the question of operations on general statements. The five operations already explained can all be applied to general statements, but the use of denial calls for special consideration. Following the syntactical rule that the denial of a statement is to be constructed by writing 'not' in front of it, the denial of

$$\text{for every } y, \text{ Tom loves } y \tag{1}$$

will be

$$\text{not (for every } y, \text{ Tom loves } y). \tag{2}$$

Now the customary English equivalent of (1) is

$$\text{Tom loves everybody,} \tag{3}$$

and the customary English equivalent of (2) is

Tom does not love everybody.　　　(4)

But this could also be stated in the form

there is someone whom Tom does not love,　　　(5)

and in this form we can construct an equivalent statement from the matrix 'Tom loves y' by first writing 'not' in front of it and then, in front of this, a new kind of prefix containing 'y':

there is a y such that, not (Tom loves y),

or, more briefly,

for some y, not (Tom loves y).　　　(6)

This is admittedly deplorable from the standpoint of English grammar, but it is good scientific syntax.*

Now (6) introduces a number of new features. First there is the application of one of the operations on statements, namely, denial, to a matrix instead of to a statement. This can also be extended to the other four operations. We can construct such compound matrices as: 'if (x is bald) then (Tom loves y)'. A second new feature is the new kind of quantifying prefix, the use of which introduces a new kind of general statement. For (6) is a general statement because it contains a dummy name. It differs from (1) in containing 'some' in the place of 'every'. To distinguish these two kinds of general statement, (1) is called a universal statement and its quantifier a universal quantifier, and (6) is called an existential statement and its quantifier an existential quantifier. But a new quantifier is not in principle necessary, since either can be defined with the help of the other and 'not'.

From the foregoing discussion it would seem that all we need in principle for constructing general statements are: (1) universal quantifiers, and (2) the application of the five operations on statements to matrices. But in practice it is convenient also to use existential quantifiers and to use the symbols '(x)' and

---

* See Note 14, p. 67.

'($\exists x$)' as abbreviations for 'for every x' and 'for some x' respectively. Let us try to formulate the biological general statement 'All rats have two parents' in accordance with these principles. This can be done as follows:

For every x, if x is a rat, then there is a y and a z such that y is distinct from z, and y is parent of x and z is parent of x.

But this can be greatly abbreviated by using single letters for the functors involved. Let us use 'R' to denote the set of rats and 'P' for 'is parent of'. Then with the other abbreviations the statement just given becomes

$$(x) \text{ (if } x \epsilon R \text{ then } (\exists y) (\exists z) (y \neq z \ \& \ yPx \ \& \ zPx)).$$

This has the form of a natural law because it contains a conditional constructed of matrices with at least one dummy name universally quantified. This formulation does not exclude the possibility of a rat having more than two parents, but neither does the original statement. Whatever may be intended it does not *say* that a rat has *only* two parents.

It will be noticed that, without explanation, I have used parentheses to indicate the scope of the quantifiers. Rules can be formulated which govern their use, but for my present purpose it is not necessary to say anything about them.

It will also be noticed that a new functor '$\neq$' has been slipped in without explanation. '$y \neq z$' is an abbreviation for 'not $(y = z)$', and '$=$' is the sign of strict identity, the kind of identity involved when we say that Paris is the capital of France. The word 'identity' is sometimes used in this sense in biology, but more commonly it is used in a totally different sense which must be discussed at a later stage.

I shall make, and in subsequent lectures test, the assumption that all theoretical statements in biology can be formulated with the help of only:

(1) the five operations on statements,
(2) universal quantification,
(3) strict identity,
(4) parentheses,

(5) dummy names which represent unshared names,

(6) the number-signs, '0', '$\frac{1}{4}$', '$\frac{1}{2}$', '1' and others where needed,

(7) dummy names representing natural and rational numbers,

(8) biological functors together with functors borrowed from other sciences when necessary,

(9) abbreviators (to be introduced and explained later),

(10) dummy names representing functors, for use in conjunction with abbreviators.

If this proves to be feasible we shall possess a thoroughly analysed basis for a biological language which is much simpler and more controllable than an untamed natural language. We shall be able to eliminate an enormous amount of unnecessary verbiage and to avoid the pitfalls, which were mentioned in the first lecture, to which the use of a natural language exposes us. It will have the merit of making errors more easily discoverable, and it will have other merits which will be clear later.

The words or other signs required for such a language can be divided into two sets: To one set belong the signs mentioned in (1), (2), (3), (4), (5), (6), (7) and (10) in the above list. They are called *formative* signs.* To the other set belong (8) and (9). These are called *descriptive* signs or subject-matter signs. We shall see that this distinction is very important.

I must now return to the problem: How can we be certain that a given statement is a consequence of one or more other statements? We have seen that it is upon this relation that the ordering of theoretical statements in a scientific theory depends. So far only a partial answer has been given. I have said that where nothing but the five operations on statements is involved we can say that either member of a tautologous biconditional follows from the other, and that the consequent of a tautologous conditional follows from the antecedent.

This applies to general statements as well as to observation records so long as the structure of the former is not involved.

---

* I borrow the term 'formative sign' from Professor Popper's article 'Logic without assumptions', see Note 20, p. 74.

But cases frequently arise when it is necessary to take this structure into account. In order to deal fully with general statements it is necessary (1) to have rules for manipulating quantifiers, and (2) to extend the truth-table principles to matrices. For the manipulating of general statements consists in first removing the quantifiers, then operating upon the exposed matrices according to the principles and metalinguistic rules already given for the five operations on statements and then replacing the quantifiers. Since there are two kinds of quantifiers in use there will be two removal rules and two insertion rules. It will suffice for my present purpose if I give only the rules for the universal quantifier (represented by '(d)', where 'd' is a dummy name):

Rule I. From any statement of the form

$$\text{If } A \text{ then } (d) \ (B),$$

we may obtain

$$\text{If } A \text{ then } B.$$

Rule II. If the dummy name d is not free in A, then from a formula of the form

$$\text{if } A \text{ then } B,$$

we may obtain

$$\text{if } A \text{ then } (d) \ (B).$$

The use of these rules and the application of the five operations on statements to matrices will be illustrated in an example to be given shortly.

It is now possible to indicate what is meant by logic within the Boole-Frege movement. First we have the system of tautologies involving only the five operations on statements, or sentential connectives as they are also called. This constitutes the calculus of statements or sentential calculus. If we add to this the system of formulas which are obtainable by the use of the additional rules for manipulating quantifiers and matrices we obtain what is called the lower functional calculus. If we admit dummy names which can have functors substituted for them, and with them form matrices with functors of higher order, to which we apply the same principles of quantification, we obtain a new crop of formulas which together form what is called the higher functional calculus. These three calculuses constitute logic.*

Now the only way to learn these calculuses is by using them, not by listening to someone talking about them. My chief motive for saying what I have said about them has been the wish to show to biologists that such a technique for deriving consequences from statements exists. At present the derivation of consequences in biology is done either by means of the more familiar parts of mathematics or by unaided intuition. In the first case some well-known mathematical formula is written down and is accompanied by semantical statements which explain that the dummy names (or some of them) occurring in the formula are to represent the results of measuring or counting some biological objects or sets of such. Then purely mathematical operations are performed upon the formula and the result reinterpreted, in accordance with the semantical statements, into biological terms. Or actual values obtained by observation are substituted for the dummy names and the result evaluated. All this presupposes that you can find a mathematical formula of the correct form for your hypothesis. When this cannot be done we are left with unaided intuition.

Now unaided intuition has certainly performed wonders in the past and nothing can take its place. But it is not infallible, and there is presumably a limit to the complexity with which even the most brilliant intuition can cope. It is therefore useful to have a means by which the scope of intuition can be extended and its results checked.

To make what I have said about the structure of biological theories more concrete I propose now to examine a part of an actual specimen. For this purpose I take the following statements from the second chapter of William Harvey's celebrated

* See Hilbert and Ackermann, *Grundzüge der theoretischen Logik* (1938). The reader who wishes to pursue this matter further is strongly recommended to consult the article by W. V. Quine entitled 'On natural deduction' in *Journ. of Symbolic Logic*, 15 (1950), pp. 93–102.

Anatomical Disquisition on the Motion of the Heart and Blood in Animals:

[G. 1] There is a time when the heart moves and a time when it is motionless.

[G. 2] During its motion the heart is erected, rises up to a point and the pulse is felt externally.

[G. 3] During its motion the heart is everywhere contracted, more drawn together.

[G. 4] During its motion the heart is felt to become harder.

[G. 5] When the heart moves it becomes paler in colour; when it is quiescent it has a deeper blood-red colour.

From these particulars it appeared evident to me that

[H. 1] The motion of the heart consists in a certain universal tension—both contraction in the line of its fibres and constriction in every sense,

[H. 2] The motion of the heart is plainly of the same nature as that of the muscles when they contract;

for

[G. 6] The muscles, when in action, acquire rigour and tenseness and from soft become hard, prominent and thickened.

We are therefore authorized to conclude that

[H. 3] The heart, at the moment of its action, is at once constricted on all sides, rendered thicker in its parieties and smaller in its ventricles and so made apt to project or expel its charge of blood.

This is indeed made sufficiently manifest by (5). *But no one need remain in doubt of the fact, for*

[G. 7] If the ventricle be pierced the blood will be seen to be forcibly projected outward upon each motion or pulsation when the heart is tense.

It will be seen that there are seven generalizations or zero-level hypotheses (G. 1–G. 7) and three explanatory hypotheses of first level (H. 1–H. 3), although these have since been so abundantly confirmed that it is difficult for us to think of them as hypotheses or to appreciate the magnitude of Harvey's achievement in introducing them. There are also the meta-theoretical statements which have been printed in italics. Now the wording of these is such as to suggest that Harvey believed that the hypotheses follow from the generalizations. But had this been the case, and were unaided intuition sufficient to determine when one statement follows from another, it would be difficult to understand why Harvey's contemporaries were so slow in adopting his theory.* This difficulty disappears when we remember that at that time the method of hypotheses was not generally understood and when we realize that the relation of *following from* holds only from a hypothesis of level n to one of level $n-1$, or of a still lower level and not vice versa.

The situation will be clearer if we rephrase Harvey in modern idiom. What he is affirming in his hypotheses is

Every heart is an intermittent muscular blood pump.
Let us split this into two hypotheses:

[H.I]   Every heart is muscular.

[H.II]   Every heart is an intermittent blood pump.

Then from H.I and G.6 (and certain other generalizations concerning muscles which Harvey takes for granted but does not mention), parts of the generalizations 2–4 follow. From H.II and certain generalizations concerning pumps (which Harvey also takes for granted without mention) the generalizations 1, 5 and 7 follow. Harvey's success largely depended on the fact that he approached his problems as an enlightened plumber might have done, and he brought to his task certain plumber's generalizations concerning pumps, and the flow of fluids through tubes, which he never mentions although they are strictly necessary to his theory. Presumably his contemporaries did not share this outlook—Galen had denied that the heart was a muscle—and that may have been an additional reason why his views were not sooner accepted.

* See Note 15, p. 68.

In order to illustrate the use of the lower functional calculus by a simple example, let us suppose that someone challenges the assertion that we can derive G.4 from H.I and G.6, and is not satisfied by being told that it is obvious. We can proceed as follows: We first adopt the following abbreviations. We use 'Mx' for 'x is muscular', 'Ax' for 'x is in action', 'Hx' for 'x is hard' and 'HTx' for 'x is a heart'. Then our premises are:

[H. I] $(x)\,(HTx \supset Mx)$,

[G. 6] $(x)\,((Mx \,\&\, Ax) \supset Hx)$,

and the statement to be derived from them is

[G. 4] $(x)\,((HTx \,\&\, Ax) \supset Hx)$.

We begin by removing the quantifiers. If S is any statement whatever, since we are assuming H. I to be true we must have

(i) $(S \text{ or } \mathrm{not}(S)) \supset (x)\,(HTx \supset Mx)$,

and from this by the use of Rule I we obtain

(ii) $(S \text{ or } \mathrm{not}(S)) \supset (HTx \supset Mx)$;

and since $(S \text{ or } \mathrm{not}(S))$ is a tautology we can, from (ii) by the rule of abruption, obtain

(iii) $(HTx \supset Mx)$;

by an exactly analogous procedure from G. 6 we obtain

(iv) $((Mx \,\&\, Ax) \supset Hx)$;

by substituting 'Mx' for 'A', 'Ax' for 'B' and 'Hx' for 'C' in principle (3) on p. 37, we obtain

(v) $((Mx \,\&\, Ax) \supset Hx) \supset (Mx \supset (Ax \supset Hx))$;

and from (iv) and (v) we can, by the rule of abruption, derive

(vi) $(Mx \supset (Ax \supset Hx))$,

by substituting 'HTx' for 'A', 'Mx' for 'B' and '$(Ax \supset Hx)$' for 'C' in principle (6) on p. 38, we obtain

(vii) $((HTx \supset Mx) \,\&\, (Mx \supset (Ax \supset Hx))) \supset (HTx \supset (Ax \supset Hx))$;

from (iii) and (vi) by the rule of adjunction we get

(viii) $(HTx \supset Mx) \& (Mx \supset (Ax \supset Hx))$;

from (vii) and (viii) by abruption we derive

(ix) $(HTx \supset (Ax \supset Hx))$;

by substituting 'HTx' for 'A', 'Ax' for 'B' and 'Hx' for 'C' in principle (4) on p. 37, we obtain

(x) $(HTx \supset (Ax \supset Hx)) \supset ((HTx \& Ax) \supset Hx)$;

and from (ix) and (x) by abruption we finally obtain

(xi) $((HTx \& Ax) \supset Hx)$.

It now only remains to reintroduce the quantifier '(x)'. Suppose S is any statement in which the dummy name 'x' is not free. Then since we have (xi) we must have

$$(S \text{ or } \text{not}(S)) \supset ((HTx \& Ax) \supset Hx),$$

and from this by Rule II we can derive

(xii) $(S \text{ or } \text{not}(S)) \supset (x)((HTx \& Ax) \supset Hx)$,

and from (xii) and the rule of abruption we obtain the desired statement,

(xiii) $(x)((HTx \& Ax) \supset Hx)$.

In giving this example I have explicitly written out each step in full. With a little practice the required transformation can be written down directly without actually making substitutions in the formulas given on p. 37, provided our statements are so constructed as to show their form. I do not wish to place a great deal of emphasis on the use of the functional calculus. I have said that logic forms only a part of the results of the Boole-Frege movement. It would be pointless to use a complicated calculus in situations for which intuition suffices. Of more general importance is the use of a simplified controllable language of the kind I am suggesting, which exhibits the form of statements and thus aids intuition and provides for the use of a calculus if this should be necessary.

But one important feature of the process of deriving consequences from statements which is illustrated by this example can hardly be overemphasized. This is the fact that this process requires attention only to the *structural* or syntactical aspect of the statements, *not to their meaning*. In obtaining G.4 from H.I and G.6, the fact that these statements speak about hearts and muscles is quite irrelevant from the point of view of the validity of the process of derivation. This depends especially on the *formative** signs, which provide, so to speak, the structural skeleton of the statements. It depends on the descriptive signs only in so far as these are of different kinds distributed in a particular way. It does not at all depend on any one meaning that we may give them.

If we analyse the whole of Harvey's theory in the way that I have described we see that it is fairly complicated and that it contains statements (apart from the methodological statements) which are neither generalizations of observation records nor explanatory hypotheses, but are *consequences* of the latter. These do not belong to the system of levels of hypotheses. Among them is the thesis that the blood circulates from the right heart through the lungs to the left heart and from the left heart through the arteries and veins back to the right heart.†

Thus we can say that a scientific theory consists of a set of hypotheses of highest level together with all their consequences. Accordingly, if we know which are the hypotheses of highest level in a theory we already possess the whole theory in an extremely compact form. If we also know the metatheoretical rules for deriving consequences we can work these out mechanically.

Moreover, it will be found that, when one statement in a scientific theory follows from one or more other statements of that theory, the conditional, constructed with the conjunction of these latter statements as its antecedent and the former as its consequent, is an *analytical conditional*.

It will be noticed that there are no observation records in a

---

* See above, p. 43.
† An analysis of Harvey's theory is given in Appendix A, p. 75.

theory. This is because such statements do not follow from general statements alone. From the hypothesis 'All rats have two parents' I cannot derive the statement 'a has two parents' unless I also have the statement 'a is a rat'.

Scientific theories are not usually expounded in the above-mentioned pyramidal form, with the highest-level hypotheses at the top and their consequences in successive layers below them. To construct them in this form usually requires a good deal of preliminary analysis. This process is called *axiomatization*. It has two aspects. First, the ordering of the statements of the theory according to their consequence relations, as already described. Secondly, there is another process which has not yet been mentioned, namely, the ordering of the functors of the theory according to their definability relations.* This relation does not appear to have received quite so much attention from experts as has been bestowed upon the consequence relation.

Let me illustrate it by reference to the five operations on statements. It can easily be shown by means of truth tables that 'A if and only if B' is analytically equivalent to the conjunction of 'if A then B' and 'if B then A'. That is why it is called a *bi*conditional. We can make use of this fact for the purpose of *defining* 'A if and only if B' by eliminating it in favour of '&' and 'if...then...'. We can do this in our meta-language by writing: 'A if and only if B' is an abbreviation for: '(if A then B) & (if B then A)'. This is not a single definition, but a definition schema with the help of which, by suitable substitutions for 'A' and 'B', we can obtain any particular abbreviation of this kind we may need. This shows that '...if and only if...' can in principle be dispensed with.

We have already learnt that '(not A) or B' is analytically equivalent to 'if A then B', so we can use this fact to eliminate 'if...then...' in an analogous manner. But 'and' can also be eliminated in favour of 'not' and 'or', because we can show that 'A & B' is analytically equivalent to 'not ((not A) or

---

* An example of this is given in Part II, Note 14, p. 211.

(not B))'. The five operations can thus be reduced to two. Finally, it is possible to reduce them to one because there is a truth combination by means of which 'or' and 'not' can be defined. This is commonly written '$A \downarrow B$'. Its truth table and those for 'not' and 'or' are as follows:

neither A nor B			not A			A or B		
A	$\downarrow$	B	A	$\downarrow$	A	$(A\downarrow B)$	$\downarrow$	$(A\downarrow B)$
T	F	T	T	F	T	F	T	F
F	F	T	F	T	F	F	T	F
T	F	F	T	F	T	F	T	F
F	T	F	F	T	F	T	F	T

It will be seen that '$A \downarrow B$' is true only when both 'A' and 'B' are false. It can therefore be called *joint denial* of 'A' and 'B'.*

This process of gradual reduction of the number of primitive operations can also be applied to functors, until we arrive finally at a *minimum vocabulary* of primitive functors which, in the system of functors of a theory, occupies a position analogous to that of the highest-level hypotheses in its system of statements. It gives us, so to speak, the conceptual content of the theory in its most concentrated form. When I said, in the first lecture, that the linguistic requirements of science prove to be surprisingly meagre, I had in mind the fact that with a suitable choice of primitive functors it is possible to construct a great many definable ones.

A few words should be added here on the subject of definition. Ordinarily a definition is a statement which is explanatory of the meaning of a word. That is to say, we have a person P who does not understand statements in which a word W occurs. We then seek a statement S which does not contain W and which P understands, and a statement S' which contains W and is such that

S' if and only if S.

S' is called the definiendum and S the definiens, the whole bi-

---

* We owe this method of reducing the number of primitive signs of the calculus of statements to one to Dr H. M. Sheffer.

conditional being called a definition. For example, suppose W is a functor of degree 1 and F and G are also functors of degree 1 with which P is already familiar. Suppose further that for every x, whenever we have Fx and Gx we also have Wx, and whenever we have Wx we also have Fx and Gx. Then we could say

$$Wx \text{ if and only if } Fx \ \& \ Gx. \tag{1}$$

Alternatively, we could proceed in the following way, using the notion of identity between sets:

W is identical with the set of all objects x such that

$$Fx \ \& \ Gx. \tag{2}$$

These are both *nominal* definitions. (1) is called a contextual definition because W is not defined in isolation but in the context 'Wx'. (2) is called an explicit definition.

This procedure, as far as the person P is concerned, presupposes that he understands the use of F and G. He may also have learnt their use in an analogous way. But sooner or later we must reach a stock of words the use of which P has learnt by means of what are called *ostensive* definitions. For example, a student beginning biology learns the use of the word 'cell' by looking through a microscope and comparing what he sees with drawings in a book which are labelled 'cell', or with the help of a teacher who points out cells to him by means of a double-viewing eyepiece, or who makes sketches and says: Do you see something like this? Then that is a cell.

In a postulate system or axiomatized theory, definitions will be either contextual or explicit definitions.* They will fix the way in which the defined signs are used in the theory, just as the postulates fix the way in which the undefined signs are used. If a reader understands the undefined signs he will be able, with the help of the definitions, to understand the defined ones. If he does not understand the undefined signs neither will he, with

---

* There is another type called recursive definitions. See the article under this head by A. Church in *The Dictionary of Philosophy*, edited by D. D. Runes (1942).

the help of the definitions alone, understand the defined ones. It may be that the undefined signs do not 'have meaning' in any intuitive sense. But if the theory is to have applications and to be testable it must be possible, at least for some of the signs which occur in the zero-level statements, to indicate their meaning either ostensively or in some other way.

From the purely syntactical point of view the definiendum is merely an abbreviation for the definiens, and this is frequently a motive for using a definition. We find in the course of our work that a certain combination of signs frequently recurs. It is then convenient to introduce a single sign by definition to replace the longer one. But it may happen that we wish to introduce a word into our theory which it does not already possess. If it is possible to find a combination of our existing signs which can be used in place of the new one, then the latter can be introduced by definition with this combination as definiens, without increasing our list of primitive or undefined signs. This process frequently requires considerable skill and ingenuity. If this cannot be done, then the new word can only be introduced as an additional primitive or undefined sign by means of new postulates.

I have already discussed the process of axiomatization in relation to biology elsewhere. I will only mention here that although axiomatization is clearly not necessary for the *development* of a theory, at least in its early stages, it is essential for the complete understanding of one, or for comparing one theory with another. But so far it has been employed very little in natural science, apart from its use in physics.

I began, in the first lecture, by saying that we could discern three activities in which biologists engage: the making and recording of observations, the invention of hypotheses and apparatus, and criticism. We have now seen that criticism, when it ceases to be purely intuitive and becomes analytical and scientific, passes into methodology, and now we see that methodology culminates in axiomatization. I should like to add that if historians of science would attempt to axiomatize the theories of the men whose work they study, they would greatly extend the scope and interest of their labours.*

I have said but little so far about the semantical aspect of theoretical statements. This raises the celebrated and difficult problems of induction. Traditionally the passage from observation records to theoretical statements is called *induction*, and the passage from one or more theoretical statements to their consequences is called deduction. I have avoided these words because, for one reason, they are frequently used in current biological literature as though they were synonymous! Thus it is possible to find the word 'deduction' used for *both* processes on one and the same page of a biological book. Indeed, the word 'induction' is rarely used in such places. The same thing happens in detective stories, where the inspector always speaks of his deductions, when he means his imaginative reconstruction of the crime, which is a hypothesis explanatory of the clues. This may be because the two processes are not distinguished, and this again because both are commonly performed intuitively. Moreover, words like 'proof', 'conclusion', 'inference', 'consequence', etc., are frequently used indiscriminately in both connexions, although with utterly different meanings in each. It is easy to see that *if* there were no distinction between deduction and induction, *all the statements of a theory, or conjunctions of them, would be analytically equivalent to one another*, we should be replacing an asymmetrical relation by a symmetrical one and the structure of the theory would be entirely altered. Moreover, there would be no need for imagination and inventiveness in scientific research; it would be as easy as falling off a log.

I have suggested that this failure to distinguish the two processes may result from the fact that the passage in either direction is performed intuitively, so that the distinction is not forced upon us until we begin to reflect. This is especially true of the passage from observation records to generalizations thereof. This seems to occur quite automatically. Sometimes

* See Appendix A, p. 75.

we get a glimpse of this in the writing of biologists. Consider, for example, the following passage from Spemann in which he is speaking about the process of lens-formation in members of the species *Rana fusca*. He says that

·lens-formation and the clearing of the deep black epidermis into cornea did not take place if the eye-rudiment in the neural plate had been removed....It seemed natural to extend this result to include all vertebrates. But soon cases of lens-formation in the complete absence of the eye-cup became known....Sure of my case with *Rana fusca* and biased by the idea that similar animal forms must behave in a similar way, I did not at first allow myself to be shaken in my conviction....Nevertheless, I repeated my experiment on another object, *R. esculenta* and now it appeared to my great surprise that, after a neat removal of the eye-rudiment from the open neural plate, lenses of great perfection can originate.*

Here then we have the process of induction in action. First there is the unconscious jump (which therefore is not mentioned) from a finite number of observations on members of the species *Rana fusca* to *all* members of this species. Then there is the great conscious jump to *all vertebrates* which 'seemed natural'. Finally, there is the great retreat from this by the discovery of a contrary instance *even within the same genus* of anuran Amphibia, a retreat which was made reluctant by the belief that 'similar animal forms must behave in a similar way'. Thus the tendency seems to be to generalize to the maximum possible extent and only to introduce restrictions on our generalizations as new observations require them. I do not propose to discuss induction because I have nothing new to add to what has already been said about it, except perhaps to say that when we already have the perfectly good word 'guessing' there seems to be little need for a technical term.†

Let me try now to sum up what I have said, implicity or explicitly, about biological statements. I have divided them

---

* H. Spemann, *Embryonic Development and Induction* (1938), p. 60.

† I do not at all wish to suggest that no distinction can be made between 'good' and 'bad' guessing. The precise formulation of the criteria upon which such a distinction may be based is the task of the theory of induction.

first into observation records and theoretical statements, and I have divided the latter further into those which belong to the successive levels reached in the process of theory-building and those which do not belong to the levels but are consequences of members of the levels.

First of all it is clear that they are *all* hypothetical, in the sense that they all *go beyond* what can strictly be said to be directly observed. What we directly observe are sensible objects in their complex relations. But observation records are statements about objects belonging to the converse domain of **OF**. We *believe in* the objects of the converse domain of **OF**, but we do not directly see them, feel them, smell them, etc., as we do the objects belonging to the domain of **OF**. But we also believe that we can *do* something to them as Dr Johnson did. If they are not too far away we can touch them, if they are not too big we can move them about and experiment with them. These beliefs are not deliberately invented by us like explanatory hypotheses, but we find ourselves already in possession of them by the time we begin to reflect.*

Theoretical statements, it is clear, cannot be verified because we can never know whether they are true. All we can do is to go on testing their consequences until an observation record turns up which contradicts them. Then we have the choice of two courses: we can say that the theoretical statement is false and reject it; or we can assume that we have been mistaken in our observations and retain the theoretical statements. If the theoretical statement has no theoretical backing it will be easily falsified. But if it has one or more levels above it, only the persistent cropping up of contradictory observation records, which cannot be satisfactorily explained away by the introduction of fresh *ad hoc* hypotheses, will lead to its falsification.

A true hypothesis would be one which is *never* falsified; but as we cannot know *which* of our existing hypotheses will never be falsified we do not know which of them are true. It is better therefore to divide hypotheses into the well confirmed, the

* See Note 16, p. 68.

confirmed, the untested and the falsified, rather than into the true and the false.* Biologists are sometimes shy of discussing untested hypotheses, but so long as they are clearly recognized as untested the practice is perfectly harmless. On the other hand, some biologists have defended and given serious credence to certain evolutionary hypotheses which are not only untested but in practice, if not in principle, untestable.†

A second very important point about hypotheses is connected with one which has already been emphasized. I have said that they do their work solely by virtue of their structure. For it is upon structure alone that the consequence relation depends, and it is with the help of this relation that the testing of hypotheses is possible, and this is independent of the meaning of the descriptive signs which occur in the *high*-level hypotheses. For this reason it is quite unnecessary that the descriptive signs in such statements should have 'meaning' in the sense that we should be able to represent them as objects which we can see or imagine. Objects which we can see or imagine belong to the domain, not to the converse domain, of **OF**. We can divide explanatory hypotheses into two kinds, (1) intelligible and (2) abstract. To the former belong those whose descriptive signs can be regarded as denoting objects which can be represented in the imagination, as is the case with the thermodynamic theory of gases, where the molecules can be pictured as little bouncing balls. To the abstract hypotheses belong the theory of energy and most theories of modern physics where the imagination is of no help. But the question whether a hypothesis is intelligible in this sense, or abstract, is strictly irrelevant, since in both cases it is the structure of the statements which is doing the work.‡ One important reservation must of course be made regarding abstract explanatory hypotheses, namely, that at *some level* they must have consequences, or contribute to the derivation of consequences, which are formulated in the language of observation records. Otherwise they would not be testable.§

---

* There is more about this in Part III, Appendix C, p. 335.
† See Note 17, p. 69.   ‡ See Note 18, p. 71.   § See Note 19, p. 72.

I should like to add a word in explanation of the mechanism of falsification of hypotheses. Suppose we have a sequence of hypotheses belonging to some theory, one from each level from n to zero

$$H_n, H_{n-1}, \ldots, H_0,$$

and such that each forms with its neighbour an analytical conditional

$$H_n \supset H_{n-1} \ \& \ H_{n-1} \supset H_{n-2} \ \& \ \ldots \ \& \ H_1 \supset H_0.$$

Then by the principle of syllogism (p.   ) we can successively eliminate all the intermediate terms and so arrive at

$$H_n \supset H_0.$$

From this, by the principle of transposition, we obtain

$$(\text{not } H_0) \supset (\text{not } H_n).$$

Now, if 'H_0' is falsified by observation so that we have '$(\text{not } H_0)$' we obtain from the above, by the use of abruption,

$$\text{not } H_n.$$

This will hold for any finite n so that no hypothesis, however remote from the observation records, is beyond the reach of falsification, provided it belongs to such a sequence.

I must apologize to biologists for devoting so much time to these abstract and general methodological problems. In the remaining lectures we shall be occupied only by methodological problems within biology itself. But in order to deal successfully with such problems in relation to biology it is necessary to have some understanding of general methodology.*

* For Bibliography to Part I, see Note 20, p. 73.

NOTES TO PART I

Note 1 (p. 3). George Boole was born on 2 November 1815 in Lincoln. He was educated locally. Opened a school of his own at the age of 20. In mathematics he was largely self-taught. In 1849 he was appointed professor of mathematics at Queen's College, Cork. He was awarded the Royal Society's Medal in 1844 for his mathematical work. He married Miss Everest in 1855. Awarded the Keith Medal of the Royal Society of Edinburgh in 1857. His first logical work, *The Mathematical Analysis of Logic*, was published in 1847 (reprinted 1947) and his principal work, *An Investigation of the Laws of Thought*, in 1854. He died on 8 December 1864.

Gottlob Frege was born in 1848 and died in 1925. He was professor of mathematics at the University of Jena from 1879 to 1918. His *Begriffschrift* was published in 1879, his *Grundlagen der Arithmetik* in 1884 and his *Grundgesetze der Arithmetik*, vol. I, in 1893 and vol. II in 1903.

Note 2 (p. 4). As Professor R. A. Fisher has said:

> Every active mind will form opinions without direct evidence, else the evidence too often would never be collected. Impartiality and scientific discipline come in in submitting the opinions formed to as much relevant evidence as can be made available. (*The Genetical Theory of Natural Selection* (1930), p. 3.)

The erroneous beliefs regarding discovery, referred to in the text, are connected with the cliché, so often used by popular writers and broadcasters on the history of science, which asserts that 'Science is based on observation and experiment'. This is like saying that health is based on good digestion. Of course science is based on observation and experiment, but *not only* on observation and experiment. Obviously, if you believe that it is only based on observation and experiment, then everything new that is introduced into science *must* be a discovery. In view of the popularity of science in these days it is deplorable that it is so little understood, even by those actively engaged in it. It is high time that the parts played in science by imagination, invention and faith—in addition to observation and experiment—were more widely recognized and understood. Ignorance in such matters breeds dogmatism and intolerance, both of which ill become the scientist. See Note 17 below, p. 69.

Note 3 (p. 6). We occasionally find, in current literature, exhortations to pay some attention to methodology. Thus Dr F. M. R. Walshe in his Harveian Oration, reported in *The Lancet*, 23 October 1948, p. 661, said:

Further, I ask how medicine can be worthily taught on its academic side unless by minds well versed in the liberal arts...understanding the principles on which knowledge is ordered and capable of expounding and of showing in action the reasoning methods involved.

Also on p. 18 of the report of the Medical Curriculum Committee of the British Medical Association, entitled *The Training of a Doctor* (1948), we find the following enlightened statement:

The fundamental purpose of the course in the basic sciences is to teach scientific method and to inculcate habits of clear and logical thinking. The scientific approach should be quite deliberately taught; it cannot be acquired as a by-product of factual instruction. This involves the training of the student in the importance of unprejudiced observation and of controlled experiment, in the evaluation of evidence and in the role of techniques and their limitations. The student should also be disciplined in *the proper use and meaning of words and the relationship of names and words to ideas and things*. At the end of the year's course he should have acquired a scientific attitude of mind and have absorbed in that attitude the atmosphere of unbiased inquiry and research. He will then no longer regard the basic sciences as collections of facts and laws, but as a constantly growing body of knowledge with potential medical applications of paramount importance.

Until teachers have themselves been trained in methodology, and the present erroneous beliefs about such matters cease to be current, it will be impossible to put the above suggestions into practice. At present, no one receives instruction in 'the proper use and meaning of words and the relationship of names and words to ideas and things', and until the results of the

Boole-Frege movement are more widely known such instruction will not be available. The words just quoted are not in italics in the original.

One reason why so little attention is paid to methodology is that our use of language is largely automatic, like breathing. But whereas when something goes wrong with our breathing we are usually warned by means of pain, there is nothing comparable to this when something goes wrong with our use of language, except when we commit some gross breach of grammar. But such errors are rare. It is the more subtle defects of language which are important in science, and these are difficult to detect and to trace to their source.

Note 4 (p. 7). In saying that thoughts can only be shared effectively by the use of language I am not taking sides about the question of telepathy. I am only assuming that even the most ardent believer in telepathy would agree that the latter does not enable us at present to dispense with language entirely.

Note 5 (p. 10). It is clear that words like 'physics', 'chemistry', 'biology', etc., are metatheoretical words, and so it comes about that the corresponding adjectives 'physical', 'chemical', etc., all have a double use: one in the object language and one in the corresponding metalanguage. Thus in the phrase 'chemical equation' the adjective belongs to the metalanguage, but in 'chemical process' it belongs to the object language. This illustrates a minor ambiguity which is easily understood when the distinction between object language and metalanguage is pointed out.

Note 6 (p. 17). In this connexion the following extracts from Otto Jespersen's *Language, Its Nature, Development and Origin* (1925) are of interest:

A child is often faced by some linguistic usage which obliges him again and again to change his notions, widen them, narrow them, till he succeeds in giving words the same range of meaning that his elders give them.

Frequently, perhaps most frequently, a word is at first for the child a proper name. 'Wood' means not a wood in general, but the particular picture which has been pointed out to the child in the dining room. The little girl who calls her mother's black muff 'muff', but refuses to transfer the word to her own white one is at this stage. Naturally, then, the word *father* when first heard is a proper name, the name of the child's own father. But soon it must be extended to other individuals who have something or other in common with the child's father. One child will use it of all *men*, another perhaps of all men with beards, while 'lady' is applied to all pictures of faces without beards; a third will apply the word to father, mother and grandfather. When the child itself applies the word to another man it is soon corrected, but at the same time it cannot avoid hearing another child call a strange man 'father' or getting to know that the gardener is Jack's 'father', etc. The word then comes to mean to the child 'grown-up person who goes with or belongs to a little one', and he will say 'See, there goes a dog with his father'. Or, he comes to know that the cat is the kittens' father, and the dog the puppies' father, and next day asks 'Wasps, are they the flies' father, or are they perhaps their mother?' (as Frans did, 4·10). Finally by such guessing and drawing conclusions he gains full understanding of the word, and is ready to make acquaintance later with its more remote applications, as 'The King is the father of his people', 'Father O'Flynn', 'Boyle was the father of chemistry', etc. (pp. 117–18).

Words with several meanings may cause children much difficulty. A Somerset child said 'Moses was not a good boy, and his mother smacked 'un and smacked 'un and smacked 'un till she couldn't do it no more, and then she put 'un in the ark of bulrushes'. This puzzled the teacher till he looked at the passage in Exodus: 'And when she could hide him no longer, she laid him in an ark of bulrushes.'

Note 7 (p. 20). Something should be added on the use of the words 'individual' and 'individual names'. In the theory of classes it was discovered by Lord Russell that certain contradictions can arise if precautions are not taken. His theory of types was devised as a formulation of these precautions. Objects which can be members of sets, but are not themselves sets, are called individuals. Their designations (individual names) are said to constitute the lowest type. Designations of sets of individuals constitute the next highest type, and designations of sets of sets of individuals the next, and so on.

What we regard as individuals depends on our starting point. Thus a wholesale dealer in fruit, who never had need to mention single oranges, might find it convenient to regard crates of oranges as individuals. But a retail dealer would find this inconvenient and would treat single fruits as individuals.

In the theory of unshared and shared names the difficulties of type do not arise, because designations corresponding to sets of sets are not regarded as names at all, but as abbreviators (see below, p. 129). For an introduction to the problems with which the theory of types deals see Quine, *Mathematical Logic* (1940), p. 128.

The suggestions concerning shared and unshared names given in the text have since been more fully worked out in my article in *The British Journal for the Philosophy of Science* (1951), **2**, and in an article by Professor Richard Martin and myself in *The Journal of Symbolic Logic* (1951), **16**.

Note 8 (p. 22). I make no distinction between objects and events because I think of all objects as being time-extended in the first instance. Momentary objects are derived from these by Whitehead's method of intensive abstraction or some other such method. The distinction made by Whitehead between objects and events I have now abandoned in accordance with my present nominalistic tendency. It does not seem to me to be useful in science.

Note 9 (p. 23). I am opposed to the popular doctrine that science is either quantitative or qualitative and that only the quantitative needs, or is capable of, precision. I reject this unclear and simple-minded antithesis and proclaim that it is possible to be precise in any branch of biology if we are prepared to take sufficient trouble. Moreover, even the quantitative treatment of a problem is only possible after it has been precisely formulated. The method of functors provides the technique for achieving this preliminary precise formulation. The situation was clearly understood by Leibniz as the following passage shows:

The progress of the art of rational discovery depends in part upon the art of characteristic (ars characteristica). The reason why people usually seek demonstrations only in numbers and lines and things represented by these is none other than that there are not, outside numbers, convenient characters corresponding to the notions. (Leibniz (G. VII, 198) quoted by B. A. W. Russell in *A Critical Exposition of the Philosophy of Leibniz* (1900).)

Professor C. I. Lewis, in his *Survey of Symbolic Logic* (1918), speaking of the work of the immediate predecessors of George Boole, writes: 'The record of symbolic logic on the continent is a record of failure, in England, a record of success. The continental students habitually emphasized intension; the English, extension' (p. 37). On p. 52 he says: 'Boole's algebra, unlike the systems of his predecessors, is based squarely upon the relations of extension.'

Note 10 (p. 24). I have myself been a victim of the word 'property'. In my *Axiomatic Method in Biology* (1937) I admitted the notion of 'genetic property' as an undefined one. Now this seems to me to have been a double error, first, in allowing the notion of property at all, and second, in taking genetic property as an undefined notion. For it is an extremely obscure notion, and the object of analysis should be to render it less obscure. In treating it as undefined all its blemishes are admitted with it. A further defect of that book is traceable to the bad example of *Principia Mathematica*. I refer to the lack of restriction on the piling up of types. Not only classes of individuals but classes of classes and classes of classes of classes are allowed. In the present work classes of classes have been admitted only in connexion with the definition of 'combined element' (see p. 101), and in a few other places (e.g. Appendix B).

The confusions connected with the notion of class (or set) are well illustrated by the following passage:

At the outset it is important to recognize the distinction between an individual and a class. A Chinese philosopher is reported to have said that if there is a dun cow and a bay horse, then there are three things; for the dun cow is one thing, and the bay horse is another thing, and the two together are a third thing. Everyone can see that there is some absurdity in this statement. The absurdity is due to the assumption that a collection of two things, i.e. a class with two members, is itself a thing of the same kind, or type, as its members. That everyone recognizes this absurdity shows that we clearly see that an individual is of a logically different type from a class. A class is not an object of which we can be directly aware. Thus we are not acquainted with the *class men*, hence 'men' is not a logically proper name for the collection of men. We must then ask what a class is. To answer this question we must inquire how we come to recognize a given class and how we do in fact use class-symbols, i.e. symbols (including words) which express classes. (S. Stebbing, *Modern Introduction to Logic* (1930), pp. 146–7.)

There is no absurdity in the Chinese philosopher's remark. There is nothing to prevent us from regarding an object consisting of a dun cow and a bay horse as one object and giving it a single name, in spite of the fact that it does not have a continuous spatial boundary. This is in principle what we do when we use the phrase 'British Empire' for an entity which consists of many geographically scattered parts. But such objects are not classes. People who use the notion of class are emphatic that a class is not the same thing as a physical collection. I should agree that we are not acquainted with the class men because there is no such thing. But this does not prevent us from *using* the theory of sets or classes. The fact that speaking of classes is only a *façon de parler* does not prevent this from being a *useful 'façon'*.

Very frequently when the phrase 'properties of so and so' is used in natural science what are meant or referred to are the laws (statements) satisfied by so and so. This is exemplified by some at least of the following passages from Einstein and Infeld's *The Evolution of Physics*:

But what is the medium through which light spreads and what are its mechanical properties?

The contradictions and inconsistencies of the old theories force us to ascribe new properties to the time-space continuum, to the scene of all events in our physical world.

From these assumptions, fully confirmed by experiment, the properties of moving rods and clocks, their changes in length and rhythm depending on velocity, are deduced.

Quantum physics formulates laws governing crowds not individuals. Not properties but probabilities are described, not laws disclosing the future of systems are formulated, but laws governing changes in time of the probabilities and relating to great congregations of individuals.

Note 11 (p. 32). In order that a statement should be an explanatory hypothesis more is usually required of it than that zero-level statements should follow from it. That this should be so is a necessary, but not always a sufficient, condition. See Part II, p. 124.

Note 12 (p. 35). By disjunction is thus meant the 'or' which does *not* exclude 'and'. It is much more commonly used than the exclusive 'or'. The interpretation of the conditional explained here by no means coincides with *all* uses of 'if...then ...' in ordinary speech. Excluded are such statements as 'If Tom had lived during the Cretaceous period then he would have seen pterodactyls', which employ the subjunctive or conditional moods.

Note 13 (p. 39). Dummy names are officially known as *variables*. Signs other than dummy names, including genuine names, are called constants. Variables 'do not possess any meaning by themselves'; see Tarski, *Introduction to Logic* (1941), p. 4, for an explanation of certain gross misunderstandings concerning variables.

Note 14 (p. 41). W. V. Quine, in his *Mathematical Logic* (1940), p. 70, gives a very good example of the vagaries of English grammar in connexion with denial. Consider the following general statements:

(1) Tom can outrun every man in the team.
(2) Tom can outrun any man in the team.

These are obviously equivalent. They both can be written in the form

$$(x) \ (\text{if } Fx \text{ then } Gx).$$

Now consider the following statements which result from inserting 'not' into corresponding places in (1) and (2):

(3) Tom cannot outrun every man in the team.

(4) Tom cannot outrun any man in the team.

We should expect (3) and (4) to be equivalent and both to be denials of (1) and (2). But this is not so. (3) can be written:
There is a man in the team whom Tom cannot outrun, and thus has the form

$$(\exists x) \ (Fx \ \& \ \text{not} \ Gx).$$

So (3) is the denial of (1). (4) can be written
There is no man in the team whom Tom can outrun, and has the form
$$\text{not} \ (\exists x) \ (Fx \ \& \ Gx),$$

from which, by eliminating the existential quantifier, we can obtain
$$(x) \ (\text{if} \ Fx \ \text{then not} \ Gx).$$

Clearly (3) and (4) are not equivalent and (4) is therefore not the denial of (1).

Note 15 (p. 47). It seems to be a rule that new and important hypotheses are at first rejected. We read, for example, that Avogadro's hypothesis was 'not accepted by the early proponents of the atomic theory' and only commanded general adherence 'after the exposition of the hypothesis some 47 years later by his fellow-countryman the Italian scientist Cannizzaro'. Also that 'Newland's Law of Octaves, 1864, an arrangement of the elements in groups of eight bringing with each eighth element a repetition of properties like the eighth note of an octave in music, aroused much ridicule and little respect, though essentially the correct formulation of periodicity' (H. S. and H. A. Taylor, *Elementary Physical Chemistry* (1937), pp. 3, 8).

Note 16 (p. 57). Whitehead, in his little book *Symbolism* (1928), maintained that we have 'two modes of direct perception of the external world'. Where one is vague, he says, the other is precise; where one is important, the other is trivial. Perception by means of sensible objects he called presentational immediacy. The other mode he called causal efficacy. He refers to this as 'the most insistent perception of a circumambient efficacious world of beings'. Sensible objects, he says, are handy, definite, and manageable, but

The sense of controlling presences has the contrary character: it is unmanageable, vague, and ill-defined.

But for all their vagueness, for all their lack of definition, these controlling presences, these sources of power, these things with an inner life, with their own richness of content, these beings, with the destiny of the world hidden in their natures, are what we want to know about. As we cross a road busy with traffic, we see the colour of the cars, their shapes, the gay colours of their occupants; but at the moment we are absorbed in using this immediate show as a symbol for the forces determining the immediate future. (p. 57.)

I have tried hard to be a phenomenalist, but I cannot conscientiously say that I have ever succeeded. Like Mr Edwards, Dr Johnson's friend, I find that something is 'always breaking in', but in my case it is not cheerfulness, it is animal faith. Nevertheless, I do not claim (with Whitehead) that the so-called external world is a directly perceived world; I feel compelled to admit that it is a hypothetical world. And this hypothesis seems unavoidable for anyone who does not believe that when he uses language he is always talking to himself.

Note 17 (p. 58). There is widespread misunderstanding about the status of scientific hypotheses. The current practice seems to be to call a hypothesis a hypothesis only when it is first propounded. After it has been before the world for some time it is called a *theory*, and when it has become well established and survived a good deal of testing it may finally be called a *fact*. But in spite of all these changes of name it has not ceased to be a hypothesis, i.e. a statement which necessarily goes far beyond any attainable data. These changes of name register changes in our attitude of belief towards the hypothesis, not changes in its own status.

The following passage illustrates a common attitude:

'Mine aren't theories', said Eugenius simply. 'They are logical deductions from known facts. They thus become facts themselves, like all the deductions and discoveries of modern science and philosophy.'

Now theories are *never* and cannot be 'logical deductions from known facts' if the phrase 'logical deduction' is used in its strict sense and if by facts is meant observation records. The above passage is not from a scientific work but from a book pointing out the extreme logical weakness of speculations concerning the life of Shakespeare and called *The Real Shakespeare* (1947) by William Bliss. But the author is unable to resist the impulse to plunge into the same trap himself. Hence the above passage. The same point is illustrated by the following passage from a paper dealing with the relation between genetics and cytology:

> By crossing two forms of *Drosophila melanogaster*, in which the X-chromosomes were visibly distinguishable at two distinct places in consequence of translocations, individuals were obtained which had 'doubly heteromorphic' X-chromosomes. In cases of exchange between the factors situated in the X-chromosomes cytological recombinations of pieces of chromosomes could be established. The Morgan theory is now no longer a theory, but a fact. (Curt Stern, 'Zytologisch-genetische Untersuchungen als Beweise für die Morgansche Theorie, u.s.w.', *Biologisches Zentralblatt*, LI (1931), p. 586.)

The experiments described constitute a valuable confirmation of Morgan's hypothesis, but it does not therefore cease to *be* a hypothesis.

The following remarks of Lord Russell are useful in this connexion:

> The actual procedure of science consists of an alternation of observation, hypothesis, experiment, and theory. The only difference between a hypothesis and a theory is subjective; the investigator believes the theory, whereas he only thinks the hypothesis sufficiently plausible to be worth testing. A hypothesis should accord with all known relevant observations, and suggest experiments (or

observations) which will have one result if the hypothesis is true, and another if it is false. This is an ideal; in actual fact, other hypotheses will always exist which are compatible with what is meant to be an *experimentum crucis*. The crucial character can only be as between *two* hypotheses, not as between one hypothesis and all the rest. When a hypothesis has passed a sufficient number of experimental tests, it becomes a theory. The argument in favour of a theory is always the formally invalid argument: '*p* implies *q*, and *q* is true, therefore *p* is true.' Here *p* is the theory, and *q* is the observed relevant facts. (*The Analysis of Matter* (1927), p. 194.)

I do not use the word 'theory' in the above sense. By a theory I mean a system of statements ordered by the consequence relation. Regarding the invalid argument referred to, see above, p. 37.

J. S. Mill, in his *Logic*, wrote:

But it is not, I conceive, a valid reason for accepting any given hypothesis that we are unable to imagine any other which will account for the facts. There is no necessity for supposing that the true explanation must be one which, with only our present experience, we could imagine. (Book III, Chap. XIV, §6.)

Nothing is explained simply because someone has been ingenious enough to invent something which he finds 'satisfying', especially if this something is not a hypothesis from which a statement describing what is to be explained can be derived. To be a genuine explanation a hypothesis must have survived *some* test.

Note 18 (p. 58). Visual sensible objects play, perhaps, an unduly large part in our thinking. When we represent something to ourselves in the imagination it is usually a visual object that we imagine. But this is not to imagine an object belonging to the converse domain of **OF**, but only a *look* of such an object and thus an object belonging to the domain of **OF**. Objects belonging to the converse domain of **OF** cannot be imagined. This confusion arises from naïve realism which does not distinguish between a look of an object and the object of which it is a look.

Some at least of our scientific statements must speak about objects which 'have' looks, feels, sounds, etc.; but so long as a theory has the right structure it is not at all necessary that all biological functors should name objects which have looks, etc. (See also next Note.)

The following passage from Frege's *Grundlagen der Arithmetik*, § 60, is interesting in this connexion:

Es ist also die Unvorstellbarkeit des Inhaltes eines Wortes kein Grund, ihm jede Bedeutung abzusprechen oder es vom Gebrauche auszuschliessen. Der Schein des Gegentheils entsteht wohl dadurch, dass wir die Wörter vereinzelt betrachten und nach ihrer Bedeutung fragen, für welche wir dann eine Vorstellung nehmen. So scheint ein Wort keinen Inhalt zu haben, für welches uns ein entsprechendes inneres Bild fehlt. Man muss aber immer einen vollständigen Satz ins Auge fassen. Nur in ihm haben die Wörter eigentlich eine Bedeutung. Die innern Bilder, die uns dabei etwa vorschweben, brauchen nicht den logischen Bestandtheilen des Urtheils zu entsprechen. Es genügt, wenn der Satz als Ganzes einen Sinn hat; dadurch erhalten auch seine Theile ihren Inhalt.

Note 19 (p. 58). In connexion with this distinction the following passages are of interest:

Indeed unless we confine ourselves altogether to mathematical symbolism it is hard to avoid dressing our symbols in deceitful clothing. When I think of an electron there rises in my mind a hard, red, tiny ball, the proton similarly is neutral grey. Of course the colour is absurd—perhaps not more so than the rest of the conception —but I am incorrigible. I can well understand that the younger minds are finding these pictures too concrete and are striving to construct the world out of Hamiltonian functions and symbols so far removed from human preconception that they do not even obey the laws of orthodox arithmetic. For myself I find some difficulty in rising to that plane of thought; but I am convinced that it has got to come. (Sir A. S. Eddington, *The Nature of the Physical World* (1944).)

If we demand from the modern physicist an answer to the question what he means by the symbol 'ψ' of his calculus, and are astonished that he cannot give an answer, we ought to realize that the situation was already the same in classical physics. There the physicist could not tell what he meant by the symbol 'E' in Maxwell's equations. Perhaps, in order not to refuse an answer, he would tell us that 'E' designates the electric field vector....We are right in demanding an interpretation of 'E', but that will be given indirectly by semantical rules referring to elementary signs together with the formulas connecting them with 'E'. This interpretation enables us to use the laws containing 'E' for the derivation of predictions. Thus we understand 'E', if 'understanding' of an expression, a sentence, or a theory means capability of its use for the description of known facts or the prediction of new facts. An 'intuitive understanding' or a direct translation of 'E' into terms referring to observable properties is neither necessary nor possible. The situation of the modern physicist is not essentially different. He knows how to use the symbol 'ψ' in the calculus in order to derive predictions which we can test by observations....He possesses that kind of understanding which alone is essential in the fields of knowledge and science. (R. Carnap, 'Foundations of Logic and Mathematics', *International Encyclopedia of Unified Science*, vol. I, no. 3.)

In Science, structure is the main study. (Lord Russell, in *Contemporary British Philosophy*.)

Alle wissenschaftlichen Aussagen sind Strukturaussagen.

Jede wissenschaftliche Aussage grundsätzlich so umgeformt werden kann, dass sie nur noch eine Strukturaussage ist.

Zunächst halten wir fest, dass es für die Wissenschaft möglich und zugleich notwendig ist, sich auf Strukturaussagen zu beschränken. (R. Carnap, *Logische Aufbau der Welt* (1928), pp. 20–1.)

...What really matters to science is not the inner nature of objects but their mutual relations and that any set of terms with the right mutual relations will answer all scientific purposes as well as any other set with the same sort of relations.... (C. D. Broad, *Scientific Thought* (1923), p. 39.)

Note 20 (p. 43). For further reading in connexion with the topics of Part I, the following works may be recommended. The best elementary introduction is A. Tarski, *Introduction to Logic and the Methodology of the Deductive Sciences* (1941). For the methodology of natural science read K. Popper, *Logik der Forschung* (1935) and C. G. Hempel and P. Oppenheim, 'Studies in the logic of explanation', in *Philosophy of Science*

(1948), vol. xv, pp. 135–75. See also my 'Technique of theory construction', *International Encyclopedia of Unified Science* (1939), vol. II, no. 5. For the concept of consequence see A. Tarski, *Über den Begriff der logischen Folgerung*, Actes du Congrès International de Philosophie Scientifique, Sorbonne, Paris, 1935. K. Popper, 'Logic without assumptions', *Proc. Aristotelian Soc.*, 5 May 1947, pp. 251–92.

For recent work on induction see: R. Carnap, 'On inductive logic', *Philosophy of Science* (1945), vol. XII, pp. 72–97; 'The two concepts of probability', *Philosophy and Phenomenological Research* (1945), vol. v, pp. 513–32; 'Remarks on induction and truth', *Philosophy and Phenomenological Research* (1946), vol. VI, pp. 590–602; 'On the application of inductive logic', *Philosophy and Phenomenological Research* (1947), vol. VIII (1947), pp. 133–48; C. G. Hempel and P. Oppenheim, 'A definition of "degree of confirmation"', *Philosophy of Science* (1945), vol. XII, pp. 98–115; W. Kneale, *Probability and Induction* (1949). In these works will be found complete bibliographies. For semantical problems see R. Carnap, *Meaning and Necessity* (1947). An interesting discussion of many points concerning the relation of mathematical logic to ordinary language will be found in H. Reichenbach, *Elements of Symbolic Logic* (1947).*

---

* Since the above list was compiled Carnap's comprehensive treatise on induction has appeared with the title *Logical Foundations of Probability*, Chicago (1950).

APPENDIX A

AN ANALYSIS OF HARVEY'S *DE MOTU CORDIS ET SANGUINIS*

I add this analysis of Harvey's *De motu* in the hope that it may interest historians of science and also in order to illustrate some of the points discussed in Part I.

I have used C. D. Leake's* and R. Willis's† translations, but the formulations of Harvey's statements here used are all from the latter translation.‡

The systematic exposition of the theory of the circulation is contained in *Chapters* II–XIV. The Introduction is devoted to combating current opinions about the heart and blood vessels. *Chapter* I gives the author's motives for writing, and the three chapters following XIV contain miscellaneous discussions confirmatory of the theory. Leake expresses the opinion that 'The last of the book seems to have been written some time after the main part of it, when long reflection on the subject had crystallized his opinion'. What follows is confined almost entirely to the systematic exposition in *Chapters* II–XIV.

As was mentioned in Part I, Harvey's statements are classifiable into (1) zero-level statements, which are here labelled with Arabic numerals, (2) first-level hypotheses, which are labelled with Roman numerals, (3) consequences of these hypotheses, other than those in (1), to which I have also given Roman numerals, (4) methodological statements, which are here given in quotation marks.

I have provided a diagram of the mammalian circulation showing the parts referred to in Harvey's hypotheses.

* Published at Springfield, Ill., U.S.A. (1928).
† Everyman's Library (1923).
‡ These formulations sometimes deviate both as regards order of words and the words themselves from Willis.

Chapter II. THE MOTION OF THE HEART

Zero-level statements

(1) There is a time when the heart moves and a time when it is motionless.

(2) In the pause, as in death, the heart is soft, flaccid, lying as it were at rest.

(3) In the motion the heart is erected and rises up to a point, so that at this time it strikes against the breast and the pulse is felt externally.

(4) In the motion the heart is everywhere contracted so that it looks narrower, relatively longer and more drawn together.

(5) In the motion the heart is felt to become harder.

(6) In cold-blooded animals the heart when it moves becomes pale in colour, when quiescent of a deeper blood-red colour.

(7) When the fore arm is grasped its tendons [i.e. muscles] are perceived to become tense and resilient when the fingers are moved.

(8) Muscles when in action contract in the line of their fibres and acquire vigour and tenseness, from soft become hard, prominent and thickened.

First-level statements

I. All hearts have muscle in their walls.

II. The muscle in any heart exhibits rhythmically alternating contractions and relaxations.

III. The muscles of any heart are so arranged that when they contract the cubic capacity of the heart is diminished.

IV. When the cubic capacity of any heart is diminished the pressure on its contents is increased.

V. Every mammalian heart has two chambers on the right and two on the left. Blood enters the right auricle through the vena cava and the left auricle through the pulmonary vein. Blood leaves the left ventricle through the aorta and the right ventricle through the pulmonary artery.

Consequences

Of I and 8:

VI. All hearts become hard during contraction. [In conformity with (4) and (5).]

VII. All hearts become soft during relaxation. [In conformity with (2).]

Of I and II:

VIII. The motion of any heart consists of rhythmical alternating contraction and relaxation. [In conformity with (1).]

Of III, IV and V:

IX. If the wall of any heart is thin enough it will appear pale during contraction and blood-coloured during relaxation. [Confirmed by (6).]

Of III and IV:

X. If a sufficiently large hole is made in the wall of any heart blood will be expelled through it.

Zero-level statement

(9) When the ventricle of a heart is pierced the blood is seen to be forcibly projected outwards upon each motion or pulsation when the heart is tense. [Confirmatory of X.]

Chapter III. THE MOTION OF THE ARTERIES
Definitions

[D.1] A heart is said to be *in systole* when it is contracting.

[D.2] An artery is said to be *in diastole* when it is dilated and yields a pulse.

Zero-level statements

(10) When the heart is in systole the arteries are in diastole.

(11) When the right ventricle contracts the pulmonary artery is distended at the same time with the other arteries of the body.

(12) The weaker the contraction of the left ventricle, the feebler is the pulse in the arteries.

(13) When the right ventricle fails to contract the pulse in the pulmonary artery ceases also.

(14) If in fishes the vessel which leads from the heart to the gills is divided then, at the moment when the heart contracts, the blood flows with force from the divided vessel.

(15) When in arteriotomy the blood is projected, now to a greater now to a less distance, we see that the greater jet corresponds to the diastole of the artery and to the systole of the heart.

(16) Wherever the motion of the blood through the arteries is impeded, then do the remote divisions of the arteries beat less forcibly.

'From these facts it is manifest that'

First-level statement

XI. The arteries are filled and distended by the blood forced into them by the contraction of the ventricles.

Chapter IV. THE MOTIONS OF THE VENTRICLES AND AURICLES

Zero-level statements

(17) In a dying heart it is seen that the auricles contract together first and this is followed by the contraction of the two ventricles together; the motion appearing to begin from the auricles and to extend to the ventricles, there being a short pause between the two motions.

(18) If, while the auricles are still alive, the ventricles are cut off, blood flows out upon each contraction of the auricles.

Chapter V

'From these and other observations of the like kind, I am persuaded it will be found that the motion of the heart is as follows:'

First-level statements

XII. The motion of any heart is such that first the auricles contract and throw the blood (which they receive from the veins) into the ventricles, which being filled then contract and send the blood into the arteries.

XIII. The right ventricle sends its charge into the lungs.

XIV. The left ventricle sends its charge into the aorta and through this by the arteries to the body at large.

Harvey next deals with the following problem: If blood reaches the right heart by way of the vena cava, but is distributed from the left heart by way of the aorta, how does it get from the right side to the left? The answer current in Harvey's time was that it did so by 'sweating through the septum of the heart'. Harvey rejects this and proceeds to seek another passage. In the Introduction he brings forward the following zero-level statements against the current view:

(i) Pores have not been demonstrated in the septum of the heart.

(ii) The septum of the heart is of a denser and more compact structure than any portion of the body, except the bones and sinews.

(iii) Both ventricles contract and dilate simultaneously.

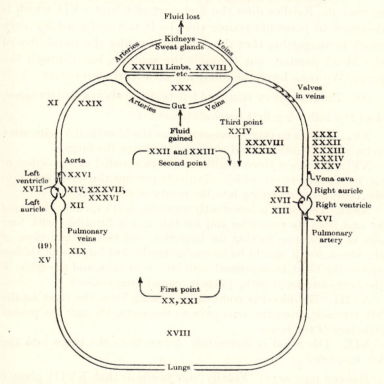

(iv) The septum of the heart is supplied with blood by the coronary artery and vein.

(v) In the foetus the foramen ovale is provided to permit the passage of blood from one side of the heart to the other.

Incidentally, (i) is not a very good point for Harvey to emphasize because his own theory requires that the blood should pass through the peripheral muscles and other organs in which in his time no 'pores' had been demonstrated.

Chapter VI begins with a plea for the study of comparative anatomy. Harvey here displays an astonishing knowledge of this subject. He describes in considerable detail points of the circulatory systems of fishes, amphibians and mammalian foetuses. But, strictly speaking, this does not advance his argument. Neither does the first part of *Chapter* VII which is designed to persuade people that he is not really asking very much in suggesting that they should consider the possibility of the blood passing, not through the septum, but through the lungs. We then have the following zero-level statement:

(19) The pulmonary veins and left ventricle always contain blood.

And the following first-level statements:

XV. There is no other passage whence the blood in the pulmonary veins and left auricle could come save through the lungs.

XVI. There are three semilunar valves situated at the orifice of the pulmonary artery which effectually prevent the blood sent into the vessel from returning into the cavity of the heart.

XVII. The heart is incessantly receiving and expelling the blood by and from its ventricles and for this end is furnished with four sets of valves two serving for induction and two for eduction, of the blood, lest it should be incommodiously sent hither and thither and so the heart be oppressed with labour in vain, and the office of the lungs interfered with. [This is quoted from Galen.]

XVIII. The blood is continually passing from the right to the left ventricle, from the vena cava to the aorta, through the porous structure of the lungs.

XIX. The blood is incessantly drawn from the lungs into the left ventricle.

Harvey now says: 'Finally, our position that XVIII plainly appears from this, that since XIII (see above) and XIX, as appears from what precedes and the position of the valves, it cannot do otherwise than XVIII.'

This concludes the passage of blood from the right heart to the left. The rest of the book is devoted to the problem of how the blood passes from the left heart to the right.

The short *Chapter* VIII contains a reference to the opposition which Harvey anticipates to his theory and also a short announcement of the argument which is worked out in subsequent chapters. This may be stated as follows:

A great quantity of blood is being pumped into the arteries through the aorta, (XIV).

(i) Why do not the arteries burst?

A great quantity of blood is passing along the veins to the vena cava.

(ii) Why do they not become drained?

Harvey mentions that fluid enters the system from the juices supplied by the aliment, but rejects this as insufficient to prevent (ii). He does not mention the loss of fluid by the sweat glands and kidneys. Presumably he rejected that as insufficient to prevent (i). These possibilities being thus excluded he maintains that there remains only the continuous passage of blood from the arteries into the veins, thus 'a motion as it were in a circle'.

In *Chapter* IX Harvey begins by saying that 'three points present themselves for confirmation which, being stated, I conceive that the truth I contend for will follow necessarily, and appear as a thing obvious to all'.

First-level statements

First point:

XX. The blood is incessantly transmitted by the action of the heart from the vena cava to the arteries in such quantity that it cannot be supplied from the ingesta.

XXI. The blood is incessantly transmitted by the action of the heart from vena cava to the arteries in such wise that the whole mass [of blood] very quickly passes through the organ.

Second point:

XXII. The blood under the influence of the arterial pulse enters and is impelled in a continuous, equable and incessant stream through every part and member of the body.

XXIII. The blood, impelled as described in XXII, is in much larger quantity than were sufficient for nutrition or than the whole mass of fluids could supply.

Third point:

XXIV. The blood, having been impelled as described in XXII through every part and member of the body, is returned incessantly by the veins to the heart from all parts and members of the body.

Harvey now says: 'These points proved, I conceive it will be manifest that'

XL. The blood circulates, revolves, propelled and then returning, from the heart to the extremities, from the extremities to the heart, and thus it performs a kind of circular motion.

The following statements are now brought forward in support of the first point:

(20) In the dead body the heart holds upwards of 2 ounces of blood.

XI. The arteries are filled and distended by the blood forced into them by the contraction of the ventricles.

XXV. At least one quarter of the total contents of the heart is thrown into the aorta at each contraction.

XXVI. At the root of the aorta are valves which prevent the return of blood from that vessel into the ventricle.

(21) During half an hour the heart makes at least 1000 beats.

Arithmetical: $\frac{1}{2}$ oz. $\times 1000 = 500$ oz.

(22) The whole body contains less than 500 oz. of blood.

'Upon this supposition, therefore, assumed merely as a ground for reasoning, we see' that

XXVII. The whole mass of blood in the body passes through the heart from the veins to the arteries, and in like manner through the lungs. And more blood passes through the heart in consequence of its action, than can either be supplied by the whole of the ingesta, or than can be contained in the veins at the same moment.

There follow a number of zero-level statements confirmatory of the above:

(23) If only a small branch of the aorta is divided the whole of the blood in the body, as well that of the veins as of the arteries, is drained away in the course of no long time.

(24) The blood mentioned in (23) comes almost exclusively from the arteries.

(25) If the aorta be tied at the base of the heart and the carotid or any other artery be opened, it is found to be empty and the veins, only, replete with blood.

(26) After death, when the heart has ceased to beat, it is impossible by dividing either the jugular or the femoral veins and arteries, by any effort to force out more than one half of the whole mass of blood.

(27) In fainting fits and in states of alarm, when the heart beats more languidly and with less force, haemorrhages are diminished or arrested.

This last statement is mentioned in confirmation of part of XVII. The next paragraph contains a statement which seems to be in contradiction to (19). Harvey discusses why 'in our dissections we usually find so large a quantity of blood in the veins, so little in the arteries'. He says that it is perhaps because 'as there is no passage to the arteries save through the lungs and heart, when an animal has ceased to breathe, and the lungs to move, the blood in the pulmonary artery is prevented from passing into the pulmonary veins, and from thence into the left ventricle of the heart'. A little further on he says

But the heart not ceasing to act at the same precise moment as the lungs, but surviving them and continuing to pulsate for a time, the left ventricle and arteries go on distributing their blood to the body at large and sending it into the veins; receiving none from the lungs, however, they are soon exhausted and left, as it were, empty.

(19) presumably refers to the *living* body.

Chapter X opens with the statement that the first point is confirmed, although that point contained the assertion that the quantity of blood passing through the heart is greater than can be supplied by the ingesta, and so far Harvey has made no further reference to this point. He seems to regard it as so obvious as to require no further support. Here he now refers to it by saying that, although a cow may give three, four or even seven gallons and more of milk in a day, yet 'the heart by computation does as much and more in the course of an hour or two'.

In this chapter he gives further zero-level statements confirmatory of the first point:

(28) If the veins in serpents and several fishes are tied some way below the heart, a space between the ligature and the heart speedily becomes empty.

(29) If, in the same experiment as described in (28) the artery is tied, the heart becomes inordinately distended.

Chapter XI is devoted to the second point. First Harvey gives the first-level statements he wishes to establish:

XXVIII. The blood enters a limb by the arteries and returns from it by the veins.

XXIX. The arteries are the vessels carrying the blood from the heart, and the veins the returning channels of the blood to the heart.

XXX. In the limbs and extreme parts of the body the blood passes either immediately by anastomosis from the arteries into the veins, or mediately by the pores of the flesh or in both ways, as in the lungs.

To these he adds XXIII which is part of the second point.

Next Harvey discusses ligatures and we are given two definitions:

[D.3] A ligature is *tight* or perfect when it is drawn so close about an extremity that no vessel can be felt pulsating beyond it.

(Harvey mentions that this type of ligature is used in castration and the removal of tumours. Nutriment and heat being cut off testes and tumours dwindle and die.)

[D.4] A ligature of *middling tightness* is one which compresses a limb firmly all round, but short of pain, and in such a way as still to suffer a certain degree of pulsation to be felt in the artery beyond it.

(This type, says Harvey, is used in blood-letting.) Note that Harvey is careful not to import anything belonging to first level into his definitions, they are strictly 'operational'. He now gives a number of zero-level statements involving the two types of ligature.

(30) If a tight ligature is thrown about an extremity no artery beyond the ligature pulsates but the artery above it begins to rise higher at each diastole and to throb more violently. The hand retains its natural colour but gradually begins to fall somewhat in temperature.

(31) If the ligature in (30) is now slackened a little so that it becomes a ligature of middling tightness, the whole hand and arm will instantly become *deeply suffused* and distended; the *veins become tumid and knotted*, and the *hand becomes gorged with blood*.

(32) At the moment of slackening mentioned in (31), if the finger is applied to the artery by the edge of the ligature blood can be felt as it were to glide through.

(33) The subject of the experiment in (32) feels a sensation of warmth and of something making its way along the course of the vessels and diffusing itself through the hand which, at the same time, begins to feel hot and becomes distended.

(34) When a ligature of middling tightness is applied, the veins below the ligature swell but never those above, whilst the arteries shrink. Only very strong pressure will force the blood beyond the ligature and cause any of the veins in the upper arm to rise.

Harvey now says: 'From these facts it is easy for every careful observer to learn that XXVIII.' After a little further detailed discussion of the connexion between D.3, D.4 (30)–(34) and XXVIII, Harvey says: 'It therefore plainly appears that'

XXXI. The ligature prevents the return of the blood through the veins to the parts above it, and maintains those beneath it in a state of permanent distension.

XXXII. The arteries, in spite of the pressure of the ligature and under the force and impulse of the heart, send on the blood from the internal parts of the body to the parts beyond the ligature.

XXXIII. The tight ligature prevents the passage of blood in both arteries and veins; the middling ligature does not prevent the passage through the arteries but only through the veins.

XXXIV. The blood which accumulates in the veins below the ligature does not come from the veins. (See (34).)

(35) When the middling ligature is removed the subject is aware of something cold making its way upward and reaching the elbow or axilla.

Harvey says that (31) is 'an obvious indication that' XXVIII (and not vice versa) and XXX, and also that

XXXV. The veins have communications with one another.

This last statement is further confirmed by:

(36) When the ligature is slackened as in (31) the veins all become turgid together.

(37) If, while the veins are turgid as in (36), any single small vein is pricked with a lancet they all speedily shrink.

Harvey next points out how his first-level hypotheses explain the procedure in phlebotomy:

(38) In phlebotomy the ligature is applied *above* the part that is punctured, not below it.

(39) In phlebotomy when the ligature is either slackened or applied too tightly the blood escapes without force.

Chapter XII concludes the discussion of the second point.

Harvey says: 'If these things be so, another point which I have already referred to, viz. XXI, will also be confirmed. We have seen that XXVIII; we have seen, farther, that almost the whole of the blood may be withdrawn from a puncture made in one of the cutaneous veins of the arm if a ligature is properly applied (not only the whole quantity in the arm but the whole that is contained in the body).' Harvey does not appear to have stated this previously, but it is presumably covered by the references to phlebotomy. He then continues:

Whence we must admit, first XXXII (on account of XI and

XXXVI. The force and motion of the blood are derived from the heart alone);

second that XX and XXI for XXXIV and

XXXVII. The arteries nowhere receive blood save and except from the left ventricle of the heart.

Nor could so large a quantity of blood be drawn from one vein (a ligature being duly applied), nor with such impetuosity, such readiness, such celerity, unless through the medium of the impelling power of the heart.

Harvey then refers again to his computations of the quantity of blood passing and says that from these 'we shall perceive that a circulation is absolutely necessary, seeing that the quantities hinted at cannot be supplied immediately from the ingesta, and are vastly more than can be requisite for the mere nutrition of the parts'.

The chapter ends with further confirmatory references to phlebotomy.

(40) When in the course of phlebotomy a state of faintness supervenes in which the heart pulsates more languidly, the blood does not flow freely, but distils by drops only.

(41) But when in (40) the patient gets rid of his fear and recovers his courage, the pulsific power is increased, the arteries begin again to beat with greater force and to drive the blood even into the part that is bound; so that the blood now springs from the puncture in the vein and flows in a continuous stream.

In *Chapter* XIII the third point is discussed. We first have a number of zero-level statements about the valves in the veins:

(42) The valves in the veins are directed upwards or towards the trunks of the veins.

(43) The parts of the valves regard each other, mutually touch and are so ready to come into contact by their edges that if anything attempts to pass from the trunks into the branches of the veins, or from the greater vessels into the less, they completely prevent it.

(44) The valves are so arranged that the horns of those that succeed are opposite the middle of the convexity of those that precede and so on alternately.

(45) The edges of the valves in the jugular veins hang downwards and are so contrived that they prevent the blood from rising upwards.

(46) The valves in the veins always look towards the seat of the heart.

XXXVIII. The valves are solely made and instituted lest the blood should pass from the greater into the lesser veins and either rupture them or cause them to become varicose.

(47) When I attempt to pass a probe from the trunk of the veins into one of the smaller branches, whatever care I take, I find it impossible to introduce it far any way, by reason of the valves, whilst it was most easy to push it along in the opposite direction.

XXXIX. The effect of the arrangement of the valves in the veins is to prevent all motion of the blood from the heart and vena cava.

(48) When a ligature is applied to the arm above the elbow as if for phlebotomy, certain knots or elevations are perceived which are formed by valves, which thus show themselves externally.

(49) When the blood is pressed from the space above one of the valves, and the finger kept on the vein inferiorly, no influx of blood takes place from above. But the vessel above the next valve upwards will continue to be distended.

(50) When pressure is applied to the distended part of the vein referred to in (49) the blood cannot be forced backwards below the valve, and the part of the vein below the valve remains empty.

Harvey says: 'It would therefore appear that XXXIX'

(51) The arm being bound as before and the veins looking full and distended, if you press at one part in the course of a vein with the point of a finger and then with another finger streak the blood upwards beyond the next valve, it is seen that this portion of the vein continues empty as before, and that the blood cannot retrograde; but the finger first applied being removed, immediately the vein is filled from below.

Harvey says 'that XXIV appears most obviously'. He then points out that the quantity of blood passing through a given length of vein when stroked as above with the finger can be computed, and then it is seen 'that so much blood has passed through a certain part of the vessel. And now I believe that you will find yourself convinced of the circulation of the blood and of its rapid motion.'

In the very brief *Chapter* XIV Harvey says: 'Since all things, both argument and ocular demonstration, show XX, XXI (first point), XXII, XXIII (second point) and XXIV (third point) it is absolutely necessary to conclude' that

XL. The blood in the animal body is impelled in a circle and is in a state of ceaseless motion.

XLI. This propulsion of the blood is the act or function which the heart performs by means of its pulse.

XLII. The propulsion of the blood is the sole and only end of the motion and contraction of the heart.

This concludes Harvey's systematic exposition of his theory. I think it is plain that we do not do justice to Harvey if we are content to call him 'the discoverer of the circulation of the blood'. Historians have devoted much effort to discussions about rival claims to this title, but they do not appear to have considered the possibility that *no one* discovered the circulation of the blood. That the blood circulates is a hypothesis to-day as much as it was in Harvey's time, but to-day it is a much better confirmed hypothesis than it was in Harvey's day. Harvey frequently asserts that his appeal is only to 'observation [or 'sense', as he calls it] and reason' as opposed to resting content with the opinions of past authorities, although he does not hesitate to quote the views of Aristotle, Galen, Columbus and others when they support his contentions. His subsequent admirers seem to have emphasized his appeal to observation and to have ignored his appeal to reason. What did Harvey mean by his 'appeal to reason'?

Harvey's procedure is clearly as follows: In each section of the work he gives a number of zero-level statements and then proceeds to enunciate the explanatory hypotheses of first level which they suggest. Sometimes he gives the hypotheses first and then the zero-level statements which suggest them. Next he proceeds to work out the logical consequences of his first-level hypotheses, among which at last we have the statement that the blood moves in a circle. It is this part of the business to which Harvey is referring when he speaks of an appeal to reason. Frequently he adds further zero-level statements by way of confirmation of these consequences, and so of the hypotheses from which they are derived. In this connexion the concluding paragraph of his book is interesting. I give it in the original Latin and in the two translations:

Haec omnia phaenomena inter dissecandum observanda et

plurima alia, si recte persensa fuerint, ante dictam veritatem viden-
tur luculenter illustrare et plane confirmare, simulque vulgaribus
opinionibus adversari; cum quam ob causam ita constituta sint et
facta haec omnia difficile cuiquam admodum sit (nisi quo nos modo)
explicare.

Leake's translation:

All these phenomena and many others noted in dissecting, if
correctly judged, seem clearly to illustrate and to confirm the truth
announced in this tract, and at the same time to refute popular
opinion. Certainly it would be hard to explain in any other way
why all these matters are so made and constituted except in a
manner conforming to my theory and to what I have expounded.

Willis's translation:

All these appearances, and many others, to be noted in the course
of dissection, if rightly weighed, seem clearly to illustrate and fully
to confirm the truth contended for throughout these pages, and at
the same time to stand in opposition to the vulgar opinion; for it
would be very difficult to explain in any other way to what purpose
all is constructed and arranged as we have seen it to be.

Our next task is to construct a map to show, if possible, how
Harvey believed his statements to be connected by the consequence relation. In constructing the accompanying map I have
done my best to connect these statements in the way he appears
to have held that they were connected, in so far as this can be
discovered from his methodological statements. It will be seen
that in some cases the consequence does *not* strictly follow from
the hypotheses as they are formulated. In many cases this is
because something is implicitly assumed which Harvey expects
the reader to supply for himself, such as familiar anatomical
data or common-sense beliefs about the passage of fluid
through tubes. But in a few cases much more seems to be
assumed, e.g. XLII. Statement XXXVII rests on an obvious
anatomical basis which I have marked '*A*' on the map.
XXXVI, on the other hand, appears to have no zero-level
support. Leake remarks that 'The sixth and seventh chapters,
on the pulmonary circulation, are puzzling. There is a good

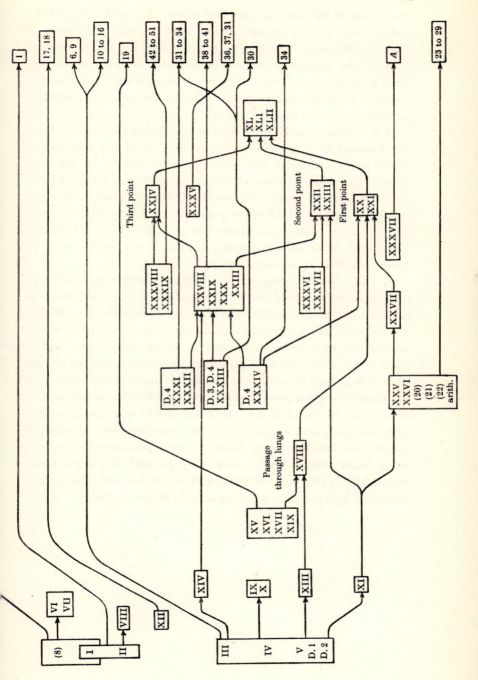

discussion of the comparative and embryological aspects of the subject, and then a peculiar use of the traditional authority of Galen as evidence.' As I have pointed out, this is the weakest part of the exposition, with the smallest zero-level support. This is easily seen from the chart. Harvey's argument here is largely a propaganda argument—a use of persuasion rather than an appeal to reason.

It is curious that Harvey does not make his statement about the amount of fluid ingested, compared with the amount of blood passing through the heart, more emphatic. If we note that at the rate of 500 oz. of blood per half-hour we shall have 24,000 oz. in 24 hours, we see that almost eight times the weight of a man of 14 stone passes in 24 hours, and no man ingests more than eight times his own weight in 24 hours! Even this is an underestimate, because 1000 heart beats in half an hour is an underestimate.

In the accompanying map, when an arrow runs from one statement to another, this means that the former statement is needed for the derivation of the latter. Thus the conditional formed with the conjunction of *all* the statements from which arrows run to a given statement A, as its antecedent, and A itself as its consequent, is an analytical conditional, or should be if A is to be a consequence of the statements conjoined. This map could be considerably enlarged by adding the confirmatory discussions in *Chapters* XV, XVI and XVII and also the more negative polemical arguments of the Introduction. More light might also be thrown on Harvey's methodological intentions by a Latin scholar who is able to cope with Harvey's Latin original from this point of view, and is familiar with the methodological beliefs which were current in Harvey's time.

PART II

METHODOLOGICAL PROBLEMS IN GENETICS

Thy reason, man?
Troth, sir, I can yield you none without words; and words
are grown so false, I am loath to prove reason with them.

Twelfth Night, iii, i.

LECTURE III

§ 1. INTRODUCTORY

I now come to the second part of my lectures. This will consist of *three* lectures: the first will show how a very simple but powerful genetical language can be constructed for the purpose of methodological analysis, and will show something of what it can do. The second will deal further with its uses and the third will explain the motives for its construction by showing how some of the difficulties of the subject are traceable to defects of the language which has been used. Geneticists, like all good scientists, proceed in the first instance intuitively and, as we shall see, their intuition has vastly outstripped the possibilities of expression in the ordinary usages of natural language. They *know* what they mean, but the current linguistic apparatus makes it very difficult for them to *say* what they mean. This apparatus conceals the complexity of the intuitions. It is part of the business of genetical methodology first to discover what geneticists mean and then to devise the simplest method of saying what they mean. If the result proves to be more complex than one would expect from the current expositions, that is because these devices are succeeding in making apparent a real complexity in the subject-matter which the natural language conceals.

We have first to discover what basic functors are involved in genetics with the help of which others may be defined, and then to show how, when these are used in combination with the few formative signs explained in previous lectures, we obtain a language which enables us to formulate genetical statements in a very precise and explicit, but at the same time compact, way.

Genetics is a science which has grown enormously in recent years, and it would be quite impossible for anyone, who has not devoted his whole time to it, to have a comprehensive grasp of the latest developments. But with these I shall not be concerned. I shall not begin at the top of the existing pyramid of genetical statements and work down; I shall begin with observation records and try to see how the levels of theoretical statements are reached. This process, which I call methodological analysis, thus proceeds in the opposite direction to that followed in axiomatization and is a necessary preliminary to it. In this procedure the necessary vocabulary is introduced piecemeal according to the requirements of each step as we proceed from one level to the level next above it. In axiomatization this whole vocabulary is given at the start, and we are at liberty to pick out whichever we choose as primitive or undefined signs, or to introduce totally new ones. In the following exposition, the undefined signs, although undefined within the system, will be explained on their first introduction with the help of metatheoretical statements outside the system. Such statements are sometimes called semantical rules. They will be prefixed by 'S'. The defined signs will be defined by means of statements within the system and prefixed by 'D'.

§ 2. PHENOTYPES AND ENVIRONMENTAL SETS

I take it to be the primary task of genetics to find answers to such questions as the following:

Given a classification of a set of parents and a classification of the environments in which they have developed, what can we say about the classification of their offspring, given the classification of the environments in which *they* have developed?

Three principal notions are involved: the relation of parent to offspring, the environment in which parents and offspring develop and their classification.

To begin with I shall not separate these constituents. I shall use a single name-forming functor which is explained in the following semantical rule:

[S. 1]   '$F_{X,Y,Z}(W_1, W_2)$' denotes the set of all offspring x such that for some u and some v, $u \in W_1$ and is a parent of x, $v \in W_2$ and is a parent of x, and u has developed in an environment belonging to the set X, v in an environment belonging to the set Y and x in an environment belonging to Z.*

I have chosen the letter '$\mathbf{F}$' for this functor in order to keep as close as possible to current usage. For it will be seen that there is a close affinity between the above and 'first filial generation' which is frequently denoted by 'F_1'. But there is (amongst others) this important point of difference: the above functor contains an explicit reference to the environmental sets for both parents and offspring. In most of its uses in the following pages the three environmental sets will not be distinct. I therefore define the following simpler form of this functor:

[D. 1] $\mathbf{F}_X(W_1, W_2) = \mathbf{F}_{X,X,X}(W_1, W_2)$.

A notation for the next generation is easily provided:

[D. 2] $\mathbf{F}^2_X(W_1, W_2) = \mathbf{F}_X(\mathbf{F}_X(W_1, W_2), \mathbf{F}_X(W_1, W_2))$.

The use of this functor, which will be called the mating functor, is governed by the following postulates:†

[H. 1] $\mathbf{F}_{X,Y,Z}(W_1, W_2) = \mathbf{F}_{Y,X,Z}(W_2, W_1)$.

[H. 2]   If $\mathbf{F}_{X,Y,Z}(W_1, W_2) \neq \Lambda$ then

$$W_1 \cap X = W_1 \cap Y = W_1 \cap Z = W_2 \cap X = W_2 \cap Y = W_2 \cap Z = \Lambda.$$

This merely states that parental sets and environmental sets have no member in common.

[H. 3]   If any of the sets X, Y, Z, W_1, W_2 is null then
     $\mathbf{F}_{X,Y,Z}(W_1, W_2)$ is null.

(I insert H. 1 to H. 3 as specimens of what might be required if we were axiomatizing and '$\mathbf{F}$' were being taken as an undefined

---

* Note that the comma in the brackets is a bold-face comma. The significance of this is explained in the next section in connexion with the *simple product* of two sets. See also Note 14, p. 212, items (2) and (6).

† All statements which are not derivable from others of the level to which we have reached, whether general postulates or specific genetical hypotheses, will be prefixed by 'H'. Consequences of such statements (theorems) will be prefixed by 'T'. Letters printed in bold-face type will always be used for biological constants, i.e. signs with a fixed biological significance, real names as opposed to dummy names. For other symbols see Note 2, p. 201.

sign, rather than as postulates which will actually be required in the sequel. In an axiom system 'F' is not likely to be treated as an undefined sign and later (Note 14, p. 214) we shall see how it can be defined and that special postulates for it are unnecessary.)

With the help of the mating functor we can formulate statements of the form $\quad \mathbf{F}_X(Y, Z) \subset W,$ \hfill (1)

which states that every member of the set $\mathbf{F}_X(Y, Z)$ is a member of the set W.

Before we consider other forms of statement containing the mating functor, something must be said about the question of the classification of environments, parents and offspring. Environmental sets are specified by reference to the composition of the soil, water or air, to the humidity and temperature of air, to the amount of exposure to sunlight, the amount and composition of food, etc.

Two kinds of classification of parents and offspring are involved in genetics. First we may specify sets of parents or offspring by means of observation records which state to which species they belong and how they are distinguished from other members of this species—either by reference to sensible objects (looks, smells, feels, tastes, etc.) or by the relation to some standard of length, weight, shape, etc., of either part or whole. For example, the matrices:

x belongs to *Drosophila melanogaster* and x has vestigial wings,
x belongs to *Pisum sativum* and x has yellow cotyledons,

specify such sets. Sets specified in this way are called *phenotypes* and the properties involved are called characters.* But as I pointed out in a previous lecture, theoretical (as opposed to applied) genetics is not interested in characters as such, and embryologists do not discuss characters but parts and the development of parts. In an agricultural show characters as

---

* I doubt whether it will suffice in *all* cases to specify phenotypes in the above way. It seems likely that some reference to the type of genetical system to which a given phenotype belongs will also be necessary in some cases, but this can only be explained later.

such are important from the point of view of winning prizes. But even here it is the plants and animals which are said to 'have' the characters which win or lose prizes, are bought and sold, and finally carried home in triumph or dejection. What both geneticists and embryologists are interested in is classifying lives *according to the way in which they develop*, and difference with respect to one or more characters is assumed to be an *index* of different modes of development. Words like 'tall', 'yellow' and 'colour-blind' will occur in applied but not in theoretical genetics. Words like 'tallness', 'yellowness' and 'colour-blindness' are best avoided altogether, for reasons explained in Part I.

'Phenotype' will be a second undefined sign, and the above remarks will, it is hoped, suffice for its semantical explanation. But a classification of parents and offspring into phenotypes is not sufficient for genetical purposes. We require a further classification of members of phenotypes into sub-sets called *genotypes* (in one, but only one, sense of that word). To discover whether a life belongs to a given genotype it is necessary to perform breeding tests. For this use of the word 'genotype' I have the authority of Professor J. B. S. Haldane who says: 'a class (of organisms) which can be distinguished from another by breeding tests is called a genotype.'* The word is also used in what appears to be a totally different sense.† But as I shall never use it in any but the above sense there will be no risk of confusion so long as this is remembered. The precise definition of 'genotype' is a somewhat difficult task which cannot be undertaken at this stage.

§3. COMBINED ALGEBRA

Statements of the form (1) above will not suffice when the members of the set of offspring are distributed in certain frequencies among *two* or more sets. In such cases geneticists, from the time of Mendel, have used expressions of the form

$$p_1 W_1 + p_2 W_2 + \ldots + p_n W_n, \tag{2}$$

* See Note 1, p. 201.
† This is discussed in the next lecture, p. 167.

where each p_i is a positive rational number and each W_i a set of lives. In Mendel's first paper, for example, we find the expression

$$1A + 2Aa + 1a.$$

(Here only the numerators of the fractions giving the proportions or frequencies are used.)

We are also sometimes told, in works on genetics, to multiply such expressions 'algebraically'. But we are not told what the plus sign means in such expressions, nor are we told anything about the laws of the algebra in question, in accordance with which the multiplication is to be carried out. This algebra cannot be the customary algebra of rational numbers, because the summands in (2) are not rational numbers, and the plus sign cannot therefore represent the addition of rational numbers.

Our next task therefore is to find definitions for these summands and for the addition and other operations involved, from which it will be possible to discover the laws which the foregoing expressions are required to obey in practice. This problem puzzled me for a long time, until at last the fact that each summand in (2) is formed by the juxtaposition of a dummy name representing a rational number in the closed interval between 0 and 1, and one representing a set, suggested to me that the algebra required must be some sort of combination of the Boolean algebra of sets and the algebra of rational numbers. George Boole, in his *Investigation of the Laws of Thought*, pointed out the very close parallel between the laws satisfied by symbols representing probabilities and the laws of the algebra of sets, which he invented; but he did not combine them into a single system.

I shall call the algebra we require *combined algebra*, the summands in (2) *combined elements*, and the whole expression (2) *a combined sum*.

It will be found that three distinct kinds of *combined multiplication* can occur in applications. If X and Y are sets, I use 'X, Y' (with bold-face comma) to denote the set of all couples one member of which belongs to X and the other to Y, order being disregarded, so that

$$X, Y = Y, X. \tag{3}$$

I call X, Y the *simple product* of the sets X and Y. It may happen that one factor is equal to the Boolean sum of two sets, e.g.

$$Y = Z \cup W.$$

The Boolean sum of Z and W is the set of all objects which belong to Z or to W or to both Z and W.* In this case we shall have

$$X, (Z \cup W) = X, Z \cup X, W. \tag{4}$$

One variety of combined product will be called *combined simple product* and written '$pX \, ; q Y$'.

I use '$X \times Y$' to denote the set of all *ordered* couples the first member of which belongs to X and the second to Y, so that unless $X = Y$ we have

$$X \times Y \neq Y \times X. \tag{5}$$

This kind of multiplication is therefore non-commutative. I call this the Cartesian product of X and Y, and the product $pX \overset{\cdot}{\times} q Y$ will therefore be called the combined Cartesian product of the two elements pX and $q Y$.†

Finally, we have the Boolean product $X \cap Y$ which is the set of all objects which belong to both X *and* Y. Corresponding to this we shall have the combined Boolean product $pX \overset{\cdot}{\cap} q Y$ of the two combined elements.

The dot in each combined product sign serves to distinguish the combined operations from the corresponding operations on sets and also to remind us that it involves arithmetical multiplication as we shall see from the definitions to be given later.

We can now proceed to the definitions. In the definition of combined element I use '$N(X)$' as an abbreviation for 'the number of members in the set X', i.e. the cardinal number of X.

[D. 3]   *Combined element*: Any combined element $p Y$ is defined as the set of all sets X such that $\dfrac{N(X \cap Y)}{N(X)} = p \; (0 \leqslant p \leqslant 1)$.

---

* See Note 2, p. 201, for a brief outline of Boolean algebra.
† See Note 3, p. 203.

[D. 4a]   *Combined sum*: If Y and Z have no member in common the combined sum of pY with qZ, i.e. $pY+qZ$, is defined as being identical with the Boolean product $pY \cap qZ$. It will therefore be the set of all sets X such that

$$\frac{N(X \cap Y)}{N(X)} = p \quad and \quad \frac{N(X \cap Z)}{N(X)} = q.$$

[D. 4b]   But if $Y = Z$, and $p+q \leqslant 1$, then $pY+qZ$ is defined as being identical with $(p+q)\,Y$.*

The definitions of the three kinds of combined product are very simple:

[D. 5] $pY \,;qZ\ = pqY\,,Z,$

[D. 6] $pY \overset{\cdot}{\times} qZ = pqY \times Z,$

[D. 7] $pY \overset{\cdot}{\cap} qZ\ = pqY \cap Z.$

Next we must define the product of a combined element into a combined sum. These are in effect distributive laws:

[D. 8] $pY \,;(qZ+rW) = pY \,;qZ+pY \,;rW,$

[D. 9] $pY \overset{\cdot}{\times}(qZ+rW) = pY \overset{\cdot}{\times} qZ+pY \overset{\cdot}{\times} rW,$

[D. 10] $pY \overset{\cdot}{\cap}(qZ+rW) = pY \overset{\cdot}{\cap} qZ+pY \overset{\cdot}{\cap} rW.$

Finally, we sometimes need to multiply a combined sum by a rational number. This is provided for in

[D. 11] $p(qZ+rW) = pqZ+prW.$

With these definitions† we can obtain the following theorems:

[T. 1] $pY+qZ = qZ+pY$ (from D. 4a and D. 4b),

[T. 2]   If $Y \cap Z = Z \cap W = W \cap Y = \Lambda$ or $Y = Z = W$ then
        $pY+(qZ+rW) = (pY+qZ)+rW$ (from D. 4a, D. 4b),

---

* For other possible relations between two sets Y and Z, the combined sum is not defined. This is because, so far as I know, the need for such other uses of combined sums does not arise in genetical calculations. The two possibilities above provided for are realized very frequently in practice. The reason for this will become clear in the sequel.

† Together with the laws of the arithmetic of rational numbers and the aws of Boolean algebra which are not explicitly referred to.

[T. 3] $pY ; qZ = qZ ; pY = qY ; pZ = pZ ; qY$ (from D. 5),

[T. 4] $pY \dot{\times} qZ = qY \dot{\times} pZ$ (from D. 6),

[T. 5] $pY \dot{\frown} qZ = qZ \dot{\frown} pY = qY \dot{\frown} pZ = pZ \dot{\frown} qY$ (from D. 7),

[T. 6] $pY ; (qZ + rW) = pqY , Z + prY , W$ (from D. 5, 8),

[T. 7] $(pY + qZ) ; (rW + sU) = prY , W + qrZ , W + psY , U$

$\qquad\qquad\qquad\qquad\qquad + qsZ , U$ (from T. 3, 6; D. 8),*

[T. 8] $(pY + qZ) ; (pY + qZ) = p^2Y , Y + 2pqY , Z + q^2Z , Z$

$\qquad\qquad\qquad\qquad\qquad\qquad$ (from T. 7, 3; D. 4b).

We are now in a position to formulate another type of statement with the mating functor

$$\mathbf{F}_X(Y , Z) \in (p_1 W_1 + p_2 W_2 + \dots + p_n W_n),$$

which may be written more briefly

$$\mathbf{F}_X(Y , Z) \in \sum_1^n p_i W_i. \qquad\qquad (6)$$

This states that the set $\mathbf{F}_X(Y , Z)$ of offspring is a member of the set $\sum_1^n p_i W_i$ of *sets* and thus contains members of W_i in the proportion p_i for each i from 1 to n.

In order to apply this combined algebra to genetics or to any other empirical subject-matter, it is convenient to have an operator on sets which is defined as follows:

[D. 12a] $\mathbf{D}_Y(X) = pY$ if and only if $X \in pY$.

The letter 'D' is taken from the word 'distribution' and '$\mathbf{D}_Y(X)$' may be read: 'the combined element expressing the frequency or distribution of Y in X.' ('D' is used in preference

---

* It is one of the peculiarities of combined algebra that a combined sum of two combined elements is not in all cases itself a combined element (see D. 4a). In order therefore to obtain T. 7 from T. 6 we require (and have tacitly used) a rule which allows us to substitute an expression representing a combined sum (e.g. '$pY + qZ$') for a dummy name representing a combined element (e.g. 'pY' in T. 6). Failing this we must turn T. 7 into a definition.

to 'F' in order to avoid confusion with the 'F' of the mating functor.)

[D. 12b] $D_{W_i}(X) = \sum_1^n p_i W_i$ if and only if $X \in \sum_1^n p_i W_i$.

'$D_{W_i}(X)$' may be read: 'the combined sum giving the distribution of W_i in X.' This notation is not indispensable but it facilitates calculation and enables certain statements to be formulated in a very simple way.*

It is easy to see that the subscripts following D are necessary. For suppose we have $D(X) = pY$ and $D(X) = qZ$, then we must have $pY = qZ$, which will not in general be the case. But in practice, so long as this danger is remembered, no ambiguity arises from dropping the subscripts, and if they are not omitted the notation becomes clumsy when many sets are involved. Moreover, when the actual distribution is given in an equation the subscripts involved are not left in any doubt.

We can now construct a *third* type of statement with the mating functor

$$D(\mathbf{F}_X(Y, Z)) = \sum_1^n p_i W_i. \tag{7}$$

Statements of the forms (1), (6) or (7) will be called *mating descriptions*.† Mating descriptions are the characteristic statements of genetics. Whenever in a biological problem mating descriptions are involved genetics is involved, and whenever genetics is involved mating descriptions are involved. We can in fact *define* genetics as:

The set of all accepted mating descriptions together with all explanatory hypotheses which have such mating descriptions

---

* Originally I interpreted '$D(X) = pY$' as asserting that the frequency of Y in X does not *deviate significantly* from p. But this interpretation raises so many and such enormous difficulties when introduced into a system which attempts otherwise to be rigorous, that it would be incompatible with an exposition which professes to be introductory (see my *Axiomatic Method in Biology*, p. 145, Note 10). I therefore proceed on the assumption that theoretical statements in genetics can be given the form they have in the text and that the problem of deviations from these laws can be dealt with within the domain of observation records.

† Note that a statement of the form $\mathbf{F}_X(Y, Z) \subset W$ can be written in the form $D(\mathbf{F}_X(Y, Z)) = 1W$.

among their consequences, together with all other consequences of such hypotheses.*

We shall find that in the course of genetical calculations situations will occur when the distribution operator 'D' and the mating functor 'F' are applied not to simple products but to *combined sums* involving such products. Consider, for example, random mating.† Suppose a set Y contains two distinct mutually exclusive genotypes Z and W and

$$D(Y) = pZ + (1-p) W. \qquad (8)$$

The distribution of couples is given by

$$D(Y, Y) = D(Y) \, ; D(Y).$$

We can now substitute for $D(Y)$ in the right-hand side according to (8) and carry out the combined simple multiplication according to T. 8, and obtain

$$D(Y, Y) = p^2 Z \, , Z + 2p(1-p) Z \, , W + (1-p)^2 W \, , W.$$

Let us now *define* $\mathbf{F}_X(D(Y, Y))$ as follows:

$$\mathbf{F}_X(D(Y, Y)) = $$
$$p^2 \mathbf{F}_X(Z, Z) + 2p(1-p) \, \mathbf{F}_X(Z, W) + (1-p)^2 \, \mathbf{F}_X(W, W).$$

On the other hand, since $Y = Z \cup W$, we have

$$\mathbf{F}_X(Y, Y) = \mathbf{F}_X(Z, Z) \cup \mathbf{F}_X(Z, W) \cup \mathbf{F}_X(W, W).$$

Now suppose that

$$D(\mathbf{F}_X(Y, Y)) = q_1 \mathbf{F}_X(Z, Z) + q_2 \mathbf{F}_X(Z, W) + q_3 \mathbf{F}_X(W, W).$$

It may be the case that the sets of offspring here involved are not homogeneous but composite. We must then be able to substitute the distributions of their components and obtain:

$$D(\mathbf{F}_X(Y, Y))$$
$$= q_1 D(\mathbf{F}_X(Z, Z)) + q_2 D(\mathbf{F}_X(Z, W)) + q_3 D(\mathbf{F}_X(W, W)).$$

---

* It might be profitable to define other sciences in an analogous way, i.e. by reference to the kinds of statement characteristic of their zero level.

† See Note 4, p. 204.

Finally, if there is an *equiproductivity* of offspring among the pairs belonging to Y, Y, i.e. if each pair of this set produces the same number of offspring as any other pair, we shall have

$$q_1 = p^2, \quad q_2 = 2p(1-p) \quad \text{and} \quad q_3 = (1-p)^2,$$

and so we obtain the formula for random mating with equi-productivity

$$\mathrm{D}(\mathbf{F}_X(Y, Y)) = p^2 \mathrm{D}(\mathbf{F}_X(Z, Z)) + 2p(1-p)\, \mathrm{D}(\mathbf{F}_X(Z, W))$$
$$+ (1-p)^2\, \mathrm{D}(\mathbf{F}_X(W, W)) = \mathbf{F}_X(\mathrm{D}(Y, Y)).$$

§ 4. THE PASSAGE FROM OBSERVATION RECORDS TO ZERO-LEVEL STATEMENTS

We can now turn to the analysis, from the methodological point of view, of what happens in a simple Mendelian experiment. By way of example we can take one of Mendel's own experiments with garden peas. Let us denote by 'Y' the set of all garden peas with yellow cotyledons, and by 'G' the set of all those with green cotyledons. Now Mendel did not experiment with $\mathbf{Y}$ and $\mathbf{G}$ but necessarily only with members of small sub-sets of these sets. Let us denote by 'A' the actual sub-set of $\mathbf{Y}$ which he used, and by 'B' the corresponding sub-set of $\mathbf{G}$, and let us denote by 'E' the set of environments then prevailing in Mendel's small garden in Brno. His observations can (in part) be recorded as follows:

[M. 1] $\mathbf{F}_E(\mathbf{A}, \mathbf{A}) \subset \mathbf{Y}$,   [M. 2] $\mathbf{F}_E^2(\mathbf{A}, \mathbf{A}) \subset \mathbf{Y}$,

[M. 3] $\mathbf{F}_E(\mathbf{B}, \mathbf{B}) \subset \mathbf{G}$,   [M. 4] $\mathbf{F}_E^2(\mathbf{B}, \mathbf{B}) \subset \mathbf{G}$,

[M. 5] $\mathbf{F}_E(\mathbf{A}, \mathbf{B}) \subset \mathbf{Y}$,   [M. 6] $\mathbf{F}_E^2(\mathbf{A}, \mathbf{B}) \in \dfrac{6{,}022}{8{,}023}\mathbf{Y} + \dfrac{2{,}001}{8{,}023}\mathbf{G}$.

Using decimal fractions M. 6 can also be written

$$\mathbf{F}_E^2(\mathbf{A}, \mathbf{B}) \in 0 \cdot 751\mathbf{Y} + 0 \cdot 249\mathbf{G}.$$

Fortunately, Mendel was not one of those who regarded science as consisting exclusively of exact reports of observations. He had the insight to regard M. 6 as an approximation to an ideal distribution of $\frac{3}{4}Y + \frac{1}{4}G$. He also showed by further breeding that one-third of the yellow peas of $F_E^2(A, B)$ behaved like members of A and two-thirds like members of $F_E(A, B)$. I call a mating description like

$$[\text{M. }6'] \quad F_E^2(A, B) \in \tfrac{3}{4}Y + \tfrac{1}{4}G$$

an observation record, because it is still confined to the restricted sets A and B. It does not represent a generalization over the whole of Y and G. To the above mating descriptions we can add the following:

[M. 7] $F_E(A, F_E(A, B)) \subset Y.$

[M. 8] $F_E(B, F_E(A, B)) \in \tfrac{1}{2}Y + \tfrac{1}{2}G.$

On further breeding half the members of Y obtained in M. 7 and all those in M. 8 behaved like members of $F_E(A, B)$. If we had begun with a different example the composite character of the corresponding sets would have been immediately evident. We could have begun with a restricted set C contained in the phenotype W of splashed white Andalusian fowls and a restricted sub-set D of the set B of black Andalusian fowls, then, using Bl to denote the phenotype blue Andalusian, to which the hybrids belong, and using K to denote the relevant environmental set, we should have the following mating descriptions:

[M. 1] $F_K(C, C) \subset W,$ [M. 2] $F_K^2(C, C) \subset W,$

[M. 3] $F_K(D, D) \subset B,$ [M. 4] $F_K^2(D, D) \subset B,$

[M. 5] $F_K(C, D) \subset Bl,$

[M. 6] $F_K^2(C, D) \in \tfrac{1}{4}W + \tfrac{1}{2}Bl + \tfrac{1}{4}B,$

[M. 7] $F_K(C, F_K(C, D)) \in \tfrac{1}{2}W + \tfrac{1}{2}Bl,$

[M. 8] $F_K(D, F_K(C, D)) \in \tfrac{1}{2}B + \tfrac{1}{2}Bl.$

The problem of generalizing these results, i.e. of passing from these observation records to zero-level statements, is complicated by the fact that we are dealing not with individuals but with sets, and our first example shows that we cannot simply replace 'A' and 'B' in the mating functor by 'Y' and 'G' respectively. What we must do is this: we must define sets corresponding to 'all peas which behave genetically like members of **A**' and 'all peas which behave genetically like members of $\mathbf{F_E(A,B)}$'. Such sets will be genotypes, and with their help we can formulate zero-level statements. It is also necessary to remove the restriction to the special environmental set **E**. We shall define the sets we require as functions of the phenotypes **Y** and **G** and a certain maximized environmental set. The problem of constructing the definitions is solved in a succession of steps, and because the conditions to be satisfied by the sets we wish to define are rather long to write, I begin by introducing an abbreviation for them.

We first write '$K_{\mathbf{Y},X}(Z)$' (or 'Z satisfies the condition $K_{\mathbf{Y},X}$') as an abbreviation for

'$Z \subset \mathbf{Y}$ and $\mathbf{F}_X(Z,Z) \subset \mathbf{Y}$ and $\mathbf{F}^2_X(Z,Z) \neq \Lambda$ and $\mathbf{F}^2_X(Z,Z) \subset \mathbf{Y}$.'

We next write '$\phi(\mathbf{Y},X)$' as an abbreviation for 'there is a U such that $K_{\mathbf{Y},X}(U)$ and for all Z and W, if $K_{\mathbf{Y},X}(Z)$ and $K_{\mathbf{Y},X}(W)$ then $K_{\mathbf{Y},X}(Z \cup W)$'. With the help of these abbreviations we now define '$\mathbf{H}(\mathbf{Y},X)$' or 'the homozygous genotype of **Y** with respect to the environmental set X' as follows:

$\mathbf{H}(\mathbf{Y},X)$ is the Boolean sum of all sets Z such that $K_{\mathbf{Y},X}(Z)$ provided that $\phi(\mathbf{Y},X)$. If $\phi(\mathbf{Y},X)$ does not hold then $\mathbf{H}(\mathbf{Y},X) = \Lambda$.

Next we proceed to *maximize* X by defining the environmental set $\mathbf{E}(\mathbf{Y})$ as follows:

[D. 13]　$\mathbf{E}(\mathbf{Y})$ is the Boolean sum of all sets X such that $\phi(\mathbf{Y},X)$.

Finally, we define the homozygous genotype $\mathbf{H}(\mathbf{Y})$ of **Y**, as follows:

[D. 14]　$\mathbf{H}(\mathbf{Y}) = \mathbf{H}(\mathbf{Y},\mathbf{E}(\mathbf{Y}))$.

$\mathbf{H}(\mathbf{Y})$ will be null unless $\phi(\mathbf{Y},\mathbf{E}(\mathbf{Y}))$, which latter is a consequence of the following postulate:

[H. 3a]　For some U, $\phi(\mathbf{Y},U)$ and for all X and Z, if $\phi(\mathbf{Y},X)$ and $\phi(\mathbf{Y},Z)$ then $\phi(\mathbf{Y},X \cup Z)$.

In an exactly analogous manner we can define $\mathbf{H}(\mathbf{G})$.

Now we can turn to the rather more difficult task of defining 'the singly heterozygous genotype of **Y** and **G**'. We again begin by writing '$M_{Y,G,X}(Z)$' as an abbreviation for

'$Z \subset Y$

and $\quad D(\mathbf{F}_X(Z,Z)) = \frac{3}{4}\mathbf{Y} + \frac{1}{4}\mathbf{G}$ and $\quad \mathbf{F}_X(\mathbf{H}(\mathbf{Y}),Z) \neq \Lambda$

and $\quad \mathbf{F}_X(\mathbf{H}(\mathbf{Y}),Z) \subset \mathbf{Y}$ and $\quad D(\mathbf{F}_X(\mathbf{H}(\mathbf{G}),Z)) = \frac{1}{2}\mathbf{Y} + \frac{1}{2}\mathbf{G}$.'

And we use '$\psi(\mathbf{Y},\mathbf{G},X)$' as an abbreviation for 'there is a U such that $M_{Y,G,X}(U)$ and for all Z and W if $M_{Y,G,X}(Z)$ and $M_{Y,G,X}(W)$ then $M_{Y,G,X}(Z \cup W)$'.
We then define $\mathbf{Ht}(\mathbf{Y},\mathbf{G},X)$ as follows:

$\mathbf{Ht}(\mathbf{Y},\mathbf{G},X)$ is the Boolean sum of all sets Z such that $M_{Y,G,X}(Z)$, provided that $\psi(\mathbf{Y},\mathbf{G},X)$. If $\psi(\mathbf{Y},\mathbf{G},X)$ does not hold then $\mathbf{Ht}(\mathbf{Y},\mathbf{G},X) = \Lambda$.

Next we maximize X as before:

$\mathbf{E}(\mathbf{Y},\mathbf{G})$ is the Boolean sum of all sets X such that $\psi(\mathbf{Y},\mathbf{G},X)$.

Finally, we define 'the singly heterozygous genotype of **Y** and **G**':

[D. 15] $\quad \mathbf{Ht}(\mathbf{Y},\mathbf{G}) = \mathbf{Ht}(\mathbf{Y},\mathbf{G},\mathbf{E}(\mathbf{Y},\mathbf{G}))$.

$\mathbf{Ht}(\mathbf{Y},\mathbf{G})$ will be null unless $\psi(\mathbf{Y},\mathbf{G},\mathbf{E}(\mathbf{Y},\mathbf{G}))$, which latter is a consequence of the following postulate:

[H. 3b] $\quad$ For some U, $\psi(\mathbf{Y},\mathbf{G},U)$ and for all X and Z, if $\psi(\mathbf{Y},\mathbf{G},X)$ and $\psi(\mathbf{Y},\mathbf{G},Z)$ then $\psi(\mathbf{Y},\mathbf{G},X \cup Z)$.

General definitions (or definition schemata) of 'the homozygous genotype of P' and of 'the singly heterozygous genotype of P and Q' can be constructed on the above lines by replacing '**Y**' and '**G**' by the dummy phenotype designations 'P' and 'Q'. In this way we get definition schemata from which any desired definition can be obtained by substituting specific phenotype designations for P and Q. But a complication arises in connexion with $\mathbf{Ht}(P,Q)$. As our second example shows, the general definition of $\mathbf{Ht}(P,Q)$ cannot be constructed on exactly the above lines. In the place of '$Z \subset P$' in the first of the conditions for which '$M_{P,Q,X}(Z)$' is an abbreviation, we must put 'for some phenotype R, $Z \subset R$'.

We can now define two familiar genetical expressions:

[D. 16]   A phenotype P is *dominant to* a phenotype Q if and only if $\mathbf{Ht}(P,Q) \subset P$.

[D. 17]   A phenotype Q is *recessive to* a phenotype P if and only if P is dominant to Q.

Thus if there is a phenotype R such that $\mathbf{Ht}(P,Q) \subset R$ and $P \cap R = Q \cap R = \Lambda$ (as in our second example), then P is not dominant to Q nor is Q dominant to P.

We assume $\mathbf{E}(Y) = \mathbf{E}(G) = \mathbf{E}(Y, G)$ because the experimental results do not require that we should assume that these environmental sets are distinct. If now we denote this common maximized environmental set by E the Boolean sums $\mathbf{H}(Y)$ and $\mathbf{Ht}(Y, G)$ satisfy the conditions $K_{Y,E}$ and $M_{Y,G,E}$ respectively by virtue of their definitions and we can derive the following generalized mating descriptions from these definitions:

[M. 1] $\mathbf{F}_E(\mathbf{H}(Y), \mathbf{H}(Y)) \subset Y$,

[M. 2] $\mathbf{F}_E^2(\mathbf{H}(Y), \mathbf{H}(Y)) \subset Y$,

[M. 3] $\mathbf{F}_E(\mathbf{H}(G), \mathbf{H}(G)) \subset G$,

[M. 4] $\mathbf{F}_E^2(\mathbf{H}(G), \mathbf{H}(G)) \subset G$,

[M. 5] $\mathbf{F}_E(\mathbf{H}(Y), \mathbf{H}(G)) \subset Y$,

[M. 6] $\mathbf{D}(\mathbf{F}_E(\mathbf{Ht}(Y, G), \mathbf{Ht}(Y, G))) = \frac{3}{4}Y + \frac{1}{4}G$,

[M. 7] $\mathbf{F}_E(\mathbf{H}(Y), \mathbf{Ht}(Y, G)) \subset Y$,

[M. 8] $\mathbf{D}(\mathbf{F}_E(\mathbf{H}(G), \mathbf{Ht}(Y, G))) = \frac{1}{2}Y + \frac{1}{2}G$,

with corresponding mating descriptions for our second example.

But having defined our genotypes we can now construct mating descriptions in purely genotypic terms. These are *not* derivable from the definitions but constitute a further generalization of the experimental results. If we let 'P' and 'Q' denote any two mutually exclusive phenotypes for which $\mathbf{H}(P) \neq \Lambda$,

$\mathbf{H}(Q) \neq \Lambda$ and $\mathbf{Ht}(P, Q) \neq \Lambda$, and if we let

$$E = \mathbf{E}(P) = \mathbf{E}(Q) = \mathbf{E}(P, Q),$$

then we can write down:

[M. 1] $\mathbf{F}_E(\mathbf{H}(P), \mathbf{H}(P)) \subset \mathbf{H}(P),$

[M. 2] $\mathbf{F}_E(\mathbf{H}(Q), \mathbf{H}(Q)) \subset \mathbf{H}(Q),$

[M. 3] $\mathbf{F}_E(\mathbf{H}(P), \mathbf{H}(Q)) \subset \mathbf{Ht}(P, Q),$

[M. 4] $\mathbf{D}(\mathbf{F}_E(\mathbf{Ht}(P, Q), \mathbf{Ht}(P, Q)))$
$$= \tfrac{1}{4}\mathbf{H}(P) + \tfrac{1}{2}\mathbf{Ht}(P, Q) + \tfrac{1}{4}\mathbf{H}(Q),$$

[M. 5] $\mathbf{D}(\mathbf{F}_E(\mathbf{H}(P), \mathbf{Ht}(P, Q))) = \tfrac{1}{2}\mathbf{H}(P) + \tfrac{1}{2}\mathbf{Ht}(P, Q),$

[M. 6] $\mathbf{D}(\mathbf{F}_E(\mathbf{H}(Q), \mathbf{Ht}(P, Q))) = \tfrac{1}{2}\mathbf{H}(Q) + \tfrac{1}{2}\mathbf{Ht}(P, Q).$

From these, with the help of the definitions, the former mating descriptions with phenotype designations on the right-hand side can be derived.

It will be noticed that in this list of mating descriptions M. 1 and M. 2 are mutually derivable from one another simply by interchange of their phenotype designations. If in M. 1 we substitute 'Q' for 'P' wherever the latter occurs we obtain M. 2; and if in M. 2 we put 'P' for 'Q' wherever the latter occurs we obtain M. 1. If the environmental set designations had been different, corresponding exchanges could have been made with them. When this relation holds between two mating descriptions I shall say that they *have the same structure*. I define a mating *type* as the set of all mating descriptions which have the same structure as any given mating description. Thus the mating types will be mutually exclusive sets of mating descriptions. In the above list M. 1 and M. 2 have the same structure and M. 5 and M. 6 have the same structure,* but between the remaining pairs of mating descriptions in this list there is no further sameness

---

* It will be noticed that in the derivation of M. 6 from M. 5 (or vice versa) we must only exchange 'Q' for 'P' (or vice versa) in the designations of the homozygous genotypes, leaving the designations of the heterozygous genotypes unchanged. In the case of M. 1 and M. 2 no heterozygous genotype designations occur. This operation can be more satisfactorily and easily defined on level 1, where we deal with a functor which, unlike $\mathbf{Ht}(P, Q)$, permits any permutation of the letters in the brackets. See below, pp. 125, 141.

of structure. Four mating types are therefore represented. I shall say that all mating descriptions having the same structure as M. 1 belong to Type 1, all those having the same structure as M. 3 belong to Type 2, all those having the same structure as M. 4 belong to Type 3, and all those having the same structure as M. 5 belong to Type 4.

I shall say that two sets of mating descriptions are *isomorphic* if and only if their members can be put into one-one correspondence in such a way that every pair of mating descriptions under the correspondence is a pair of descriptions having the same structure, i.e. belonging to the same mating type. Thus the zero-level mating descriptions for our two original examples are not isomorphic if they have phenotype designations on the right-hand side, but they are isomorphic if they are stated in purely genotypic terms.

§ 5. GENETICAL SYSTEMS OF ORDER 1
AND ALLELIC INDEX (*n*)

We now take a step further in generalization. The two examples described above form but two members of an enormous set of known examples which is characterized by the fact that each member has two mutually exclusive homozygous genotypes and a singly heterozygous genotype in which the offspring from the two homozygous genotypes are included. Each member will satisfy a set of six mating descriptions which is isomorphic with the set of six given in the last list above (p. 111).

It seems desirable to have a numerical characterization for this great and genetically important assemblage which will admit of generalization to other assemblages. I propose to call it the set of all *genetical systems of order* 1 *and allelic index* (2). I say they are genetical systems because (in the absence of mutation) they are genetically closed, i.e. the offspring from any two members of such a set themselves belong to the set. I say they are of order 1 because every heterozygous genotype which is included in the system is *singly* heterozygous, and I say they

have allelic index (2) because each contains exactly *two* homozygous genotypes. The significance of the brackets in the allelic
index cannot be explained until later.

In order to express this more systematically and precisely,
let us call the Boolean sum $H(P) \cup H(Q) \cup Ht(P, Q)$, the system
generated by the phenotypes P and Q, and let us denote it by
'$S(P, Q)$', thus:

[D. 18] $S(P, Q) = H(P) \cup H(Q) \cup Ht(P, Q)$.

We have so far only defined *singly* heterozygous genotype.
We now require:

[D. 18a] Y is a *heterozygous genotype* if and only if for some
phenotype P, some environmental set X and some rational
number p such that $0 < p < 1$, we have

$$Y \neq \Lambda \quad \text{and} \quad Y \subset P \quad \text{and} \quad D(F_X(Y, Y)) = pP.$$

Now we can say

[D. 19] $S(P, Q)$ is a genetical system of order 1 and allelic index
(2) if and only if: $P \cap Q = \Lambda$ and $H(P) \neq \Lambda$, $H(Q) \neq \Lambda$ and
$Ht(P, Q) \neq \Lambda$, every heterozygous genotype included in the
system is singly heterozygous and $E(P) = E(Q) = E(P, Q)$.

The set of all genetical systems of order 1 and allelic index (2)
has two sub-sets. First, there are those in which each of the three
genotypes is included in a distinct phenotype, as in our second
example. This sub-set can be denoted by (1, 1, 1). Secondly,
there are those which resemble our first example in having one
phenotype containing two genotypes and the other containing
only one. This sub-set can therefore be denoted by (2, 1). I call
a set of natural numbers giving the number of genotypes included in each of the phenotypes of a genetical system the
partition of the system, because the sum of these numbers will
be equal to the total number of genotypes. Thus the set of all
genetical systems of order 1 and allelic index (2) has only two
sub-sets distinguished by their partitions, because such a system
could not be of partition (3).

It is now not difficult to generalize further to systems of order 1 and allelic index (n). First we define

[D. 20] $S(P_1, P_2, ..., P_n) = \sum\limits_{1}^{n} H(P_i) \cup \sum\limits_{i=1}^{n-1} \sum\limits_{j=2}^{n} Ht(P_i, P_j)$ with $i < j$

(the summation being Boolean throughout). Next we define

[D. 21] $S(P_1, P_2, ..., P_n)$ is a genetical system of order 1 and allelic index (n) if and only if

(i) $P_i \cap P_j = \Lambda$ for $i, j = 1, 2, ..., n$ and $i \neq j$,

(ii) every heterozygous genotype contained in $S(P_1, P_2, ..., P_n)$ is singly heterozygous,

(iii) $H(P_i) \neq \Lambda$ for each $i = 1, 2, ..., n$,

(iv) $Ht(P_i, P_j) \neq \Lambda$ for each $i = 1, 2, ..., n-1$; $j = 2, 3, ..., n$ and $i < j$,

(v) $E(P_i) = E(P_j) = E(P_i, P_j)$ for each $i = 1, 2, ..., n$; $j = 2, 3, ..., n$ and $i < j$.

We have already given examples of mating types 1, 2, 3 and 4 (see p. 112). We now proceed to define three more types.

Type 5 is the set of all mating descriptions having the same structure as the following (using 'E' to denote the common maximized environmental set):

$$D(F_E(H(P), Ht(Q, R))) = \tfrac{1}{2}Ht(P, Q) + \tfrac{1}{2}Ht(P, R)$$

(P, Q and R being mutually exclusive).

Type 6 is the set of all mating descriptions having the same structure as the following:

$$D(F_E(Ht(P, Q), Ht(P, R)))$$
$$= \tfrac{1}{4}H(P) + \tfrac{1}{4}Ht(Q, P) + \tfrac{1}{4}Ht(P, R) + \tfrac{1}{4}Ht(Q, R)$$

(P, Q and R being mutually exclusive).

Type 7 is the set of all mating descriptions which have the same structure as the following:

$$D(F_E(Ht(P, Q), Ht(R, S)))$$
$$= \tfrac{1}{4}Ht(P, R) + \tfrac{1}{4}Ht(Q, R) + \tfrac{1}{4}Ht(P, S) + \tfrac{1}{4}Ht(Q, S)$$

(P, Q, R and S being all mutually exclusive).

We can now formulate the following hypotheses:

[H. 4] Every mating description, in which the mating functor contains only genotype designations of genotypes which belong to a genetical system of order 1 and allelic index (2), belongs to one of the types 1, 2, 3 or 4.

[H. 5] Every mating description, in which the mating functor contains only genotype designations of genotypes which belong to a genetical system of order 1 and allelic index (3), belongs to one of the types 1, 2, 3, 4, 5 or 6.

[H. 6] Every mating description, in which the mating functor contains only genotype designations of genotypes which belong to a genetical system of order 1 and allelic index (n) with $n > 3$, belongs to one of the types 1, 2, 3, 4, 5, 6 or 7.

These hypotheses thus assert that the mating descriptions for a system of order 1 all belong to one of seven and only seven mating types. This concludes the theory of genetical systems of order 1.*

§ 6. GENETICAL SYSTEMS OF ORDER GREATER THAN 1

The next step in generalization consists in removing the restriction to systems of order 1. For this purpose we make use of the notion of the *genetical product* of two genetical systems. In some cases this is identical with their Boolean product; but, as this is not always so, a distinction in terminology is unavoidable. I will illustrate the procedure first of all by means of an example.

As one of the factor systems we can take our original example, $S(\mathbf{Y}, \mathbf{G})$. As our second factor we can take the system $S(\mathbf{R}, \mathbf{W})$, where $\mathbf{R}$ is the set of all garden peas with round (or smooth) cotyledons, and $\mathbf{W}$ is the set of all those with wrinkled cotyledons. Our two systems of order 1 will thus be

$$S_1 = H(\mathbf{Y}) \cup H(\mathbf{G}) \cup Ht(\mathbf{Y}, \mathbf{G}), \quad S_2 = H(\mathbf{R}) \cup H(\mathbf{W}) \cup Ht(\mathbf{R}, \mathbf{W}).$$

* See Note 5, p. 206. It will be noticed that H. 4–H. 6 are stated in meta-theoretical terms, because they speak about mating descriptions, etc.; this is done here simply for the sake of ease and brevity of exposition. If we were axiomatizing it would not be difficult to formulate corresponding statements in purely genetical terms.

Let us first take the Boolean product of the Boolean sum of the phenotypes of S_1 into the corresponding sum for S_2:

$$(Y \cup G) \cap (R \cup W) = (Y \cap R) \cup (G \cap R) \cup (Y \cap W) \cup (G \cap W).*$$

In order to abbreviate the formulas let us agree to write the Boolean products simply by juxtaposition of the symbols, thus: $Y \cap R = YR$. Then the Boolean sum of our four phenotypes can be written

$$YR \cup GR \cup YW \cup GW.$$

The system generated by these phenotypes will be denoted by '$S_1 \times S_2$', thus:

$$S_1 \times S_2 = S(YR, GR, YW, GW).$$

I have used the same sign for this multiplication as for Cartesian multiplication in order to avoid a multiplicity of symbols, but the two operations must not be confused.

Let us suppose that we have available for experiment sub-sets **A**, **B**, **C** and **D** of these four phenotypes respectively, and let us denote the set of environments available by '**E**'. Then it is found by experiment that

$$F_E(A, A) \subset YR \quad \text{and} \quad F_E^2(A, A) \subset YR.$$

A thus behaves like a homozygous genotype. In fact it behaves as though it were contained in the Boolean product $H(Y) \cap H(R)$. Corresponding results are obtained with $F_E(B, B)$, $F_E(C, C)$ and $F_E(D, D)$. We have, in fact, four homozygous genotypes which we can write

$$H(YR), \quad H(GR), \quad H(YW) \quad \text{and} \quad H(GW).$$

It is also found by experiment that

$$F_E(A, B) \subset YR$$

and

$$D(F_E^2(A, B)) = \tfrac{3}{4}YR + \tfrac{1}{4}GR = (\tfrac{3}{4}Y + \tfrac{1}{4}G) \cap 1R,$$

so that $F_E(A, B)$ behaves like the Boolean product of a singly heterozygous genotype $Ht(Y, G)$ and a homozygous genotype

---

* See Note 2, p. 202, formula (8 a).

H(R). We shall denote the genotype in which $F_E(A, B)$ is included by $Ht(YR, GR)$. Correspondingly we obtain three more singly heterozygous genotypes:

$$Ht(YR, YW), \quad Ht(GR, GW) \quad \text{and} \quad Ht(YW, GW).$$

Finally, it is found that

$$F_E(A, D) \subset YR$$

and

$$D(F_E^2(A, D)) = \tfrac{9}{16}YR + \tfrac{3}{16}GR + \tfrac{3}{16}YW + \tfrac{1}{16}GW$$

$$= (\tfrac{3}{4}Y + \tfrac{1}{4}G) \wedge (\tfrac{3}{4}R + \tfrac{1}{4}W).$$

$F_E(A, D)$ thus behaves as though it were contained in the Boolean product of two singly heterozygous genotypes:

$$Ht(Y, G) \cap Ht(R, W).$$

It will be denoted by $Ht(YR, GW)$. If we take $F_E^2(B, C)$, we obtain a mating description which is identical on its right-hand side with the above description for $F_E^2(A, D)$, and we can therefore say that the two genotypes concerned are *genetically equivalent*. The doubly heterozygous genotype in which $F_E(B, C)$ is included will be written $Ht(GR, YW)$. Geneticists regard $Ht(YR, GW)$ and $Ht(GR, YW)$ as one and the same doubly heterozygous genotype, although in a strict set-theoretical sense they are not identical. They are distinguished by their parental sets but not by their offspring.

We can now see what we have to do in order to obtain the genetical product of two genetical systems of order 1 and allelic index (2). First we obtain the phenotypes of the system by taking the Boolean products of the phenotypes of the one system with those of the other. We then write down the Boolean sum of the homozygous genotypes of these four phenotypes. To these we add the Boolean sum of all the singly heterozygous genotypes in which are contained the offspring from the mating of two of these homozygous genotypes when they differ with respect to only *one* phenotype. Finally, we add to this the two doubly heterozygous genotypes in which are contained the offspring from the mating of two homozygous genotypes when they differ with respect to *two* phenotypes.

It is easy to see that, at least in the case of our example, the resulting sum is identical with the Boolean product of the two systems. Let us denote the homozygous genotypes of the factor systems by adding a single prime to the phenotype designations and the singly heterozygous genotypes by adding two primes to the designations of the phenotypes in which they are contained. Then, by the laws of Boolean algebra, we have

$$(Y' \cup Y'' \cup G') \cap (R' \cup R'' \cup W') = Y'R' \cup Y''R' \cup G'R' \cup$$
$$Y'R'' \cup Y''R'' \cup G'R'' \cup$$
$$Y'W' \cup Y''W' \cup G'W'.$$

The square array on the right-hand side of this equation is the Boolean algebraical analogue of the chequer-board diagrams which are found in genetical books. This notation obliterates the distinction between the two doubly heterozygous genotypes. They are both included in $Y''R''$. It therefore suffices for those systems in which they are genetically equivalent and the total number of genotypes is counted as 9.

I shall say that the genetical product of two systems of order 1 formed in the above way is a genetical system of order 2. The set of all such systems has two sub-sets distinguished as follows:

(1) The two doubly heterozygous genotypes are genetically equivalent, the total number of genotypes is equal to 9 and the genetical product is identical with the Boolean product.

I call such systems *Mendelian* because all the systems of order 2 investigated by Mendel were of this kind. The allelic index is written $(n_1)(n_2)$, if the allelic indices of the factor systems are (n_1) and (n_2), and the two factor systems are then said to be *independent*.

(2) The two doubly heterozygous genotypes are *not* genetically equivalent, the total number of genotypes is equal to 10 and the genetical product is *not* identical with the Boolean product of the two factor systems.

I call such systems *Batesonian* because they were first recorded by the celebrated Cambridge geneticist William Bateson. The allelic index is written (n_1, n_2) if the indices of the factor systems are (n_1) and (n_2), and the two factor systems are then said to *belong to the same linkage group*.

The partition of the genetical product will depend upon the partitions of the factor systems. In our example each factor system has the partition $(2, 1)$ and the partition of their genetical product is $(4, 2, 2, 1) = (2 \times 2, 2 \times 1, 2 \times 1, 1 \times 1)$. If the product had been Batesonian, the partition would have been $(5, 2, 2, 1)$.

Something more must now be said about the distinction between Mendelian and Batesonian systems of order 2. Suppose we have two mutually exclusive phenotypes P and Q, and two other mutually exclusive phenotypes A and B such that the products PA, QA, PB and QB are not null, the homozygous genotypes $\mathbf{H}(PA)$, $\mathbf{H}(QA)$, $\mathbf{H}(PB)$ and $\mathbf{H}(QB)$ are not null and there is a maximized environmental set E common to both systems. Then the doubly heterozygous genotypes $\mathbf{Ht}(PA, QB)$ and $\mathbf{Ht}(QA, PB)$, such that

$$\mathbf{F}_E(\mathbf{H}(PA), \mathbf{H}(QB)) \subset \mathbf{Ht}(PA, QB)$$

and

$$\mathbf{F}_E(\mathbf{H}(QA), \mathbf{H}(PB)) \subset \mathbf{Ht}(QA, PB),$$

will be genetically equivalent if the system is Mendelian and not if it is Batesonian. The distinction is most simply shown by a mating description in which each genotype designation appears in the mating functor with that of one of the homozygous genotypes, say $\mathbf{H}(QB)$. If the system is Mendelian we have

$$\mathbf{D}(\mathbf{F}_E(\mathbf{Ht}(PA, QB), \mathbf{H}(QB)))$$
$$= \tfrac{1}{4}\mathbf{Ht}(PA, QB) + \tfrac{1}{4}\mathbf{Ht}(QA, QB) + \tfrac{1}{4}\mathbf{Ht}(PB, QB) + \tfrac{1}{4}\mathbf{H}(QB),$$

and the corresponding mating description with

$$\mathbf{F}_E(\mathbf{Ht}(QA, PB), \mathbf{H}(QB))$$

on the left-hand side will be the same on the right-hand side. But if the system is Batesonian, there will be a positive rational number p, such that $0 < p < \tfrac{1}{2}$ and

$$\mathbf{D}(\mathbf{F}_E(\mathbf{Ht}(PA, QB), \mathbf{H}(QB)))$$
$$= \tfrac{1}{2}(1-p)\,\mathbf{Ht}(PA, QB) + \tfrac{1}{2}p\mathbf{Ht}(QA, QB)$$
$$+ \tfrac{1}{2}p\mathbf{Ht}(PB, QB) + \tfrac{1}{2}(1-p)\,\mathbf{H}(QB),$$

and

$$D(\mathbf{F}_E(\mathbf{Ht}(QA, PB), \mathbf{H}(QB)))$$
$$= \tfrac{1}{2}(1-p)\,\mathbf{Ht}(QA, QB) + \tfrac{1}{2}p\mathbf{H}(QB)$$
$$+ \tfrac{1}{2}\mathbf{Ht}(PA, QB) + \tfrac{1}{2}(1-p)\,\mathbf{Ht}(PB, QB).$$

This number p is called the *recombination value** of the two factor systems S_1 and S_2. Symbolically this can be written

$$\mathbf{rc}(S_1, S_2) = p.$$

We can now proceed to the last step in generalization by removing the restriction to genetical systems of order 2 and defining systems of order m. For this purpose it is necessary to give the phenotype designations two subscripts: the first to indicate to which of the m factor systems it belongs, the second to distinguish it from other phenotypes of the same factor system. Thus P_{ij} is the jth phenotype of the ith factor system, and $S(P_{m1}, P_{m2}, ..., P_{mn_m})$ denotes the mth factor system if it has allelic index (n_m) in accordance with definition D. 21. Next we must construct certain other preliminary definitions. First, we define the common maximized environmental set for a genetical system of order 1 and allelic index (n):

[D. 22] $\mathbf{E}(S)$ is the set of all environments x such that for some X, some P_1, some P_2, ..., some P_n we have $S = S(P_1, P_2, ..., P_n)$; $X = \mathbf{E}(P_i) = \mathbf{E}(P_i, P_j)$ for $i = 1, 2, ..., n$; $j = 2, 3, ..., n$ and $i < j$ and $x \in X$.

Secondly, we shall say:

[D. 23] X is *genetically equivalent* to Y if and only if for some Z which is the common maximized environmental set of the genetical system in which both X and Y are included, and for any genotype W contained in that system we have

$$D_W(\mathbf{F}_Z(X, X)) = D_W(\mathbf{F}_Z(Y, Y)).$$

---

* It should be stated that the value of p may be different for the two sexes. In *Drosophila*, for example, the above would hold if the members of $\mathbf{Ht}(PA, QB)$ and $\mathbf{Ht}(QA, PB)$ were females; if they were males, the result would be the same as in Mendelian systems.

Thirdly, we must remove the restriction to singly heterozygous genotypes. To this end we define:

[D. 24] $\mathbf{Ht}(P_{1i_1}P_{2i_2}\ldots P_{mi_m}, P_{1j_1}P_{2j_2}\ldots P_{mj_m})$ is the set of all lives x such that for some X, some Y and some genetical systems $S_1, S_2, \ldots, S_m$ $(m>1)$ each of order 1 with $P_{ki_k} \subset S_k$ and $P_{kj_k} \subset S_k$ with $1 \leqslant k \leqslant m$ and $Y = \mathbf{E}(S_1) = \mathbf{E}(S_2) = \ldots = \mathbf{E}(S_m)$, we have

$$\mathbf{F}_Y(\mathbf{H}(P_{1i_1}P_{2i_2}\ldots P_{mi_m}), \mathbf{H}(P_{1j_1}P_{2j_2}\ldots P_{mj_m}))$$

is genetically equivalent to X and $x \in X$.

And then we can say:

[D. 25] $\mathbf{Ht}(P_{1i_1}P_{2i_2}\ldots P_{mi_m}, P_{1j_1}P_{2j_2}\ldots P_{mj_m})$ is a k-ply heterozygous genotype, if and only if it is not null and for exactly k pairs $(1 \leqslant k \leqslant m)$ of phenotypes P_{ri_r}, P_{rj_r} we have $\mathbf{Ht}(P_{ri_r}, P_{rj_r}) \neq \Lambda$ with $1 \leqslant r \leqslant m$.

We can now define the genetical product of m genetical systems each of order 1:

[D. 26] $\mathbf{S}(P_{11}, P_{12}, \ldots, P_{1n_1}) \times \mathbf{S}(P_{21}, P_{22}, \ldots, P_{2n_2}) \times \ldots$

$$\times \mathbf{S}(P_{m1}, P_{m2}, \ldots, P_{mn_m}) = \sum_1^{n_1}\sum_1^{n_2}\ldots\sum_1^{n_m}\mathbf{H}(P_{1i_1}P_{2i_2}\ldots P_{mi_m})$$

$$\cup \sum_{i_1,j_1=1}^{n_1}{}'\sum_{i_2,j_2=1}^{n_2}{}'\ldots\sum_{i_m,j_m=1}^{n_m}{}'\mathbf{Ht}(P_{1i_1}P_{2i_2}\ldots P_{mi_m}, P_{1j_1}P_{2j_2}\ldots P_{mj_m}),$$

the summation being Boolean throughout, the primes indicating that those terms are to be omitted for which $i_1, i_2, \ldots, i_n = j_1, j_2, \ldots, j_n$.

Finally, we can say:

[D. 27] S is a genetical system of order m if and only if it is the genetical product of m $(m>1)$ systems $S_1, S_2, \ldots, S_m$, each of order 1, each of its genotypes is non-null and there is a non-null environmental set X such that

$$X = \mathbf{E}(S_1) = \mathbf{E}(S_2) = \ldots = \mathbf{E}(S_m),$$

which will be called the common environmental set $\mathbf{E}(S)$ of S.

A genetical system S of order m is Mendelian if all its factor systems are independent. If the allelic indices of its m factor systems are $(n_1), (n_2), \ldots, (n_m)$, then the allelic index of S will be $(n_1)(n_2)\ldots(n_m)$ with m pairs of parentheses. Juxtaposition of the phenotype designations in the designations of its genotypes will represent Boolean multiplication, as in the example given above of a system of order 2.

A genetical system S of order m is Batesonian if all its factor systems belong to the same linkage group. If the allelic indices of its m factor-systems are $(n_1), (n_2), \ldots, (n_m)$ then the allelic index of S will be $(n_1, n_2, \ldots, n_m)$ with one pair of parentheses. When $m > 2$ juxtaposition of the phenotype designations in the designations of its genotypes must be interpreted as representing not Boolean but *Cartesian* multiplication (see p. 101). This has the effect (Cartesian multiplication being non-commutative) of establishing an order among the factor systems. Thus with $m = 3$ we shall have: $S_1 \times S_2 \times S_3 \neq S_2 \times S_3 \times S_1 \neq S_3 \times S_1 \times S_2$, etc. It is sometimes said that the factor systems have the order $S_1 \times S_2 \times S_3$ if and only if $\mathbf{rc}(S_1, S_2) + \mathbf{rc}(S_2, S_3) \geqslant \mathbf{rc}(S_1, S_3)$.

A genetical system S of order m (with $m > 2$) may be said to be *mixed*, if and only if at least two but less than m of its factor systems belong to the same linkage group. If there are k distinct linkage groups with $1 < k < m$, then there will be k pairs of parentheses in the allelic index of the system. Thus if $m = 3$ and S is mixed, we can have allelic indices $(n_1)(n_2, n_3)$ or $(n_1, n_2)(n_3)$ or $(n_1, n_3)(n_2)$.

Thus if we are given the allelic index of a genetical system we know its order and the number of its linkage groups, and we know the number of homozygous genotypes in each of its factor systems. If we are given its partition we know the total number of its phenotypes and how many genotypes are contained in each.

If we write 'g' in front of an allelic index in order to have a designation for the total number of genotypes included in any system having that allelic index we can say

$$g(n) = \tfrac{1}{2}n(n+1),$$

$$g(n_1)(n_2) = g(n_1).g(n_2),$$

$$g(n_1, n_2) = g(n_1.n_2),$$

$$g(n_1)(n_2, n_3) = g(n_1).g(n_2, n_3), \text{ etc.}$$

A Mendelian system of allelic index $(n_1)(n_2)\ldots(n_m)$ will contain

$$n_1 n_2 \ldots n_m$$

homozygous genotypes, and

$$\binom{n_1}{2} n_2 n_3 \ldots n_m + \binom{n_2}{2} n_1 n_3 \ldots n_m + \ldots + \binom{n_m}{2} n_1 n_2 \ldots n_{m-1}$$

singly heterozygous genotypes, and

$$\binom{n_1}{2}\binom{n_2}{2} n_3 n_4 \ldots n_m$$

$$+ \binom{n_1}{2}\binom{n_3}{2} n_2 n_4 \ldots n_m + \ldots + \binom{n_{m-1}}{2}\binom{n_m}{2} n_1 n_2 \ldots n_{m-2}$$

doubly heterozygous genotypes, and so on to

$$\binom{n_1}{2}\binom{n_2}{2}\ldots\binom{n_m}{2}$$

m-ply heterozygous genotypes.

In a Batesonian system with allelic index $(n_1, n_2, \ldots, n_m)$, the number of k-ply heterozygous genotypes is 2^{k-1} times as many as in the corresponding Mendelian system of order m, for every k from 1 to m inclusive.

We can also formulate the following hypothesis concerning Mendelian systems:

[H. 7]　If $X_1 X_2 \ldots X_m$ and $Y_1 Y_2 \ldots Y_m$ are both Boolean products of m distinct genotypes, and each is included in a Mendelian system of order m with common environmental set E, then

$$D(\mathbf{F}_E(X_1 X_2 \ldots X_m, Y_1 Y_2 \ldots Y_m))$$

$$= D(\mathbf{F}_E(X_1, Y_1))\dot\cap D(\mathbf{F}_E(X_2, Y_2))\dot\cap \ldots \dot\cap D(\mathbf{F}_E(X_m, Y_m)),$$

provided that genotypes whose designations share the same subscript belong to the same factor system of order 1. From this and H. 6 we shall have:

[T. 9]　The right-hand side of any mating description in a Mendelian system of order m $(m > 1)$ is the combined Boolean product of m factors each of which belongs to one of the seven mating types 1, 2, 3, 4, 5, 6 or 7.*

Although the foregoing remarks by no means exhaust the theory of genetical systems of order m at zero level, and are not intended to, because this is not a text-book of genetics, they will nevertheless suffice to illustrate the principles of Part I when applied to observation records and zero-level statements of genetics. For up to this point we have remained on the theoretical level of statistical generalizations of observation records, i.e. on zero level. All the functors used have been defined with the help of 'phenotype' and the mating functor '$F_X(Y, Z)$'. The only other undefined signs used have been the specific phenotype designations 'Y', 'G', etc., which have been introduced purely for illustrative purposes and do not belong to theoretical genetics. The notion of genotype, in the sense in which it has been used here, has been defined and does not take us beyond zero level. Upon this single theoretical level Mendel himself placed a level of first-order explanatory hypotheses which must now be considered.

§ 7. FUNCTORS REQUIRED FOR FIRST-LEVEL STATEMENTS

It is characteristic of scientific theories that passing to a new higher level involves changing the subject, talking about something new and hence introducing new words or other descriptive or subject-matter signs. Why this is so becomes obvious when we reflect that one of the purposes of passing to a higher level is to widen the scope of our theory so that it embraces more of the subject-matter of the science to which it belongs. In order that statements belonging to this wider scope should be derivable from hypotheses of higher levels, the latter must contain signs belonging to the branches of the science over which we wish to extend the scope of our theory, or signs with the help of which such signs are definable.

* See Note 6, p. 207.

On the new level of genetical theory we do not speak in the first instance of parents and offspring and mating, but about *gametes* and their *union* to form *zygotes*. It therefore becomes necessary to enlarge our vocabulary by the addition of some new undefined functors.

I shall use, to begin with, small Greek letters as dummy names for sets of gametes. With this convention and the comma notation for the simple product of two sets, the expression 'α, β' will denote the set of all pairs of gametes, one member of which belongs to α and the other to β. By writing 'U' in front of this we obtain an expression which is explained in the following semantical rule:

[S. 2]   '$U(\alpha, \beta)$' denotes the set of all zygotes formed by the union of a gamete belonging to the set α with one belonging to the set β.

The use of this new functor will conform to the following postulate:

[H. 8] $U(\alpha, \beta) = U(\beta, \alpha)$.

In what follows I shall always mean, by a zygote, a *cell* formed by the union of two gametes. If this cell divides into two cells I shall cease to speak of a zygote and call the object composed of these two cells an embryo in the two-celled stage, if they both form parts of one life.

So far the notion of development has only been introduced implicitly through the unanalysed mating functor. We now require a functor of degree three which will play the part of an abbreviation for

x develops in y into z.

Instead of beginning with an undefined functor of degree 3 for this purpose I introduce two undefined functors with the help of which it can be defined:

[S. 3]   '$x\mathbf{En}y$' is true if and only if x is the environment of y.*

* For a brief discussion of the notion of environment and a set of postulates for **En** see Note 8, p. 208.

[S. 4]   '$\mathbf{B}(x)$' denotes the first moment or beginning of x, the time-slice of x which precedes all others in time.*

We can now define the required functor of degree 3 as follows:

[D. 28] $\mathbf{dlz}(x, y, z)$ if and only if, for some sets α and β, $x \in \mathbf{U}(\alpha, \beta)$,

$$\mathbf{B}(x) = \mathbf{B}(z) \quad \text{and} \quad y\mathbf{En}z.$$

$\mathbf{dlz}(x, y, z)$ may be read 'The zygote x develops in the environment y into the life z'.

As functors of degree 3 are not so familiar as those of degree 2, it will perhaps be desirable to point out some of their peculiarities when expressed in English. If we have the statement

Tom sits between Dick and Harry,

we are in no danger of losing sight of the fact that it is constructed with the help of a functor of degree 3. We are not tempted to write

Tom sits between Dick

and so to forget Harry, because this simply does not form a statement. But if we begin with

Stanley met Livingstone in Central Africa,

we see that   Stanley met Livingstone

is a perfectly good statement containing a functor of degree 2 although it is extracted from one containing a functor of degree 3. Now when we consider

a develops in b into c

(supposing 'a', 'b' and 'c' to be names, not dummies), we find we have a statement containing a functor of degree 3 from which we can extract three perfectly good statements, *each* containing a functor of degree 2, namely,

a develops in b,

b is the environment of c,

a develops into c.

* See my *Axiomatic Method in Biology*, p. 66.

It is extremely easy therefore, in this instance, to overlook the fact that we are really dealing with a functor of degree 3 and so to forget one of the three terms. I believe that this has been an important source of the misunderstandings which have occasioned controversies about heredity and environment. Obvious though this functor is when it is pointed out, I have been very slow myself in stumbling upon it. If I had used it in my book on the axiomatic method in biology, that book would have been much improved.

It may also be useful to point out here that when we are using a symbolic language we can always define three functors of degree 2 if we are given one of degree 3. Thus starting with $\mathbf{dlz}(x, y, z)$ we can define

(i) A two-termed relation $\mathbf{d}$ as that in which x stands to y when *for some z* we have $\mathbf{dlz}(x, y, z)$.

(ii) A two-termed relation $\mathbf{d}'$ as that in which y stands to z when *for some x* we have $\mathbf{dlz}(x, y, z)$. (Assuming as we do that this is a one-many relation, we can use '$\mathbf{en}(z)$' to denote *the* environment which stands in $\mathbf{d}'$ to z.)

(iii) A two-termed relation $\mathbf{d}''$ as that in which x stands to z when *for some y* we have $\mathbf{dlz}(x, y, z)$. (Assuming as we do that this is also a one-many relation, we can use '$\mathbf{z}(z)$' to denote *the* zygote which stands in $\mathbf{d}''$ to z.)

It will be noticed that, although these are two-termed relations, thanks to the use of the existential quantifier ('*for some z*', etc.) in their definitions, their connexion with a functor of degree 3 is preserved.

By a life I am meaning the whole time-extent of what develops from the moment of fertilization to some moment later. If this moment is the moment of death I speak of a complete life. Where it is necessary to be very precise, the time-length of the life in question could be specified.* With the usual assumptions regarding time, there will be an infinity of parts which are lives in every life. Consequently, we can have, with a given zygote a,

$$\mathbf{dlz}(a, b, c) \quad \text{and} \quad \mathbf{dlz}(a, b', c'), \tag{9}$$

* See Note 3, Part III, p. 322.

although $$b \neq b' \quad \text{and} \quad c \neq c', \tag{10}$$

and $\qquad\qquad b$ is part of b' $\quad$ and $\quad c$ part of c',

or $\qquad\qquad b'$ is part of b $\quad$ and $\quad c'$ part of c.

But it is also possible to have (9) and (10), although c is not part of c' and c' not part of c. When this happens we say that c and c' are monozygotic or identical twins.

Regarding what we are to understand by the environment y in $\mathbf{dlz}(x, y, z)$, I propose to say nothing in these lectures. The word is in common use in biology, although there the distinction is not always made explicit between particular environments and sets of environments; 'y' of course is a dummy name representing some particular environment.

With the help of the matrix '$\mathbf{dlz}(x, y, z)$' we can formulate embryological laws of a type which is presupposed in genetics. The reason for this presupposition of embryological laws is as follows: In natural science, if an investigator reports an experiment which cannot be repeated by his colleagues with the same result, his observation records relating to this experiment do not become generalized and incorporated in the body of accepted scientific statements. But a given zygote can only develop *once*. Consequently *no* embryological experiment which involves the development of zygotes can be repeated. In order to escape from this difficulty we are driven to assume that we have at our disposal *sets* of zygotes, and also *sets* of environments, such that if we take *any* member of the set of zygotes and let it develop in *any* member of the set of environments, then we shall get, in some respects at least, the same result as if we took any other of the zygotes and let it develop in any other of the environments. For example, suppose Z is some specific set of zygotes and E some specific set of environments and P some specific phenotype. Then *if* we find that, whenever a member of Z develops in a member of E it develops into a member of P, we can say that Z is *developmentally homogeneous* with respect to E and P. The relativization 'with respect to E and P' is necessary as will be apparent by taking the following instance. Suppose members of *P* are either male or female but not both, and we denote by '*MP*' those which are male, then it would not be the case that *Z* was developmentally homogeneous with respect to *E* and *MP*, because some members of *Z* would develop in members of *E* into females.

In this connexion we can say something about the use of the word 'identity' in biology which was referred to in a previous lecture. If *Z* is developmentally homogeneous with respect to *E* and *P* we can also say that any two members of *Z* are *developmentally identical* with respect to *E* and *P*. Here again the relativization with respect to *E* and *P* is essential. Just to say that two zygotes are identical would seem to be either meaningless or metaphysical, unless you mean strict identity. But in the latter case you have not two zygotes but one. Paris is identical with the capital of France, but these are not two cities. Thus identity in biology, apart from strict identity, is always identity relative to some set or sets. Later it will be necessary to distinguish between *developmental* identity and *genetical* identity.*

In order to express briefly what has been said about the sets *Z*, *E* and *P*, I write '**Dlz**(Z, E, P)' as an abbreviation for '*Z* is developmentally homogeneous with respect to *E* and *P*'. I use a capital '**D**' to indicate that sets, not individuals, are concerned, because '**dlz**' occurs in the strict definition of '**Dlz**' which is as follows. I shall say:

[D. 29]   **Dlz**(Z, E, P) if and only if, for every *x*, *y* and *z*, if **dlz**(x, y, z) and $x \in Z$ and $y \in E$ then $z \in P$.†

It must be understood that '**Dlz**' is not to be regarded as a shared name. It is what I call an *abbreviator*. With its help we construct an abbreviation for the universal general statement on the right-hand side of the definition. If '*Z*', '*E*' and '*P*' are not names but dummy names we obtain a definition schema from which a definition results if we replace these letters by names.

To complete our vocabulary of first-level expressions we still

* See below, p. 197.   † See Note 9, p. 209.

need two more signs. The phrase, 'the set of all lives which have developed from some member of the set Z of zygotes in some member of the set E of environments', will frequently occur, and it is therefore desirable to have an abbreviation for it. For this purpose I use '$\mathbf{L}_E(Z)$' which is defined:

[D. 30]　$\mathbf{L}_E(Z)$ is the set of all lives w such that for some x and some y, $x \epsilon Z$ and $y \epsilon E$ and $\mathbf{dlz}(x, y, w)$.

Finally, we shall need the undefined sign '$\mathbf{G}_X(Y)$' which is explained in the following semantical rule:

[S. 5]　'$\mathbf{G}_X(Y)$' denotes the set of all gametes which are produced by members of the genotype Y when they develop in members of the environmental set X.

It may also be desirable to give formal expression to the following *syntactical* rule:

[S. 6]　The blank spaces in the functors '$\mathbf{F}_X(\ ,\ )$' and '$\mathbf{G}_X(\ )$' can only be occupied by genotype designations.

Another useful notion is that of the P-environmental range of a set Z of zygotes, P being a phenotype. We can denote it by '$\mathbf{Er}(P, Z)$', it is defined as follows:

[D. 31]　$\mathbf{Er}(P, Z)$ is the set of all environments y such that for some Y, $\mathbf{Dlz}(Z, Y, P)$ and $y \epsilon Y$.

The P-environmental range of Z will thus be the set of environments in which members of Z will develop into members of P. Suppose that every member of P has a time-length of at least t units and let 'W' denote the set of all lives which have a time-length of at least t units. Then $\mathbf{Er}(W, Z)$ will be the set of environments in which members of Z develop into members of W. If now $\mathbf{Er}(W, Z)$ is included in $\mathbf{Er}(P, Z)$ then every environment in which a member of Z develops into a member of W will also be one in which a member of Z develops into a member of P. Important use will be made of this notion in Lecture V in the special case when W is the set of all adult lives. (See pp. 183 and 187. For more information about the notion of time-length see Part III, Note 3, p. 322.)

By means of our enlarged vocabulary we can now formulate the following identity:

$$\mathbf{F}_X(Z, W) = \mathbf{L}_X(\mathbf{U}(\mathbf{G}_X(Z), \mathbf{G}_X(W))).$$

If we were proceeding axiomatically we could use this to define $\mathbf{F}$ by means of $\mathbf{L}$, $\mathbf{U}$ and $\mathbf{G}$. It states that the set of all offspring from the mating of members of Z with members of W, when both parents and offspring have developed in members of X, is identical with the set of all lives which have developed in members of X from zygotes formed by the union of a gamete produced by a member of Z which has developed in a member of X with a gamete produced by a member of W when it also has developed in a member of X.

Our three new signs, $\mathbf{U}$, $\mathbf{L}$ and $\mathbf{G}$, which, like $\mathbf{F}$, are all name-forming functors, can be applied not only to single sets, but also to Boolean sums and to combined sums. For example, $\mathbf{L}_X(Z_1 \cup Z_2)$ is identical with $\mathbf{L}_X(Z_1) \cup \mathbf{L}_X(Z_2)$. We can say in the language of algebraists that the operator $\mathbf{L}_X$ is *distributive* into a Boolean sum. Corresponding identities hold for $\mathbf{F}_X$, $\mathbf{G}_X$ and $\mathbf{U}$.

We must now consider what conditions must be satisfied if these operators are to be distributive into *combined* sums. As the same principles apply, *mutatis mutandis*, to all four operators, it will suffice if we explain the procedure for $\mathbf{L}_X$. What does it mean in *biological* terms to say that $\mathbf{L}_X$ is distributive into a combined sum? First we must *define* $\mathbf{L}_X$ when it is applied to a combined sum. Suppose W is the Boolean sum of n mutually exclusive sets of zygotes (with $n > 0$)

$$W = Z_1 \cup Z_2 \cup \ldots \cup Z_n,$$

and suppose the distribution of the n sets composing W is given by

$$\mathrm{D}(W) = p_1 Z_1 + p_2 Z_2 + \ldots + p_n Z_n = \sum_1^n p_i Z_i. \tag{11}$$

We now define '$L_X\left(\sum\limits_1^n p_i Z_i\right)$' as follows:

$$L_X\left(\sum\limits_1^n p_i Z_i\right) = \sum\limits_1^n p_i L_X(Z_i). \tag{12}$$

Then with the above constitution of W we shall have

$$L_X(W) = L_X(Z_1)\cup L_X(Z_2)\cup ...\cup L_X(Z_n);$$

let the distribution of these sub-sets in $L_X(W)$ be given by

$$D(L_X(W)) = q_1 L_X(Z_1) + q_2 L_X(Z_2) + ... + q_n L_X(Z_n)$$
$$= \sum\limits_1^n q_i L_X(Z_i). \tag{13}$$

Now (13) gives us the relative proportions of certain sets of lives classified according to the set of zygotes (a sub-set of W) from which they have developed (X being common to all). If each member of W develops into the same number (m) of lives of a given time-length as any other member we shall have $q_i = p_i$ for each $i = 1, 2, ..., n$ and consequently we shall, by (11) and (12), have

$$L_X(D(W)) = D(L_X(W)). \tag{α}$$

Let us say that any set W of zygotes which satisfies this requirement is *equiproductive* with respect to L_X.

Now clearly, although equiproductivity with respect to L_X (for some X) frequently happens, we cannot assert that it *always* happens. In the case of human zygotes, for example, there is no fixed m. It is commonly assumed that some zygotes develop into one, some into two and some into no lives of a given time-length. Consequently we cannot allow (α) to stand as an independent statement which is to hold for *any* set W of zygotes and some set X of environments. It can only form part of the antecedent in a genetical law, as will be seen in the next lecture.

Corresponding remarks apply to the operators F_X, G_X and U. Each of these will be distributive into $D(W)$, if W is equiproductive with respect to the operation in question.

This rather complicated discussion on the distributivity of 'L_X' illustrates the way in which a symbolic language enables us to embody the fruits of our thinking in a formula so that we can operate with the symbols without the necessity of going through the same processes of thought again each time we use them. Having established the equation (α) we can apply it in subsequent developments without each time thinking of the complicated discussion connected with it. We may recall the words of Whitehead when he said:

It is a profoundly erroneous truism, repeated by all copy-books and by eminent people when they are making speeches, that we should cultivate the habit of thinking of what we are doing. The precise opposite is the case. Civilization advances by extending the number of important operations which we can perform without thinking about them. Operations of thought are like cavalry charges in a battle—they are strictly limited in number, they require fresh horses, and must only be made at decisive moments.

LECTURE IV

§1. FIRST-LEVEL HYPOTHESES

At the end of the last lecture I had completed explaining the new functors which are required for formulating first-level explanatory hypotheses in a genetical theory. We introduced four new undefined signs $U(\alpha, \beta)$, $x\mathbf{Eny}$, $\mathbf{B}(x)$ and $\mathbf{G}_X(Y)$. With the help of these we defined $\mathbf{dlz}(x, y, z)$, $\mathbf{Dlz}(X, Y, Z)$, $\mathbf{L}_X(Z)$ and $\mathbf{Er}(P, Z)$. We also formulated an identity connecting the old signs of zero level with the new ones of first level. We shall now write this in the more general form:

[H. 9] $\quad \mathbf{F}_{X, Y, Z}(W_1, W_2) = \mathbf{L}_Z(U(\mathbf{G}_X(W_1), \mathbf{G}_Y(W_2)))$.

This has the status of a hypothesis at the present stage of our analysis because '$\mathbf{G}_X(Y)$' is undefined. From this, with the help of D. 1 (p. 97), we obtain the simpler form

[T. 10] $\quad \mathbf{F}_X(W_1, W_2) = \mathbf{L}_X(U(\mathbf{G}_X(W_1), \mathbf{G}_X(W_2)))$.

We also reached a result concerning the distribution of 'L' into a combined sum. This does not have the status of an independent hypothesis; we shall call it condition (α)

$$D(\mathbf{L}_X(W)) = \mathbf{L}_X(D(W)),$$

since it holds when W is an equiproductive set of zygotes with respect to $\mathbf{L}$ and the environmental set X, or when some more complicated condition is satisfied by W.

We are now ready to consider the more special first-level hypotheses that are required for deriving the mating descriptions of genetical systems. Our problem will be to find a set of statements, formulated with the help of first-level functors, from which the mating descriptions for such systems follow.

Mendel assumed that, as it is commonly expressed, the union of the gametes takes place at random. In order not to rule out the possibility of selective union of gametes in some cases we shall refrain from asserting this as an independent hypothesis, just as we refrained in the case of condition (α). We shall call the assumption of the random union of the gametes condition (β) and formulate it in our language as follows:

$$D(U(G_X(Y), G_X(Z))) = U(D(G_X(Y)); D(G_X(Z))).$$

This is reached in a succession of steps analogous to those followed in the case of L_X, except that in the present case we are dealing with sets of pairs and the notion of random pairing is involved. We first note that the distribution of pairs is expressed by

$$D(X, Y) = D(X); D(Y).$$

Next we have the condition of random pairing and equi-productivity with respect to U,

$$D(U(X, Y)) = U(D(X, Y)).$$

If we now substitute for '$D(X, Y)$' in the right-hand side of the second equation in accordance with the first, we obtain

$$D(U(X, Y)) = U(D(X); D(Y)).$$

Finally from this, by substitutions for 'X' and 'Y', we obtain condition (β).

But this does not suffice for the derivation of mating descriptions, because the latter are statements about mating and offspring, and condition (β) only gives us distributions of sets of zygotes. To obtain what we want we must therefore apply the operator L and make use of condition (α). If in the latter we substitute '$U(G_X(Y), G_X(Z))$' for 'W' we obtain

$$D(L_X(U(G_X(Y), G_X(Z)))) = L_X(D(U(G_X(Y), G_X(Z)))).$$

Substituting in the right-hand side of this according to condition (β) we obtain

$$D(L_X(U(G_X(Y), G_X(Z)))) = L_X(U(D(G_X(Y)); D(G_X(Z)))).$$

Substituting in the left-hand side according to T. 10 we finally obtain

$$D(F_X(Y, Z)) = L_X(U(D(G_X(Y)); D(G_X(Z)))),$$

which we shall call condition (γ). This is the formula we require. It includes in one statement conditions (α) and (β) as well as the assumption of the equiproductivity of the set of gamete-pairs with respect to **U**. (See Note 10, p. 210.)

We shall also require a gamete set designation for sets specified, not according to the genotypes which produce them, but according to the genotypes to which the lives belong which develop from the zygotes which result from their union in pairs. Thus we say

[D. 32]   **Gm**(P), for any phenotype P, is the set of all gametes x such that, for some α, $\alpha \neq \Lambda$ and **Dlz**$(\mathbf{U}(\alpha , \alpha), \mathbf{E}(P), \mathbf{H}(P))$ and $x \in \alpha$.*

With this definition we shall have the following consequence:

[T. 11]   For any phenotype P such that $\mathbf{H}(P) \neq \Lambda$

$$\mathbf{Dlz}(\mathbf{U}(\mathbf{Gm}(P) , \mathbf{Gm}(P)), \mathbf{E}(P), \mathbf{H}(P)).$$

The next statement will not follow from the definition but must be asserted as an independent first-level hypothesis:

[H. 10]   For any phenotypes P and Q such that $\mathbf{Ht}(P, Q) \neq \Lambda$

$$\mathbf{Dlz}(\mathbf{U}(\mathbf{Gm}(P) , \mathbf{Gm}(Q)), \mathbf{E}(P, Q), \mathbf{Ht}(P, Q)).$$

Next we require two hypotheses concerning the production of such gamete sets:

[H. 11]   If P is any phenotype and $X = \mathbf{E}(P)$, then

$$\mathbf{G}_X(\mathbf{H}(P)) \subset \mathbf{Gm}(P).$$

* For reasons which are given in Note 9, p. 210, D. 32 is not a satisfactory definition. A better one is easily obtained by the use of the functor '$\mathbf{u}(x, y)$' which is defined in Note 14 (1), p. 211, as denoting *the* zygote which is formed by the union of gamete x with gamete y. Thus '$\mathbf{u}$' is the analogue for individuals of '$\mathbf{U}$' for sets, and the latter can easily be defined by means of the former. From the axiomatic point of view this would be the proper procedure to follow. This has not been done in the text because '$\mathbf{u}$' is rarely needed there and it was desired to restrict the number of definitions as far as possible. To obtain a better definition of '$\mathbf{Gm}(P)$' let us first define $\mathbf{Z}(P)$ as the set of all zygotes x such that, for some X we have $x \in X$ and $\mathbf{Dlz}(X, \mathbf{E}(P), \mathbf{H}(P))$ and $\mathbf{H}(P) \neq \Lambda$. We can then easily define $\mathbf{Gm}(P)$ as the set of all gametes u such that for some v, $\mathbf{u}(u, v) \in \mathbf{Z}(P)$. Or, we can combine the two steps into one and write the definition as follows: $\mathbf{Gm}(P)$ is the set of all gametes u such that, for some v and some X, we have $\mathbf{u}(u, v) \in X$ and $\mathbf{Dlz}(X, \mathbf{E}(P), \mathbf{H}(P))$ and $\mathbf{H}(P) \neq \Lambda$.

[H. 12]   If P and Q are any phenotypes such that $\mathbf{Ht}(P, Q) \neq \Lambda$ and $X = \mathbf{E}(P, Q)$, then

$$D(\mathbf{G}_X(\mathbf{Ht}(P, Q))) = \tfrac{1}{2}\mathbf{Gm}(P) + \tfrac{1}{2}\mathbf{Gm}(Q).$$

This is a way of formulating Mendel's hypothesis that the hybrids produce two kinds of gametes in approximately equal numbers. For the derivation of mating descriptions two more statements will be required:

[T. 12]   For any X, Y and Z, if $\mathbf{Dlz}(X, Y, Z)$ then $\mathbf{L}_Y(X) \subset Z$.

This is simply a consequence of D. 29 and D. 30.

[H. 13]   For any α, β, γ and δ, if $\alpha \subset \gamma$ and $\beta \subset \delta$, then

$$\mathbf{U}(\alpha, \beta) \subset \mathbf{U}(\gamma, \delta).$$

This is merely necessitated by the fact that 'U' is at present an undefined sign. If we were axiomatizing and had adopted the definition of 'U' which will be given later, then H. 13 would be a consequence of the definition.

Before we proceed to examples of derivations we must deal with a difficulty which arises on level 1. We have seen that certain of the formulas needed on this level (e.g. condition (γ)) cannot be asserted as independent hypotheses but only if certain states of affairs are realized. But our hypotheses on zero level were stated unconditionally. They cannot therefore, as they stand, be derived from our first-level hypotheses. There seem to be two ways out of this difficulty. We can modify our definitions of genetical systems so that only those are called genetical systems which satisfy condition (γ), or we can define a special sub-set of the genetical systems, namely those which satisfy condition (γ) and then reformulate our zero-level hypotheses so that they are asserted only for such special genetical systems. The latter is the course adopted here.*

* In this connexion I am a little doubtful about the formulation of hypothesis H. 12. Perhaps some restriction should be placed on P and Q in its antecedent. This is a point for expert geneticists to decide.

[D. 33] We shall say that a genetical system S satisfies condition (γ) if the latter condition holds when 'Y' and 'Z' are replaced by any of the phenotype designations of S. And we call a genetical system *regular* if and only if it satisfies condition (γ).

Now suppose lists or catalogues were published of the genetical systems so far investigated. Each entry would specify the generating phenotypes, would state whether the system was regular or not and would give the allelic index and partition. Such a catalogue would contain the whole of zero-level genetics at the time of its publication. The rest of genetics would be first and higher level genetics and would contain no specific phenotype designation. How would the entries in the catalogue be tested? We can now illustrate the procedure by a simple example, letting 'Y' and 'G' have the same significance they had in our example on p. 106. We should find the following entry in the catalogue:

$S(Y, G)$ is a regular genetical system of allelic index (2) and partition (2, 1), with Y dominant to G.

From this statement, together with our first-level statements we can now derive all the characteristic mating descriptions for a system of allelic index (2). For illustrative purposes it will suffice if we carry out the derivation for only two of these descriptions. First we will derive

$$F_E(H(Y), H(Y)) \subset H(Y)$$

(where 'E' is an abbreviation for '$E(Y)$'). We begin by substituting '$H(Y)$' for both 'W_1' and 'W_2' in T. 10, obtaining

(1) $F_E(H(Y), H(Y)) = L_E(U(G_E(H(Y)), G_E(H(Y))))$.

From D. 19 we know that $H(Y) \neq \Lambda$ and therefore from H. 11 we get

$$G_E(H(Y)) \subset Gm(Y),$$

and from this and H. 13 and D. 30 we are entitled to write

(2) $L_E(U(G_E(H(Y)), G_E(H(Y)))) \subset L_E(U(Gm(Y), Gm(Y)))$.

By T. 11 we have

$$\mathbf{Dlz}(\mathbf{U}(\mathbf{Gm}(\mathbf{Y}),\mathbf{Gm}(\mathbf{Y})),E,\mathbf{H}(\mathbf{Y})),$$

and from this and T. 12 we obtain

(3) $$\mathbf{L}_E(\mathbf{U}(\mathbf{Gm}(\mathbf{Y}),\mathbf{Gm}(\mathbf{Y})))\subset\mathbf{H}(\mathbf{Y}).$$

Finally, from (1), (2) and (3) with the help of formulas (3) and (4) in Note 2, p. 201, we obtain

$$\mathbf{F}_E(\mathbf{H}(\mathbf{Y}),\mathbf{H}(\mathbf{Y}))\subset\mathbf{H}(\mathbf{Y}),$$

which is the required mating description; and since $\mathbf{H}(\mathbf{Y})\subset\mathbf{Y}$, we can obtain the corresponding mating description with a phenotype designation on the right-hand side.

Next let us substitute '$\mathbf{Ht}(\mathbf{Y},\mathbf{G})$' for both '$Y$' and '$Z$' in condition ($\gamma$) on p. 135 and put '$E$' ($=\mathbf{E}(\mathbf{Y},\mathbf{G})$) for '$X$', obtaining

(1) $$\mathbf{D}(\mathbf{F}_E(\mathbf{Ht}(\mathbf{Y},\mathbf{G}),\mathbf{Ht}(\mathbf{Y},\mathbf{G})))$$
$$= \mathbf{L}_E(\mathbf{U}(\mathbf{D}(\mathbf{G}_E(\mathbf{Ht}(\mathbf{Y},\mathbf{G})));\mathbf{D}(\mathbf{G}_E(\mathbf{Ht}(\mathbf{Y},\mathbf{G}))))));$$

we are entitled to do this by D. 33 and the information that $\mathbf{S}(\mathbf{Y},\mathbf{G})$ is regular. Substituting '$\mathbf{Y}$' for 'P' and '$\mathbf{G}$' for 'Q' in H. 12 we get

(2) $$\mathbf{D}(\mathbf{G}_E(\mathbf{Ht}(\mathbf{Y},\mathbf{G}))) = \tfrac{1}{2}\mathbf{Gm}(\mathbf{Y})+\tfrac{1}{2}\mathbf{Gm}(\mathbf{G}).$$

It will simplify the remaining formulas if we let '$\mathbf{y}$' stand for '$\mathbf{Gm}(\mathbf{Y})$' and '$\mathbf{g}$' for '$\mathbf{Gm}(\mathbf{G})$'. Using these abbreviations and (2), the right-hand side of (1) becomes

(3) $$\mathbf{L}_E(\mathbf{U}(\tfrac{1}{2}\mathbf{y}+\tfrac{1}{2}\mathbf{g};\tfrac{1}{2}\mathbf{y}+\tfrac{1}{2}\mathbf{g}));$$

carrying out the combined simple multiplication according to T. 8 of combined algebra this becomes

(4) $$\mathbf{L}_E(\mathbf{U}(\tfrac{1}{4}\mathbf{y},\mathbf{y}+\tfrac{1}{2}\mathbf{y},\mathbf{g}+\tfrac{1}{4}\mathbf{g},\mathbf{g})).$$

And since the system is regular the zygote set will be equiproductive with respect to $\mathbf{L}_E$ and the gametes with respect to $\mathbf{U}$, and we can therefore transform (4) into

(5) $$\tfrac{1}{4}\mathbf{L}_E(\mathbf{U}(\mathbf{y},\mathbf{y}))+\tfrac{1}{2}\mathbf{L}_E(\mathbf{U}(\mathbf{y},\mathbf{g}))+\tfrac{1}{4}\mathbf{L}_E(\mathbf{U}(\mathbf{g},\mathbf{g})).$$

From this, with the help of T. 11, H. 10, T. 12, and another principle which has not been formulated in the text,* we obtain

(6) $$\tfrac{1}{4}\mathbf{H(Y)} + \tfrac{1}{2}\mathbf{Ht(Y, G)} + \tfrac{1}{4}\mathbf{H(G)}.$$

Finally, from (1) and the successive transformations of its right-hand side we obtain

(7) $$D(\mathbf{F}_E(\mathbf{Ht(Y, G)}, \mathbf{Ht(Y, G)}))$$
$$= \tfrac{1}{4}\mathbf{H(Y)} + \tfrac{1}{2}\mathbf{Ht(Y, G)} + \tfrac{1}{4}\mathbf{H(G)},$$

which is another mating description of a type characteristic of a regular genetical system of allelic index (2). If we know that **Y** is dominant to **G** the corresponding mating description with phenotypes on the right-hand side can be obtained. All the other mating descriptions are obtainable in an analogous manner.

It is easy to see how these hypotheses are to be generalized to enable us to deal with any genetical system of order 1:

[H. 14] If $S = S(P_1, P_2, ..., P_n)$ is any genetical system of order 1 then

    (i) $\mathbf{Dlz}(\mathbf{U}(\mathbf{Gm}(P_i), \mathbf{Gm}(P_j)), \mathbf{E}(S), \mathbf{Ht}(P_i, P_j))$,

    (ii) $\mathbf{G}_E(\mathbf{H}(P_i)) \subset \mathbf{Gm}(P_i)$ (where $E = \mathbf{E}(S)$),

    (iii) $D(\mathbf{G}_E(\mathbf{Ht}(P_i, P_j))) = \tfrac{1}{2}\mathbf{Gm}(P_i) + \tfrac{1}{2}\mathbf{Gm}(P_j)$,

for each $i, j = 1, 2, ..., n$ and $i < j$.

From this and the more general hypothesis, H. 9, and condition (γ), we can, for regular systems, derive the generalized mating descriptions on p. 114. In order to obtain the corresponding mating descriptions with phenotypes on the right-hand side we must be able to derive the dominance relations between the phenotypes from the partition of the system.

---

* This principle may be formulated as follows. Suppose $W = Z_1 \cup Z_2 \cup ... \cup Z_n$ and $Z_i \cap Z_j = \Lambda$ for $i, j = 1, 2, ..., n$, $i \neq j$, suppose further that we have sets U_i such that $Z_i \subset U_i$ for every $i = 1, 2, ..., n$ and also $U_i \cap U_j = \Lambda$ for $i, j = 1, 2, ..., n$ and $i \neq j$. Then if $D_{Z_i}(W) = \sum_1^n p_i Z_i$, we also have

$$D_{U_i}(W) = \sum_1^n p_i U_i.$$

We can also derive hypotheses H. 4, H. 5 and H. 6 concerning the seven mating types for a regular system of order 1. It is easy to see, on level 1, why only seven mating types are possible in a regular genetical system of allelic index (n). For suppose we have the following matrix, using, within the mating functor, expressions belonging to level 1,

$$\mathbf{F}_X(\mathbf{L}_X(\mathbf{U}(\alpha,\beta)),\mathbf{L}_X(\mathbf{U}(\gamma,\delta))).$$

It is at once evident that at most four distinct gamete-sets can be represented, and four can only be represented if $n > 3$ (since n is equal to the total number of distinct gamete-sets characteristic of the system). Now suppose that only one set is represented, so that $\alpha = \beta = \gamma = \delta$, then we shall have the left-hand side of a mating description of Type 1.* If $\alpha = \beta$ and $\gamma = \delta$, but $\beta \neq \gamma$ so that two distinct sets are represented, we shall have Type 2. If $\alpha = \gamma$ and $\beta = \delta$ but $\alpha \neq \beta$ then we shall have Type 3. If $\alpha \neq \beta$ but $\beta = \gamma = \delta$ we shall have Type 4, and these are the only possibilities if $n = 2$. If $n = 3$ we have two more possibilities, namely, $\alpha \neq \beta$ and $\alpha \neq \gamma$ and $\beta \neq \gamma$ but $\gamma = \delta$, which yields Type 5, and $\alpha \neq \beta$, $\alpha = \gamma$, $\alpha \neq \delta$, $\beta \neq \delta$ which yields Type 6. Finally, with $n > 3$ we have Type 7 with all four gamete-sets distinct.

Now we come to genetical systems of order greater than 1. These are more easily dealt with on level 1 than on zero level, thus illustrating the simplifying and clarifying effect of an explanatory hypothesis.†

Suppose we have two systems S_1 and S_2 each of allelic index (2) and common environmental set E. Let

$$S_1 = \mathbf{L}_E(\mathbf{U}(\alpha\cup\beta,\alpha\cup\beta)),$$

$$S_2 = \mathbf{L}_E(\mathbf{U}(\gamma\cup\delta,\gamma\cup\delta)),$$

then their genetical product (using juxtaposition of set desig-

---

* The mating-type designations are those explained on pp. 112, 114.

† Very roughly speaking we may say that observation records are intelligible but vague, explanatory hypotheses are clear but (often) unintelligible (in the sense of 'abstract', see p. 58).

nations to indicate Boolean product) will be

$$S_1 \times S_2 =$$
$$= \mathbf{L}_E(\mathbf{U}((\alpha \cup \beta) \cap (\gamma \cup \delta), (\alpha \cup \beta) \cap (\gamma \cup \delta)))$$
$$= \mathbf{L}_E(\mathbf{U}(\alpha\gamma \cup \beta\gamma \cup \alpha\delta \cup \beta\delta, \alpha\gamma \cup \beta\gamma \cup \alpha\delta \cup \beta\delta))$$
$$= \mathbf{L}_E(\mathbf{U}(\alpha\gamma, \alpha\gamma)) \cup \mathbf{L}_E(\mathbf{U}(\beta\gamma, \alpha\gamma)) \cup \mathbf{L}_E(\mathbf{U}(\alpha\delta, \alpha\gamma)) \cup \mathbf{L}_E(\mathbf{U}(\beta\delta, \alpha\gamma))$$
$$\cup \mathbf{L}_E(\mathbf{U}(\beta\gamma, \beta\gamma)) \cup \mathbf{L}_E(\mathbf{U}(\alpha\delta, \beta\gamma)) \cup \mathbf{L}_E(\mathbf{U}(\beta\delta, \beta\gamma))$$
$$\cup \mathbf{L}_E(\mathbf{U}(\alpha\delta, \alpha\delta)) \cup \mathbf{L}_E(\mathbf{U}(\beta\delta, \alpha\delta))$$
$$\cup \mathbf{L}_E(\mathbf{U}(\beta\delta, \beta\delta)).$$

Now if $\mathbf{L}_E(\mathbf{U}(\beta\delta, \alpha\gamma))$ is genetically equivalent to $\mathbf{L}_E(\mathbf{U}(\alpha\delta, \beta\gamma))$, then $S_1 \times S_2$ is a Mendelian system of allelic index (2) (2) and with nine distinct genotypes. If $\mathbf{L}_E(\mathbf{U}(\beta\delta, \alpha\gamma))$ and $\mathbf{L}_E(\mathbf{U}(\alpha\delta, \beta\gamma))$ are not genetically equivalent, then $S_1 \times S_2$ is a Batesonian system with allelic index (2, 2) and ten distinct genotypes.

This procedure for expressing and expanding the product can be extended to any number of factors with any allelic index.[*]

In the case of Mendelian systems the gamete-set frequencies for the genotypes in the genetical product of two or more systems are obtainable from those of the single factor systems by combined Boolean multiplication. Thus in the above example

$$\mathbf{D}(\mathbf{G}(\mathbf{L}_E(\mathbf{U}(\alpha, \beta)))) = \tfrac{1}{2}\alpha + \tfrac{1}{2}\beta,[\dagger]$$
$$\mathbf{D}(\mathbf{G}(\mathbf{L}_E(\mathbf{U}(\gamma, \delta)))) = \tfrac{1}{2}\gamma + \tfrac{1}{2}\delta,$$

and we find that

$$\mathbf{D}(\mathbf{G}(\mathbf{L}_E(\mathbf{U}(\alpha\gamma, \beta\delta)))) = (\tfrac{1}{2}\alpha + \tfrac{1}{2}\beta) \dot\cap (\tfrac{1}{2}\gamma + \tfrac{1}{2}\delta)$$
$$= \tfrac{1}{4}\alpha\gamma + \tfrac{1}{4}\beta\gamma + \tfrac{1}{4}\alpha\delta + \tfrac{1}{4}\beta\delta.$$

We can express this, which requires a new hypothesis, as follows: if XZ is any one of the Boolean products which is a genotype in a Mendelian system of order 2 with environmental set E, then

$$\mathbf{D}(\mathbf{G}_E(XZ)) = \mathbf{D}(\mathbf{G}_E(X)) \dot\cap \mathbf{D}(\mathbf{G}_E(Z)).$$

With the help of this new hypothesis we can derive the rule already given for multiplying offspring frequencies in mating

---

[*] See Notes 7 and 11, p. 208 and p. 210.

[†] I omit the subscript after 'G' when the latter is immediately followed by '(L' showing the required subscript.

descriptions belonging to systems of order 1 in order to obtain mating descriptions of systems of order 2 of which they are factors.*

With this example before us it is not a difficult task to formulate a very general hypothesis corresponding to the above for any Mendelian system of order m $(m > 1)$.

[H. 15]   If $X_1 X_2 \ldots X_m$ is any one of the Boolean products which is a genotype in a Mendelian system of order m and with environmental set E, then

$$D(\mathbf{G}_E(X_1 X_2 \ldots X_m))$$
$$= D(\mathbf{G}_E(X_1)) \,\dot\frown\, D(\mathbf{G}_E(X_2)) \,\dot\frown\, \ldots \,\dot\frown\, D(\mathbf{G}_E(X_m)).$$

This is the most general hypothesis for gamete-set frequencies in Mendelian systems, additional to hypotheses H. 11 and H. 12. Hypothesis H. 9 and condition (γ) are required for both Mendelian and Batesonian systems.

This is a complete generalization of what can strictly be called Mendelism. We see that it demands no hypotheses above the first level, which was the level reached by Mendel.

In Batesonian systems, although H. 9 and condition (γ) are still required, H. 15 does not hold. This corresponds to the fact that each Batesonian system is a law unto itself as far as the gamete-set frequencies are concerned. Thus with reference to the above scheme, for each system of allelic index $(2, 2)$, there will be a rational number p within the open interval 0 to $\frac{1}{2}$ such that

$$D(\mathbf{G}(\mathbf{L}_E(\mathbf{U}(\alpha\gamma, \beta\delta)))) = \tfrac{1}{2}(1-p)\,\alpha\gamma + \tfrac{1}{2}p\alpha\delta + \tfrac{1}{2}p\beta\gamma + \tfrac{1}{2}(1-p)\,\beta\delta,$$

and

$$D(\mathbf{G}(\mathbf{L}_E(\mathbf{U}(\alpha\delta, \beta\gamma)))) = \tfrac{1}{2}(1-p)\,\alpha\delta + \tfrac{1}{2}p\alpha\gamma + \tfrac{1}{2}p\beta\delta + \tfrac{1}{2}(1-p)\,\beta\gamma.$$

The connexion between Mendelian and Batesonian systems can only be explained at a higher theoretical level than the first. But before that level is reached another type of genetical system must be considered.

* See H. 7, p. 123.

§ 2. SECOND- AND THIRD-LEVEL HYPOTHESES.
SEX SYSTEMS

The passage to explanatory hypotheses of higher levels is best illustrated by certain systems belonging to what I shall call *sex systems*. These differ in several respects from those which have so far been described. Perhaps the simplest type is that which is exemplified by *Bonellia*. I call this the set of *environmental* sex systems.

In genetical systems of this type we have two mutually exclusive sets called sexes, namely, **M** of males and **F** of females. These may be treated as genotypes as far as the syntactical rule S. 6 is concerned, but strictly speaking they do not satisfy the definitions of 'genotype' previously given. For this system there are at least two mutually exclusive environmental sets, E_1 and E_2. The sex system has the following peculiar mating descriptions:

(1) For all X, Y and Z: $F_{X,Y,Z}(M,M) = F_{X,Y,Z}(F,F) = \Lambda$,

(2) $F_{E_1,E_1,E_1}(M,F) = \Lambda$,   (3) $F_{E_1,E_1,E_2}(M,F) = \Lambda$,

(4) $F_{E_1,E_2,E_1}(M,F) \subset M$,   (5) $F_{E_2,E_1,E_1}(M,F) = \Lambda$,

(6) $F_{E_1,E_2,E_2}(M,F) \subset F$,   (7) $F_{E_2,E_1,E_2}(M,F) = \Lambda$,

(8) $F_{E_2,E_2,E_1}(M,F) = \Lambda$,   (9) $F_{E_2,E_2,E_2}(M,F) = \Lambda$.

These zero-level statements are derivable from the following first-level hypotheses:

[H. 16] $G_{E_2}(M) = \Lambda$,   [H. 17] $G_{E_1}(F) = \Lambda$,

[H. 18] $U(G_{E_1}(M), G_{E_1}(M)) = U(G_{E_2}(F), G_{E_2}(F)) = \Lambda$,

[H. 19]   for all X, $U(X, \Lambda) = \Lambda$,

[H. 20]   for all X, $Dlz(\Lambda, X, \Lambda)$,

[H. 21] $Dlz(U(G_{E_1}(M), G_{E_2}(F)), E_1, M)$,

[H. 22] $Dlz(U(G_{E_1}(M), G_{E_2}(F)), E_2, F)$.

From H. 9, H. 18, H. 19, H. 20 and T. 12 we obtain mating description (1). If we substitute 'E_1' for 'X', 'Y' and 'Z' and 'M' for 'W_1' and 'F' for 'W_2' in H. 9, we obtain

$$F_{E_1, E_1, E_1}(M, F) \subset L_{E_1}(U(G_{E_1}(M), G_{E_1}(F))).$$

By H. 17 the right-hand side of this inclusion becomes

$$L_{E_1}(U(G_{E_1}(M), \Lambda)),$$

and by H. 19 this becomes

$$L_{E_1}(\Lambda).$$

From this, T. 12 and H. 20 we obtain

$$L_{E_1}(\Lambda) = \Lambda,$$

whence $$F_{E_1, E_1, E_1}(M, F) = \Lambda,$$

which is mating description (2). By analogous substitutions we can obtain the remaining mating descriptions of the system.

But such systems are quite exceptional. Nearly all sex systems belong to what may be called simple zygotic sex systems. In these we again have two mutually exclusive sub-sets M and F (to simplify the notation I use the same symbols)* and a single environmental set E. The mating descriptions are as follows:

(1) $F_E(M, M) = \Lambda,$

(2) $F_E(F, F) = \Lambda,$

(3) $D(F_E(M, F)) = \frac{1}{2}M + \frac{1}{2}F.$

In order to formulate first-level hypotheses for such a system we must first define three sets of gametes which I will denote by f, m and m'.

[D. 34] f is the set of all gametes x which are produced by members of F when they develop in members of E, i.e.

$$f = G_E(F).$$

---

* Thus 'F' and 'M' are not to be interpreted as denoting *all* females and males respectively, but only those which are contained in some (unspecified) genetical system.

[D. 35] **m** is the set of all gametes x such that for some β

$$\mathbf{Dlz}(\mathbf{U}(\mathbf{f},\beta),\mathbf{E},\mathbf{F}) \quad \text{and} \quad x\epsilon\beta.$$

[D. 36] **m'** is the set of all gametes x such that for some set β

$$\mathbf{Dlz}(\mathbf{U}(\mathbf{f},\beta),\mathbf{E},\mathbf{M}) \quad \text{and} \quad x\epsilon\beta.$$

It will then follow that

(i) $\mathbf{Dlz}(\mathbf{U}(\mathbf{f},\mathbf{m}),\mathbf{E},\mathbf{F})$ and (ii) $\mathbf{Dlz}(\mathbf{U}(\mathbf{f},\mathbf{m'}),\mathbf{E},\mathbf{M})$.

We can now formulate the following first-level hypotheses:

[H. 24] $\mathbf{D}(\mathbf{G_E}(\mathbf{M})) = \frac{1}{2}\mathbf{m} + \frac{1}{2}\mathbf{m'}$,

[H. 25] $\mathbf{U}(\mathbf{f},\mathbf{f}) = \mathbf{U}(\mathbf{m},\mathbf{m}) = \mathbf{U}(\mathbf{m},\mathbf{m'}) = \mathbf{U}(\mathbf{m'},\mathbf{m'}) = \Lambda$.

Thus as far as D. 34 and H. 24 are concerned **F** resembles a homozygous and **M** a heterozygous genotype in a genetical system of allelic index (2). **M**, because its members produce two kinds of gametes, is said to be heterogametic. But in some simple zygotic sex systems these relations are reversed, **F** is heterogametic producing two distinct kinds of gametes, and **M** produces only one kind.

In passing to explanatory hypotheses of the *second* level we require, as before, a new functor—again a name-forming functor, which I call the *composition* functor. This functor is one of very wide applicability. It has two forms, one for individuals and a derived form for sets. If we add to our list of undefined signs the letter **P**, to denote the relation 'part of', so that $x\mathbf{P}y$ reads x is part of y, we can define the composition functor for individuals—written $\mathbf{c}(R,x,y)$—as follows:

[D. 37] $\mathbf{c}(R,x,y)$ is *the* object u such that $x\mathbf{P}u$ and $y\mathbf{P}u$ and $x R y$, and for every w, if $w\mathbf{P}u$, then w and x have parts in common or w and y have parts in common.

Thus we can say that $\mathbf{c}(R,x,y)$ is the object composed of x and y when x stands in relation R to y. For example, if x is a man and y a horse and R is the relation between man and horse when the former is riding the latter, then $\mathbf{c}(R,x,y)$ will be the single object composed of x and y when x is riding y. If x is *not* riding y then there will be no such object. This is the composition functor for individuals. The corresponding functor for sets—written $\mathbf{C}(R, X, Y)$—is easily defined as follows:

[D. 38] $\mathbf{C}(R, X, Y)$ is the set of all objects u such that for some x and y, $x \in X$ and $y \in Y$ and $u = \mathbf{c}(R, x, y)$.

The composition functor for sets will be frequently used in the sequel.

So far, although we have spoken about zygotes and gametes, it has not been necessary to say anything about their composition. On level 2 the composition functor enables us to construct designations for sets of cells and of parts of cells. For this purpose we must adopt certain letters as constant designations for the relations involved, in place of the dummy 'R'. I shall use '$\mathbf{S}$' as explained in the following rule:

[S. 7]   '$x\mathbf{S}y$' is true if and only if x is a nucleus and y a cytoplasm and each is a part of the same living cell.

The following postulates will govern the use of '$\mathbf{S}$':

[H. 26]   For all x and y, if $x\mathbf{S}y$, then $x \neq y$.

[H. 27]   For all x and y, if $x\mathbf{S}y$, then not $(y\mathbf{S}x)$.

[H. 28]   For all x, y and z, if $x\mathbf{S}y$ and $z\mathbf{S}y$, then $x = z$.*

[H. 29]   For all x, y and z, if $x\mathbf{S}y$ and $x\mathbf{S}z$, then $y = z$.

Thus if N is a set of nuclei and K a set of cytoplasms, then $\mathbf{C}(\mathbf{S}, N, K)$ will be the set of all cells having a nucleus belonging to N and a cytoplasm belonging to K.

---

* This postulate involves the convention that every cell has but one nucleus and thus involves regarding every so-called multinucleate cell as a syncytium, or as having a single nucleus divided into discrete parts. The other convention which admits multinucleate cells involves regarding the whole musculature of the heart of a mammal, for example, as a gigantic multinucleate cell or as a syncytium. The convention here adopted is simpler from the notational point of view, it suffices for genetical purposes and is perhaps preferable on physiological grounds.

It must be understood that, when I speak of a cell (or of a part of a cell), I mean that cell (or that part) throughout its time-extent, just as in the case of a complete life. If a cell x arises by division of a cell and itself divides, I shall mean by 'the complete cell x' the whole time-extent of the object from the end of one division to the end of the next.

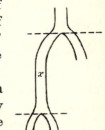

The hypothesis of level 1 of the sex system which is derivable from the new explanatory hypotheses of level 2 is H. 24, which states the gamete-set frequencies characteristic of **M**. In order to formulate these second-level hypotheses we require to define two mutually exclusive sets of nuclei and two mutually exclusive sets of cytoplasms. The general rule seems to be that, when you have two mutually exclusive sets at level n, you require at least two mutually exclusive sets at level $n+1$. We began with two mutually exclusive sets, **F** and **M**, at zero level; we have required three, **f**, **m** and **m′**, at first level. We now require four (two pairs of) mutually exclusive sets at second level: two of nuclei ($\mathbf{N}_f$ and $\mathbf{N}_m$), to distinguish **f** and **m** from **m′**, and two of cytoplasms ($\mathbf{K}_f$ and $\mathbf{K}_m$), to distinguish **f** from **m** and **m′**. Using the composition functor and our new undefined sign **S** we proceed as follows.

[D. 39] $\mathbf{N}_f$ is the set of all nuclei x such that, for some y,
$$\mathbf{c(S},x,y)\,\epsilon\,\mathbf{f}\cup\mathbf{m}.$$

[D. 40] $\mathbf{N}_m$ is the set of all nuclei x such that, for some y,
$$\mathbf{c(S},x,y)\,\epsilon\,\mathbf{m'}.$$

[D. 41] $\mathbf{K}_f$ is the set of all cytoplasms y such that, for some $x\,\epsilon\,\mathbf{N}_f$, we have
$$\mathbf{c(S},x,y)\,\epsilon\,\mathbf{f}.$$

[D. 42] $\mathbf{K}_m$ is the set of all cytoplasms y such that, for some $x\,\epsilon\,\mathbf{N}_f\cup\mathbf{N}_m$, we have
$$\mathbf{c(S},x,y)\,\epsilon\,\mathbf{m}\cup\mathbf{m'}.$$

With these definitions it will follow that

(i) $\mathbf{C(S},\mathbf{N}_f,\mathbf{K}_f)\subset\mathbf{f}$;   (ii) $\mathbf{C(S},\mathbf{N}_f,\mathbf{K}_m)\subset\mathbf{m}$;

(iii) $\mathbf{C(S},\mathbf{N}_m,\mathbf{K}_m)\subset\mathbf{m'}$;   (iv) $\mathbf{C(S},\mathbf{N}_m,\mathbf{K}_f)=\Lambda$;

and since $\mathbf{f} \cap \mathbf{m} = \Lambda$ and $\mathbf{f} \cap \mathbf{m}' = \Lambda$ we must have $\mathbf{K}_f \cap \mathbf{K}_m = \Lambda$; and since $\mathbf{m} \cap \mathbf{m}' = \Lambda$ we must have $\mathbf{N}_f \cap \mathbf{N}_m = \Lambda$. But the two kinds of zygotes $\mathbf{U}(\mathbf{f}, \mathbf{m})$ and $\mathbf{U}(\mathbf{f}, \mathbf{m}')$ will *not* differ with respect to their cytoplasms (and this is important for subsequent developments). For we have

$$\mathbf{U}(\mathbf{C}(\mathbf{S}, \mathbf{N}_f, \mathbf{K}_f), \mathbf{C}(\mathbf{S}, \mathbf{N}_f, \mathbf{K}_m)) \subset \mathbf{U}(\mathbf{f}, \mathbf{m}),$$

and $$\mathbf{U}(\mathbf{C}(\mathbf{S}, \mathbf{N}_f, \mathbf{K}_f), \mathbf{C}(\mathbf{S}, \mathbf{N}_m, \mathbf{K}_m)) \subset \mathbf{U}(\mathbf{f}, \mathbf{m}').$$

Consequently each zygote of each set will receive its cytoplasm from a member of $\mathbf{K}_f$ and a member of $\mathbf{K}_m$, and so members of the two sets of zygotes will not differ in this respect.*

We require a designation for the relation in which a cell x stands to a cell y, when x has divided and y is one of its daughter cells. For this purpose I use '$\mathbf{D}$'. We also require a designation for the relation in which a cell x stands to a cell y when there is a third cell z such that $x\mathbf{D}z$ and $z\mathbf{D}y$. This is written $x\mathbf{D}^2y$ and called the square or second power of $\mathbf{D}$. This process can obviously be repeated. We may have a fourth cell w such that $x\mathbf{D}^2y$ and $y\mathbf{D}w$; x is then said to stand in the third power of $\mathbf{D}$ to w, written $x\mathbf{D}^3w$. $\mathbf{D}$, $\mathbf{D}^2$ and $\mathbf{D}^3$ are all called powers of $\mathbf{D}$, and they are obviously only the first three terms of a sequence which has many more higher terms which are exemplified by dividing cells. If we wish to state that a cell x stands in an unspecified power of $\mathbf{D}$ to another cell y we write $x\mathbf{D}_{po}y$. Clearly $\mathbf{D}$, $\mathbf{D}^2$ and $\mathbf{D}^3$ are all special cases of $\mathbf{D}_{po}$.†

Cells in which the first reduction division occurs will be called reduction cells (and denoted by $\mathbf{rc}$), and the cells in which the next division occurs can be called post-reduction cells. If we confine attention to animal cells the set $\mathbf{rc}$ is easily definable (for genetical purposes) with our present vocabulary as the set of all cells x, such that x stands in $\mathbf{D}$ to exactly two cells and each

---

* For the genetical product of a zygotic sex system with a genetical system of allelic index (2), see Note 13, p. 211.

† A strict definition of R_{po} for any two-termed relation R can easily be given with the help of natural numbers. For the subtle definition of Frege without the help of natural numbers, see Quine's *Mathematical Logic* (1940), p. 215. See also Appendix B, p. 221.

of these stands in **D** to exactly two gametes, or one stands in **D** to exactly one gamete and the other does not stand in **D** to any gamete.

By the nucleus of a cell x (written $\mathbf{n}(x)$) I shall mean *the* object y such that for some z, $\mathbf{c}(\mathbf{S}, y, z) = x$. And by the cytoplasm of a cell x I shall mean *the* object z such that for some y, $\mathbf{c}(\mathbf{S}, y, z) = x$.

So far only sets of gamete nuclei have been defined. We can now define three other sets:

[D. 43] I shall say that the nucleus of a cell y belongs to the set $\mathbf{N}_{fm}$, if and only if y is a zygote belonging to $\mathbf{U}(\mathbf{f}, \mathbf{m}')$, or a member of $\mathbf{U}(\mathbf{f}, \mathbf{m}')$ stands in $\mathbf{D}_{po}$ to y, but no reduction cell stands in that relation to y.

[D. 44] I shall say that the nucleus of a cell y belongs to the set $\mathbf{N}_{ff}$, if and only if y is a zygote belonging to $\mathbf{U}(\mathbf{f}, \mathbf{m})$, or a member of $\mathbf{U}(\mathbf{f}, \mathbf{m})$ stands in $\mathbf{D}_{po}$ to y, but no reduction cell stands in that relation to y, or a reduction cell having a nucleus belonging to $\mathbf{N}_{fm}$ stands in **D** to y and y stands in **D** to a member of **m**.

[D. 45] I shall say that the nucleus of a cell y belongs to the set $\mathbf{N}_{mm}$, if and only if a reduction cell having a nucleus belonging to $\mathbf{N}_{fm}$ stands in **D** to y and y stands in **D** to a member of **m**'.

We can now formulate the hypotheses which are necessary for the derivation of H. 24 (see p. 146). First we require five hypotheses belonging to level 1. Because $\mathbf{G}_Y(X)$ is an undefined sign in the present theory the following hypothesis containing it is necessary:

[H. 30] If X is any genotype and x is any member of $\mathbf{G}_Y(X)$, then there exist y, z and w such that $\mathbf{dlz}(y, z, w)$ and $w \in X$ and $z \in Y$ and $y \mathbf{D}_{po} x$.*

Then we require the following quite general hypotheses concerning **dlz** and $\mathbf{D}_{po}$:

* With the definition of $\mathbf{G}_Y(X)$ given in Note 14, p. 214, H. 30 ceases to have the status of a hypothesis and becomes a consequence of the definition. This would be the situation if we were following the axiomatizing procedure when the signs necessary for defining $\mathbf{G}_Y(X)$ would have been available from the beginning.

[H. 31] For every x, y, z, u and v, if $\mathbf{dlz}(x, y, z)$ and $\mathbf{dlz}(u, v, z)$, then $x = u$.*

[H. 32] For every x and y, if x is a zygote and y a gamete and $x\mathbf{D}_{\mathrm{po}}y$, then there is one and only one reduction cell z such that $x\mathbf{D}_{\mathrm{po}}z$ and $z\mathbf{D}^2y$.†

The next two are special hypotheses about the sex system.

[H. 33] If x is any member of $\mathbf{F}$, then there are u and v such that $\mathbf{dlz}(u, v, x)$ and $v \in \mathbf{E}$ and $u \in \mathbf{U}(\mathbf{f}, \mathbf{m})$.

[H. 34] If x is any member of $\mathbf{M}$, then there are u and v such that $\mathbf{dlz}(u, v, x)$ and $v \in \mathbf{E}$ and $u \in \mathbf{U}(\mathbf{f}, \mathbf{m}')$.

The remaining hypotheses belong to level 2 and deal with reduction cells.

[H. 35] If z is any reduction cell and $\mathbf{n}(z) \in \mathbf{N}_{ff}$, then there is one and only one gamete to which z stands in $\mathbf{D}^2$ and it is a member of $\mathbf{f}$.

[H. 36] For all z, y and w, if $z \in \mathbf{rc}$ and $\mathbf{n}(z) \in \mathbf{N}_{fm}$ and $z\mathbf{D}y$ and $z\mathbf{D}w$ and $y \neq w$, then $\mathbf{n}(y) \in \mathbf{N}_{ff}$ or $\mathbf{n}(w) \in \mathbf{N}_{ff}$.

[H. 37] For all z, y and w, if $z \in \mathbf{rc}$ and $\mathbf{n}(z) \in \mathbf{N}_{fm}$ and $z\mathbf{D}y$ and $\mathbf{n}(y) \in \mathbf{N}_{ff}$ and $y\mathbf{D}w$, then $w \in \mathbf{m}$.

[H. 38] For all z, y and w, if $z \in \mathbf{rc}$ and $\mathbf{n}(z) \in \mathbf{N}_{fm}$ and $z\mathbf{D}y$ and $\mathbf{n}(y) \in \mathbf{N}_{mm}$ and $y\mathbf{D}w$, then $w \in \mathbf{m}'$.

With these hypotheses, and the relevant definitions, H. 24 will follow. But if that were all that could be accomplished, there would be little point in adding this further layer to our pyramid of hypotheses. We should have increased its height without widening its base. Our genetical predictions would still only be made through mating descriptions. But the merit of level 2 lies in the fact that it is a step towards widening the base

---

* The literature of experimental embryology may contain references to artificially induced exceptions to this statement.

† '$z\mathbf{D}^2y$' suffices for animals; for the general case we should write '$z\mathbf{D}_{\mathrm{po}}y$'.

of the pyramid of genetical statements. This is because the members of the sets of nuclei that have been defined can sometimes be identified by observing certain of their parts microscopically. Consequently, a new method of making and testing genetical predictions becomes available, namely, through cytology and cytochemistry. But so long as we have only one level above zero level the overlap of genetics with other branches of biology remains negligible.

To illustrate this it is necessary to take a further step in analysis and to speak about the parts of nuclei called chromosomes, and this involves another application of the composition functor. For the relation required I shall use the letter 'Q' as explained in the following semantical rule:

[S. 8]   '$Q(x_1, x_2, ..., x_n)$' is true, if and only if $x_1, x_2, ..., x_n$ are n chromosomes all parts of one and the same nucleus which has only n chromosomes.

The use of this new undefined sign will be governed by the following postulates:

[H. 39]   If $Q(x_1, x_2, ..., x_n)$, then for any x_i and x_j where $i, j = 1, 2, ..., n$ and $i \neq j$ we must have $x_i \neq x_j$.

[H. 40]   If $Q(x_1, x_2, ..., x_n)$, then $Q(x_n, x_1, x_2, ..., x_{n-1})$ and so on for all the remaining permutations of the n letters. (Thus Q is not an ordering relation.)

[H. 41]   If $c(Q, x_1, x_2, ..., x_n)$ is a nucleus and $c(Q, x_1, y_2, y_3, ..., y_n)$ is a nucleus, then $(x_2, x_3, ..., x_n)$ is a permutation of $(y_2, y_3, ..., y_n)$.

The problem of defining chromosome sets has proved to be a very difficult one, so before we deal with the special problem of defining the chromosome sets concerned in sex systems it will be desirable to say something first about the general problem. The difficulties are chiefly connected with the fact that Q is not an ordering relation. For that reason most of the more obvious methods of definition fail.*

* See Note 15, p. 214.

Suppose 'A' and 'B' are two statements such that 'if A then B' expresses a natural law. Then we can say that 'A' expresses a *sufficient* condition for the occurrence of what is asserted by 'B'. If we also have 'if (not A) then (not B)' we can say that 'A' expresses a *necessary* condition for the occurrence of what is asserted by 'B'. But by the principle of transposition (see p. 37) 'if (not A) then (not B)' may be written 'if B then A'. Consequently we have 'if A then B and if B then A', and so by the definition of the biconditional (see p. 51) we have 'A if and only if B'. Thus when the biconditional holds 'A' asserts both a necessary and sufficient condition for the occurrence of what is asserted by 'B'.

Now suppose that both 'A' and 'B' are conjunctions of *two* statements, e.g. $A \equiv (C \, \& \, D)$ and $B \equiv (E \, \& \, F)$. What information must we have in order that we may say that 'C' expresses a necessary *and* sufficient condition for the occurrence of what 'E' asserts, and that 'D' expresses a necessary and sufficient condition for the occurrence of what 'F' asserts? In order that this inference should be possible we need the following four statements:

(1) If $C \, \& \, D$, then $E \, \& \, F$.

(2) If (not C) $\& \, D$, then (not E) $\& \, F$.

(3) If $C \, \&$ (not D), then $E \,\&$ (not F).

(4) If (not C) $\&$ (not D), then (not E) $\&$ (not F).

From the conjunction of (1), (2), (3) and (4) it can easily be shown, by means of truth tables, that $C \equiv E$ and $D \equiv F$ follow. But $C \equiv E$ cannot be obtained from less than the conjunction of all four statements. It cannot be derived from (1) and (2) alone.

There are still other preliminaries to be dealt with. The notion of allelic index has already been explained. It will promote brevity if we use these allelic indices as set designations of the sets of genetical systems which they characterize. Thus instead of saying 'S has the allelic index (2) (2) (2)' we can simply write '$S \in$ (2) (2) (2)'. The notion of belonging to the same linkage group has also been defined, but 'linkage group' itself has not yet been defined. The relation of belonging to the same linkage group between two factor systems (i.e. having a recombination value) is obviously symmetrical and is found to be transitive and so gives rise to what are called abstractive sets.* That is to say, if we take any factor system S' of a genetical system S, the set of all factor systems of S which stand in the relation in question to S' will constitute a linkage group of S. If any factor systems remain outside this set (if the system S is mixed) we must take any one of these and repeat the process to form another linkage group of S, and so on until no factor system remains outside. But linkage groups defined in this way would be sets of sets; and, as we wish to avoid sets of sets as far as possible, we must take, not these sets of sets, but their Boolean sums as the linkage groups. Thus suppose we have a system

$$S \in (n_1, n_2, n_3) (n_4, n_5) (n_6),$$

such that $\quad S = (S_1 \times S_2 \times S_3) \times (S_4 \times S_5) \times (S_6).$

This has three linkage groups: $S_1 \cup S_2 \cup S_3$, $S_4 \cup S_5$ and S_6. How the numbers are assigned is partly arbitrary and partly not. It is arbitrary *between* the brackets because this involves Boolean multiplication, it is not arbitrary *within* the brackets because this involves Cartesian multiplication (see p. 101).† Factor systems within a pair of brackets must be numbered consecutively, but it is arbitrary which bracket pair comes first. Thus S could have been described as $S = (S_1 \times S_2) \times (S_3 \times S_4 \times S_5) \times (S_6)$. But having adopted a certain numbering we can define $\mathbf{L}_1(S)$ or the first linkage group of S as the Boolean sum of all factor systems of S which belong to the same linkage group as S_1, and we can define $\mathbf{L}_{n+1}(S)$ as the Boolean sum of all factor systems of S which belong to the same linkage group as S_{m+1} if S_m is the factor system of $\mathbf{L}_n(S)$ with the greatest subscript. These definitions suffice to

---

* See my *Axiomatic Method in Biology*, p. 41.

† That is to say the sign '×' *between* brackets represents the genetical multiplication of two independent systems, the same sign *within* a bracket-pair represents Cartesian multiplication between linked factor systems.

determine all the linkage groups of a given system S. Finally, we need designations for sets of nuclei $N(P)$ and sets of cytoplasms $K(P)$ for any phenotypes P such that $H(P) \neq \Lambda$. These are provided for in the following:

[D. 46] $N(P)$ is the set of all nuclei x, such that P is a phenotype for which $H(P) \neq \Lambda$, and for some y, $c(S, x, y) \in Gm(P)$.

[D. 47] $K(P)$ is the set of all cytoplasms y, such that P is a phenotype for which $H(P) \neq \Lambda$, and for some x, $c(S, x, y) \in Gm(P)$.

Now we can proceed to some examples of correlations between chromosome sets and phenotypes.

First we must lay down the following general postulate:

[H. 42]   If S is a genetical system with k linkage groups and X is the Boolean sum of all nuclear sets $N(P)$, where P is any phenotype such that $H(P) \neq \Lambda$ and $H(P) \subset S$, then there is a natural number n, such that $k \leqslant n$ and every member of X contains exactly n chromosomes. n will be called the gametic chromosome number of S.*

Now we have a succession of postulates† concerning special genetical systems:

[H. 43]   If $S \in (2)$ and $S = S(P, Q)$, i.e. S is the system generated by P and Q, and the gametic chromosome number of S is 2, then there exist sets X, Y and Z of chromosomes such that $Z \cap X = Z \cap Y = \Lambda$ and

(1) $(x)(y)((Q(x, y) . x \in X . y \in Z) \supset c(Q, x, y) \in N(P))$,

(2) $(x)(y)((Q(x, y) . x \in Y . y \in Z) \supset c(Q, x, y) \in N(Q))$.

These statements suffice to establish that the presence of a member of X together with a member of Z in a nucleus is a sufficient condition for that nucleus to be a member of $N(P)$, and that the presence of a member of Y with a member of Z is

---

* This postulate will not always hold for a genetical system which contains a sex system as a factor system, because in some such systems each member of N_f contains one more chromosome than each member of N_m (see p. 159).

† I state the formulas in these postulates entirely in symbols, using a dot in place of 'and', because they are rather long. For other symbols used see Part I, pp. 35 and 41.

a sufficient condition for the nucleus to be a member of $N(Q)$. But they do not at all suffice to establish that these are necessary conditions. We can now define the set of chromosomes correlated with P relatively to the set Z, denoting it by $\chi_Z(P)$ in the following way:

[D. 48] $\chi_Z(P)$ is the set of all chromosomes x, such that for some y, $Q(x, y)$ and $y \in Z$ and $c(Q, x, y) \in N(P)$.

We could equally well call it the set of chromosomes correlated with P in the system S, denoting it by $\chi_S(P)$. The important point is that it must be defined relatively to one or more fixed sets of chromosomes of the system, the number depending upon the gametic chromosome number of the system. If this had been 3 in the present example, then it would have been necessary to relativize the set we wish to define with respect to two sets. It then becomes preferable to write $\chi_S(P)$ instead of $\chi_{Z,W}(P)$, supposing Z and W to be the sets concerned. The definition would then be

[D. 49] $\chi_S(P)$ is the set of all chromosomes x such that for some y and some z, $Q(x, y, z) . y \in Z . z \in W . c(Q, x, y, z) \in N(P)$.

In order to establish that the presence of a member of $\chi_S(P)$ with a member of Z in a nucleus is a *necessary* condition for the membership of that nucleus in $N(P)$, we should require the following addition to the postulate:

(3) $(x)(y)((Q(x, y) . x \in \overline{X} . y \in Z) \supset c(Q, x, y) \in \overline{N(P)}).$*

Thus we must know that if a member of Z occurs in a nucleus with *any* chromosome which does not belong to X, then that nucleus does not belong to $N(P)$, and this we are not told. We are only told what happens when a member of Z is in a nucleus with a member of Y. We know that Y is included in $\overline{X}$ but not that it is identical with $\overline{X}$. For from the fact that $S \in (2)$ and $S = S(P, Q)$ it follows that $P \cap Q = \Lambda$, and from this it follows that $N(P) \cap N(Q) = \Lambda$ and hence that $X \cap Y = \Lambda$ and

$$\chi_S(P) \cap \chi_S(Q) = \Lambda.$$

* See Note 2, p. 201.

We must now turn to a more complicated example, introduced by another postulate.

[H. 44]   If $S \in (2)(2)$ and $S = \mathrm{S}(P, Q) \times \mathrm{S}(A, B)$ and the gametic chromosome number of S is 2, then there exist sets X_1, X_2, Y_1, Y_2 such that

$$(x)(y)((\mathbf{Q}(x,y) . x \in X_1 . y \in Y_1) \supset \mathbf{c}(\mathbf{Q}, x, y) \in \mathbf{N}(P) \cap \mathbf{N}(A)),$$

$$(x)(y)((\mathbf{Q}(x,y) . x \in X_2 . y \in Y_1) \supset \mathbf{c}(\mathbf{Q}, x, y) \in \mathbf{N}(Q) \cap \mathbf{N}(A)),$$

$$(x)(y)((\mathbf{Q}(x,y) . x \in X_1 . y \in Y_2) \supset \mathbf{c}(\mathbf{Q}, x, y) \in \mathbf{N}(P) \cap \mathbf{N}(B)),$$

$$(x)(y)((\mathbf{Q}(x,y) . x \in X_2 . y \in Y_2) \supset \mathbf{c}(\mathbf{Q}, x, y) \in \mathbf{N}(Q) \cap \mathbf{N}(B)).$$

We can now define $\chi_S(P)$ for this system as follows:

[D. 50] $\chi_S(P)$ is the set of all chromosomes x such that, for some y, $\mathbf{Q}(x, y)$ and $y \in Y_1 \cup Y_2$ and $\mathbf{c}(\mathbf{Q}, x, y) \in \mathbf{N}(P)$.

$\chi_S(P)$ must thus be defined relatively to the Boolean sum of Y_1 and Y_2. If the gametic chromosome number had been n $(n > 2)$ it would have been necessary to define it relatively to $n - 2$ constant sets $Z_1, Z_2, ..., Z_{n-2}$ as well as to $Y_1 \cup Y_2$. Corresponding definitions can be constructed for $\chi_S(Q)$, $\chi_S(A)$ and $\chi_S(B)$.

The next example involves a Batesonian sub-system.

[H. 45]   If $S \in (2, 2)(2)$ and $S = (\mathrm{S}(P, Q) \times \mathrm{S}(A, B)) \times \mathrm{S}(K, L)$ and the gametic chromosome number is 2, then there exist sets X_1, X_2, X_3, X_4 and Y_1, Y_2 such that

$$(x)(y)((\mathbf{Q}(x,y) . x \in X_1 . y \in Y_1) \supset \mathbf{c}(\mathbf{Q}, x, y) \in \mathbf{N}(PA) \cap \mathbf{N}(K)),$$

$$(x)(y)((\mathbf{Q}(x,y) . x \in X_1 . y \in Y_2) \supset \mathbf{c}(\mathbf{Q}, x, y) \in \mathbf{N}(PA) \cap \mathbf{N}(L)),$$

$$(x)(y)((\mathbf{Q}(x,y) . x \in X_2 . y \in Y_1) \supset \mathbf{c}(\mathbf{Q}, x, y) \in \mathbf{N}(PB) \cap \mathbf{N}(K)),$$

$$(x)(y)((\mathbf{Q}(x,y) . x \in X_2 . y \in Y_2) \supset \mathbf{c}(\mathbf{Q}, x, y) \in \mathbf{N}(PB) \cap \mathbf{N}(L)),$$

$$(x)(y)((\mathbf{Q}(x,y) . x \in X_3 . y \in Y_1) \supset \mathbf{c}(\mathbf{Q}, x, y) \in \mathbf{N}(QA) \cap \mathbf{N}(K)),$$

$$(x)(y)((\mathbf{Q}(x,y) . x \in X_3 . y \in Y_2) \supset \mathbf{c}(\mathbf{Q}, x, y) \in \mathbf{N}(QA) \cap \mathbf{N}(L)),$$

$$(x)(y)((\mathbf{Q}(x,y) . x \in X_4 . y \in Y_1) \supset \mathbf{c}(\mathbf{Q}, x, y) \in \mathbf{N}(QB) \cap \mathbf{N}(K)),$$

$$(x)(y)((\mathbf{Q}(x,y) . x \in X_4 . y \in Y_2) \supset \mathbf{c}(\mathbf{Q}, x, y) \in \mathbf{N}(QB) \cap \mathbf{N}(L)).$$

We can now define

[D. 51] $\chi_S(K)$ is the set of all chromosomes y such that, for every x, if $\mathbf{Q}(x,y)$ and $x \in X_1 \cup X_2 \cup X_3 \cup X_4$, then $\mathbf{c}(\mathbf{Q}, x, y) \in \mathbf{N}(K)$.

The definition for $\chi_S(L)$ will be on similar lines. Next we define

[D. 52] $\chi_S(PA)$ is the set of all chromosomes x such that, for some y, $\mathbf{Q}(x,y)$ and $y \in Y_1 \cup Y_2$ and $\mathbf{c}(\mathbf{Q}, x, y) \in \mathbf{N}(PA)$.

If we denote and number the two linkage groups of S by

$$\mathbf{L}_1(S) = \mathrm{S}(P, Q) \times \mathrm{S}(A, B) \quad \text{and} \quad \mathbf{L}_2(S) = \mathrm{S}(K, L)$$

(which we call first and which second is of course quite arbitrary), then we can see that there will be a set of chromosomes correlated with each. We can call these sets $\chi_1(S)$ and $\chi_2(S)$ respectively. Then

$$\chi_1(S) = \chi_S(PA) \cup \chi_S(PB) \cup \chi_S(QA) \cup \chi_S(QB)$$

and
$$\chi_2(S) = \chi_S(K) \cup \chi_S(L).$$

From these examples we can see that, for a system

$$S \in (n_1, n_2, n_3)(n_4, n_5)(n_6),$$

the corresponding postulate will require to assert the existence of $n_1 . n_2 . n_3$ sets X_i correlated with the first linkage group, $n_4 . n_5$ sets Y_j correlated with the second and n_6 sets Z_k correlated with the third, so that the total number required is

$$(n_1 . n_2 . n_3) + (n_4 . n_5) + (n_6).$$

To establish the correlations $n_1 . n_2 . n_3 . n_4 . n_5 . n_6$, formulas of the form

$$(x)(y)(z)((\mathbf{Q}(x, y, z) . x \in X_i . y \in Y_j . z \in Z_k)$$
$$\supset \mathbf{c}(\mathbf{Q}, x, y, z) \in \mathbf{N}(P_{11}P_{21}P_{31}) \cap \mathbf{N}(P_{41}P_{51}) \cap \mathbf{N}(P_{61}))$$

will be needed.

We must now say a little about the chromosome sets for sex systems. It will suffice for purposes of illustration if we consider a common type of system without attempting to treat the subject in full generality. Suppose, then, that

$$S = \mathbf{M} \cup \mathbf{F}$$

is a simple zygotic sex system with **M** heterogametic and that the gametic chromosome number is 3 in one set N_f and 2 in the other N_m. Then we require the following postulate regarding S:

[H. 46]　There exist sets X, Z_1 and Z_2 such that

$$(x)\,(y)\,(z)\,(\mathbf{Q}(x,y,z)\,.\,x\epsilon X\,.\,y\epsilon Z_1\,.\,z\epsilon Z_2\,.\,\supset\,.\,\mathbf{c}(\mathbf{Q},x,y,z)\epsilon N_f),$$

$$(x)\,(y)\,(z)\,(\mathbf{Q}(x,y)\,.\,x\epsilon Z_1\,.\,y\epsilon Z_2\,.\,\supset\,.\,\mathbf{c}(\mathbf{Q},x,y)\epsilon N_m).$$

In such a system the set commonly denoted by '**X**' and called the set of **X**-chromosomes would be definable as follows:

[D. 53]　$\mathbf{X}(S)$ is the set of all chromosomes x such that for some y and some z, $y\epsilon Z_1$ and $z\epsilon Z_2$ and $\mathbf{Q}(x,y,z)$ and $\mathbf{c}(\mathbf{Q},x,y,z)\epsilon N_f$.

But in many systems the gametic chromosome number is the same in both sets of nuclei and the postulate requires four sets X, Y, Z_1 and Z_2 (if the gametic chromosome number is 3) and contains the statement

$$(x)\,(y)\,(z)\,(\mathbf{Q}(x,y,z)\,.\,x\epsilon Y\,.\,y\epsilon Z_1\,.\,z\epsilon Z_2\,.\,\supset\,.\,\mathbf{c}(\mathbf{Q},x,y,z)\epsilon N_m).$$

From this we obtain a definition of the set called the set of **Y**-chromosomes. *Drosophila* conforms to this plan (except that the gametic chromosome number is 4), but experiment shows that $\mathbf{C}(\mathbf{Q},Z_1,Z_2)\subset N_m$, even though no member of **Y** (specified cytologically) is present.

The remaining chromosome sets in a sex system S with gametic chromosome number equal to 4 cannot be separately defined unless S is a factor system in a system of order 4. But we can define them collectively as sets of *triples*. They are usually called autosomes, so we can say (relatively to such a system S):

[D. 54]　$\mathbf{A}(S)$ is the set of all triples x, y, z such that for some w, $\mathbf{Q}(x,y,z,w)$ and $w\epsilon\mathbf{X}(S)\cup\mathbf{Y}(S)$ and $\mathbf{c}(\mathbf{Q},x,y,z,w)\epsilon N_f\cup N_m$.

It may be helpful if we display the mutually exclusive sets involved in a sex system of the type described above in the form of a table.

Level 0	$F \cap M = \Lambda$		Sets of
Level 1	$L_E(U(f, m)) \cap L_E(U(f, m')) = \Lambda$		lives
Level 1	$f \cap m = \Lambda$	$m \cap m' = \Lambda$	Sets of
Level 2	$C(S, N_f, K_f) \cap C(S, N_f, K_m) = \Lambda$	$C(S, N_f, K_m) \cap C(S, N_m, K_m) = \Lambda$	gametes
Level 2	$K_f \cap K_m = \Lambda$ Sets of cytoplasms	$N_f \cap N_m = \Lambda$	Sets of
Level 3		$C(Q, A, X) \cap C(Q, A, Y) = \Lambda$	nuclei
Level 3		$X \cap Y = \Lambda$	Sets of chromosomes

§ 3. FOURTH-LEVEL HYPOTHESES. THE DISTINCTION BETWEEN MENDELIAN AND BATESONIAN SYSTEMS

Sex systems were introduced to illustrate explanatory hypotheses belonging to levels 2 and 3. Examples of those belonging to level 2 have already been given. The next task would be to formulate hypotheses on level 3 which speak about the behaviour of chromosomes, especially those in reduction cells and post-reduction cells, which are explanatory of hypotheses H. 35 to H. 38. This would require (according to current beliefs) the introduction of new functors to express the pairing, duplicating, separating, breaking and joining of chromosomes. I shall not attempt to do this here. Instead I shall return to the problem of the distinction between Mendelian and Batesonian systems in order to illustrate the passage to level 4.

From the examples given above in the previous section it will be seen that if $S = S(P, Q) \times S(A, B)$ is Mendelian $\chi_S(P)$ and $\chi_S(A)$ are distinct sets, but when S was Batesonian we defined $\chi_S(PA)$ but did not define $\chi_S(P)$ and $\chi_S(A)$ separately. In the former case the two sets of chromosomes are correlated with distinct linkage groups, in the latter with the same one. Since a gamete contains only one member from the set correlated with each linkage group we require an explanation of the manner in which a member of $\chi_S(PA)$ differs from a member of $\chi_S(PB)$

and from a member of $\chi_S(QA)$. This involves an appeal to a higher theoretical level on which we can speak about the *parts* of chromosomes, and thus involves a further application of the composition functor. Genetics is indebted to the celebrated American geneticist, T. H. Morgan, for the invention of a hypothesis which speaks about *separable* parts of chromosomes called *genes*. Consequently we need a new relation in which the parts of chromosomes stand to one another. For this new relation the letter '**R**' will be used. This will be a further addition to our primitive vocabulary of undefined signs.

Our treatment of nuclei by means of the composition functor has carried with it the assumption that every part of a nucleus (considered, like everything else, as a time-extended object) is a part of a chromosome.* When we come to the analysis of chromosomes it will not suffice to make the corresponding assumption that every part of a chromosome is part of a gene, because, according to cytology, some parts of chromosomes are not genes. Account must therefore be taken of such parts and our definitions must be relativized with respect to them, otherwise we may sooner or later get into difficulties. If we ignore them in the interests of simplicity we shall be shirking our task. When, therefore, we write a statement of the form

$$c(\mathbf{R}, x_1, x_2, ..., x_m) \in \chi_S(P),$$

we shall not assume that each x_i is a gene, but only that it is one of m elements which together stand in the multigrade relation **R** to one another to constitute a chromosome. These elements might be called *chromosome bands*. Thus we can define the set of all such bands as follows:

[D. 55] **bnd** is the set of all objects x such that, for some $y_1, y_2, ..., y_{i-1}, y_{i+1}, ..., y_m$, and natural numbers m and i ($m > 1$), $\mathbf{R}(y_1, y_2, ..., y_{i-1}, x, y_{i+1}, ..., y_m)$ and

$$c(\mathbf{R}, y_1, y_2, ..., y_{i-1}, x, y_{i+1}, ..., y_m) \in \mathbf{chr} \dagger$$

and $1 \leqslant i \leqslant m$.

---

* If anyone is unwilling to adopt this assumption he must make provision, in his use of the composition functor, for whatever other categories of parts he wishes to mention. † See Note 14, (10), p. 214.

We adopt the following postulates governing the relation $\mathbf{R}$:

[H. 47]   If $\mathbf{R}(x_1, x_2, \ldots, x_m)$, then $x_i \neq x_j$ for each $i, j = 1, 2, \ldots, m$ and $i \neq j$.

[H. 48]   If $\mathbf{R}(x_1, x_2, \ldots, x_m)$, then not $(\mathbf{R}(x_m, x_1, x_2, \ldots, x_{m-1}))$.

And so on for all the remaining permutations of the m letters. $\mathbf{R}$ is thus an ordering relation.

First consider a Batesonian system $S = \mathrm{S}(P, Q) \times \mathrm{S}(A, B)$. On zero level we shall have the homozygous genotypes

$$\mathbf{H}(PA), \quad \mathbf{H}(QA), \quad \mathbf{H}(PB), \quad \mathbf{H}(QB);$$

on level 1 the gamete-sets

$$\mathbf{Gm}(PA), \quad \mathbf{Gm}(QA), \quad \mathbf{Gm}(PB), \quad \mathbf{Gm}(QB);$$

on level 2 the nuclear sets, and constant cytoplasmic sets

$$\mathbf{N}(PA), \mathbf{N}(QA), \mathbf{N}(PB), \mathbf{N}(QB) \text{ and } K = \mathbf{K}(PA) = \mathbf{K}(QA), \text{ etc.};$$

on level 3 the chromosome sets

$$\chi_S(PA), \quad \chi_S(QA), \quad \chi_S(PB), \quad \chi_S(QB).$$

Thus we begin with four mutually exclusive phenotypes, and at each level we have four corresponding, mutually exclusive sets. We now seek a corresponding set of four mutually exclusive sets on level 4.

We require a postulate which asserts that there exist sets X_1, X_2, Y_1 and Y_2 and Z and natural numbers m, i and j, such that $m > 2$ and $i, j = 1, 2, \ldots, m$ with $i < j$ and for all $x_1, x_2, \ldots, x_m$, if $\mathbf{R}(x_1, x_2, \ldots, x_i, \ldots, x_j, \ldots, x_m)$ and $x_i \in X_1$ and $x_j \in Y_1$, and for every x_k, such that $1 \leqslant k \leqslant m$ but $k \neq i$ and $k \neq j$, we have $x_k \in Z$, then

$$\mathbf{c}(\mathbf{R}, x_1, x_2, \ldots, x_i, \ldots, x_j, \ldots, x_m) \in \chi_S(PA);$$

and if $x_i \in X_1$ and $x_j \in Y_2$, then

$$\mathbf{c}(\mathbf{R}, x_1, x_2, \ldots, x_i, \ldots, x_j, \ldots, x_m) \in \chi_S(PB);$$

and if $x_i \in X_2$ and $x_j \in Y_1$, then

$$\mathbf{c}(\mathbf{R}, x_1, x_2, \ldots, x_i, \ldots, x_j, \ldots, x_m) \in \chi_S(QA);$$

and if $x_i \in X_2$ and $x_j \in Y_2$, then

$$\mathbf{c}(\mathbf{R}, x_1, x_2, ..., x_i, ..., x_j, ..., x_m) \in \chi_S(QB).$$

Z is thus a constant factor which can be thought of as the Boolean sum of sets $Z_1, Z_2, ..., Z_m$ (but without Z_i, Z_j) to which every $x_1, x_2, ..., x_m$ (except x_i and x_j) belongs respectively.

We can now define the set of chromosome bands (which in this case would be called genes) which is correlated with P relatively to the sets Y_1, Y_2 and Z, denoting it by $\Gamma_S(P)$.

[D. 56] $\Gamma_S(P)$ is the set of all bands x, such that for some $x_1, x_2, ..., x_m$ (x_i and x_j having the same significance as in the postulate for S), $x = x_i$ and $x_j \in Y_1 \cup Y_2$ and for all x_k with $1 \leqslant k \leqslant m$ and $k \neq i$ and $k \neq j$ we have $x_k \in Z$ and

$$\mathbf{c}(\mathbf{R}, x_1, x_2, ..., x_i, ..., x_j, ..., x_m) \in \chi_S(PA) \cup \chi_S(PB).$$

Corresponding definitions can be constructed for $\Gamma_S(Q)$, $\Gamma_S(A)$ and $\Gamma_S(B)$. If we now put $S(P, Q) = S_1$ and $S(A, B) = S_2$, then $\chi_1(S)$ will be the chromosome set of the single linkage group of the system. Then we can define:

[D. 57] $\Gamma_{11}(S) = \Gamma_S(P) \cup \Gamma_S(Q)$.

We can call $\Gamma_{11}(S)$ the *first locus* of $\chi_1(S)$ and the correspondingly defined $\Gamma_{12}(S) = \Gamma_S(A) \cup \Gamma_S(B)$ will be the second locus of $\chi_1(S)$.*

Returning now to the question of how a member of $\chi_S(PA)$ differs from one of $\chi_S(PB)$ and from one of $\chi_S(QA)$, we can say that a member of $\chi_S(PA)$ will differ from one of $\chi_S(PB)$ with respect to the first locus of $\chi_1(S)$, and from one of $\chi_S(QA)$ with respect to the second locus of $\chi_1(S)$. But if S were Mendelian the two loci concerned would belong to distinct linkage groups, $\Gamma_{11}(S) = \Gamma_S(P) \cup \Gamma_S(Q)$ and $\Gamma_{21}(S) = \Gamma_S(A) \cup \Gamma_S(B)$, and of course the required postulate for S would be correspondingly different.

So much for the distinction, expressible on level 4, between Mendelian and Batesonian systems. The foregoing analysis has

---

* If S were a sub-system of a larger system S', the first locus of S' would not necessarily be the first of S. This would depend upon the order of S in S' established by the recombination values between the factor systems.

provided a basis upon which we can now discuss certain expressions in common use in genetics. It seems clear that $\Gamma_S(P)$, as I have defined it, is what geneticists have in mind when they use the expression 'the gene for P', and $\Gamma_S(Q)$ is what they are referring to when they speak about the gene for Q, relatively to a given system S. But if this is so, then we have succeeded in formulating a correct analytical definition for this somewhat complicated and, at first sight, rather obscure idea. And here I think we have a good example of the way in which the intuition of geneticists has outstripped the ordinary possibilities of natural language. They have *known* what they meant but their language has made it very difficult for them to *say* what they meant. Without the help of a symbolic language and the theory of sets it would be exceedingly difficult to formulate an adequate definition of 'the gene for P'. Even with such aids much time and labour was expended before I succeeded in hitting upon the chain of definitions leading from P through $\mathbf{H}(P)$, $\mathbf{Gm}(P)$, $\mathbf{N}(P)$ and $\chi_S(P)$ to $\Gamma_S(P)$, and even now further work with them may still reveal unsuspected defects in these definitions. It is no wonder then that the notion 'the gene for P' should seem obscure and should have occasioned some controversy even among geneticists themselves. As long ago as 1911 W. Johannsen was raising objections to the phrase, and Professor C. H. Waddington mentions the same objection when he writes: 'Any gene, in fact, has not only a main effect by which it is usually recognized but also a host of smaller effects which may be difficult to detect in the normal organism but may be apparent as modifying effects of mutant genes.'*

But this difficulty disappears when we recognize the distinction between the intensional and the extensional points of view (see p. 24), and adhere to the extensional method by regarding phenotypes as sets. From the intensional point of view our phenotype P may be specified by reference to as many characters as you please; but any two characters which have the same extension (like *rational animal* and *featherless biped*) will determine the

* *An Introduction to Modern Genetics* (1939), p. 162.

same set, in this case the same phenotype. So long as they all characterize members of P, and only members of P, they may be as numerous as you please.

Another difficulty is also mentioned by Professor Waddington when he writes: 'There is, therefore, no simple one-one relation between a gene and a phenotypic character, but such a relation only exists between the phenotype and the genotype as a whole.'*

But again if we adhere to the extensional method there *is* such a one-one relation all the way down the levels, between a given phenotype P and one of the sets at each level, so long as we have another distinct phenotype Q with which to contrast it.† This is shown in the following table:

L	
0	$P \cap Q = \Lambda$
1	$\mathbf{Gm}(P) \cap \mathbf{Gm}(Q) = \Lambda$
2	$\mathbf{N}(P) \cap \mathbf{N}(Q) = \Lambda$
3	$\chi_S(P) \cap \chi_S(Q) = \Lambda$
4	$\Gamma_S(P) \cap \Gamma_S(Q) = \Lambda$

This fact also illustrates another curious point about genetical terminology. Geneticists sometimes use the letters A and a, and their combinations AA, Aa and aa, ambiguously. That is to say, it is not *always* perfectly clear whether these symbols are denoting sets belonging to one level or another. Thus AA may sometimes represent a genotype (in the sense in which I have been using that word) or a set of zygotes or a pair of sets of nuclei or of chromosomes or of genes. But just because of the above one-one relation running through the levels this ambiguity does not have harmful consequences in genetical calculations, although it may sometimes puzzle the inexperienced reader.

---

* Ibid. p. 163.

† The relation of gene set to phenotype *need* not be one-one; it may be two-one as in the example $S(\mathbf{W, R, P, S})$ in Note 6, p. 207.

Finally, another point mentioned by Professor Waddington can also be expressed with the help of the foregoing analysis. In the same paragraph as that from which the last quotation was taken he writes:

Thus it is strictly incorrect to say that w^+ corresponds to red eyes, and w to white eyes in *Drosophila melanogaster*: we should say that, in the usual genotypes met with in *Drosophila melanogaster* a substitution of w^+ for w will change the eyes from white to red. The whole of the genotype other than the particular gene in which we are interested can be referred to as the genotypic milieu or the genetic background.

He then mentions examples of the way in which by altering this background 'the degree of expression, the penetrance and the actual mode of expression of certain genes' may be altered. Now all this is provided for in our chain of definitions, or at least these definitions have been formulated with the intention of making such provision. Because the set $\Gamma_S(P)$ in our examples is by definition the set of *all* genes x such that if x, together with a member from *each* of the remaining $m-1$ constant sets of chromosome bands referred to in the appropriate postulate for S, stand in **R** to one another, and if the chromosome so constituted stands together with $n-1$ chromosomes, one from each of the chromosome sets specified by the postulates of S, in the relation **Q** to constitute a nucleus belonging to $\mathbf{N}(P)$, and if this nucleus stands in **S** to a member of $\mathbf{K}(P)$ so as to constitute a member of $\mathbf{Gm}(P)$, and if this gamete unites with another member of the same set, then the resulting zygote, if it develops in a member of $\mathbf{E}(P)$ will develop into a member of $\mathbf{H}(P)$ and so into a member of P. Thanks to the chain of definitions all this is expressed by saying that x is a member of $\Gamma_S(P)$.

The genetic milieu of $\Gamma_S(P)$ will be the Boolean sum of all the constant sets (other than $\Gamma_S(P)$) of chromosome bands specified by the postulate of S involved in the definition of $\Gamma_S(P)$ and of all the constant chromosome sets (other than $\chi_S(P)$) specified by the postulate of S which is involved in the definition of $\chi_S(P)$. We can only make predictions so long as we remain within S.

Changing the genetic milieu means changing S, and then what happens can only be discovered by making new experiments, unless of course the new system is one which has already been investigated.

It will be noticed that Professor Waddington uses the word 'genotype' in the above passages, not in the sense in which I have been using it (following the precedent of Professor J. B. S. Haldane), but in another and totally different sense, although in a sense which is very widely current in genetical writing. What do geneticists mean by 'genotype' in this second sense? One thing they *might* mean by 'the genotype of P' is simply $\mathbf{N}(P)$, or, if it is desired to refer to zygotic nuclei, it would be the set of all nuclei x such that, for some y,

$$y \in \mathbf{U}(\mathbf{C}(\mathbf{S}, \mathbf{N}(P), \mathbf{K}(P)), \mathbf{C}(\mathbf{S}, \mathbf{N}(P), \mathbf{K}(P)))$$

and x is the nucleus of y. This would be a homozygous zygotic genotype. By introducing a second phenotype Q together with $\mathbf{N}(Q)$, a heterozygous zygotic genotype could be defined. But I think many (perhaps all) geneticists would repudiate such a definition in second-level terms and would insist that this notion must be formulated in terms belonging to level 4. This is much more complicated because not only have all the gene sets to be mentioned but also the $\mathbf{R}$-relations between their members. If only the gene sets need be considered, it would suffice to say that a set X belongs to the genotype of P in the system S if, and only if, X contains just one member (one of which belongs to $\Gamma_S(P)$) from each of the sets $\Gamma_{ij}(S)$, where i ranges from 1 to n (the total number of chromosomes in each member of $\mathbf{N}(P)$), and j ranges from 1 to m_i (the total number of bands on the ith chromosome). This procedure, plausible though it may seem, is open to the objection that it presupposes that you can define each chromosome set separately, and, as we have seen, that would only be possible by reference to a genetical system of relatively high order, namely, to one whose order is at least equal to the number of chromosomes in each member of the gamete set concerned. But even if this difficulty were overcome there would still remain the problem of the relations between the genes. To cope with this problem it would be necessary to define sets of sequences of genes, and not only sets of sequences but sets of sets of sequences—one for each chromosome. This second sense of 'genotype' is thus somewhat obscure and complicated, and as I have not used the word in this sense I do not feel under any obligation to define it. That is a task that must be left to the experts who use it, if they wish to make clear in precisely what sense they use it. One thing seems quite clear: when Johannsen wrote 'A "genotype" is the sum total of all the "genes" in a gamete or in a zygote' he was not defining 'genotype' (although he called this statement a definition); he was only mentioning a *member* of one, and then without reference to the ordering relation **R**, about which nothing was known in his time.

When geneticists say (as they sometimes do) that 'a complete set of genes is all that is necessary for normal development', what they mean is, I think, that it is biologically possible for a cell containing a nucleus belonging to $N(P)$, if it stands in **S** to a suitable cytoplasm, to develop, provided it has the appropriate environment, into a member of P. This statement is therefore somewhat misleading to the non-expert.

There is one minor ambiguity which should be mentioned in connexion with the use of such phrases as 'the gene for P'. It is not *always* clear whether a *set* of genes is being referred to or some particular *individual* gene. Usually it is the former but not always. This is because 'the' is habitually used in two quite different senses. When someone says 'the mathematician would use logarithms for this purpose', he means (usually) *any* mathematician would use logarithms for this purpose. But when someone says 'the mathematician who invented the differential calculus also wrote philosophy', his intention will be to refer to one particular individual mathematician. He may have been thinking of Leibniz. But in fact he would fail in his intention. For there is no such mathematician, because Newton also independently invented the differential calculus. These two senses of 'the' occur together in the phrase 'the heart of the dog-fish', because this phrase refers to the set of all objects x such that for some y, y is a dogfish and x is *the* (one and only) heart of y. But any danger of ambiguity from this source is easily avoided if we speak of 'the gene set of P' instead of 'the gene for P'.*

It will, I hope, be clear from the foregoing analysis that in relation to any phenotype P, such that $\mathbf{H}(P) \neq \Lambda$, there are three fundamental sets to be considered from the genetical point of view: $\mathbf{N}(P)$, $\mathbf{K}(P)$ and $\mathbf{E}(P)$. For various reasons which will be explained in detail in the next lecture, $\mathbf{K}(P)$ and $\mathbf{E}(P)$ tend to be forgotten or neglected. This has been the primary source of most of the controversies and misunderstandings in the history of genetics.

Having dealt with the distinction between Mendelian and Batesonian systems as expressible on level 4, I turn now to consider what hypotheses are required in order that the hypothesis given on p. 143, regarding gamete-set frequencies in a Batesonian system, should be derivable.

In the genetical product $S_1 \times S_2$ of our two systems of allelic index (2), which we are now supposing to be Batesonian, so that its allelic index will be (2, 2), we shall have four mutually exclusive chromosome sets to consider:

$$\chi_S(AP), \quad \chi_S(AQ), \quad \chi_S(BP) \quad \text{and} \quad \chi_S(BQ).$$

The remaining chromosome sets, which cannot be separately defined, will be represented by $\mathbf{M}(AP, BQ)$.† I shall also use K to represent the Boolean sum of all the cytoplasm sets concerned in the cell sets involved in what follows, since differences between cytoplasm sets do not have to be considered. With this notation

---

* It should also be mentioned that 'the gene set of $\mathbf{P}$' will not always be a set of single genes, but may be a set of ordered n-tuples of genes. For example, for the system S($\mathbf{W}$, $\mathbf{R}$, $\mathbf{P}$, $\mathbf{S}$), mentioned in Note 6, p. 207, we should have sets of couples of genes.

† The letter '$\mathbf{M}$' is chosen because these represent the genetic *milieu* mentioned above.

the four gamete sets in our example on p. 143 can be represented as follows:

$$\alpha\gamma = \mathbf{C}(\mathbf{S}, \mathbf{C}(\mathbf{Q}, \mathbf{M}(AP, BQ), \chi_S(AP)), K),$$
$$\alpha\delta = \mathbf{C}(\mathbf{S}, \mathbf{C}(\mathbf{Q}, \mathbf{M}(AP, BQ), \chi_S(AQ)), K),$$
$$\beta\gamma = \mathbf{C}(\mathbf{S}, \mathbf{C}(\mathbf{Q}, \mathbf{M}(AP, BQ), \chi_S(BP)), K),$$
$$\beta\delta = \mathbf{C}(\mathbf{S}, \mathbf{C}(\mathbf{Q}, \mathbf{M}(AP, BQ), \chi_S(BQ)), K).$$

Using K with the same significance as above we next define five sets of diploid *cells* quite generally as follows:

$$C_{ap,bq} =$$
$$\mathbf{C}(\mathbf{S}, \mathbf{C}(\mathbf{Q}, \mathbf{M}(AP, BQ), \mathbf{M}(AP, BQ), \chi_S(AP), \chi_S(BQ)), K),$$

$$C_{ap,ap} =$$
$$\mathbf{C}(\mathbf{S}, \mathbf{C}(\mathbf{Q}, \mathbf{M}(AP, BQ), \mathbf{M}(AP, BQ), \chi_S(AP), \chi_S(AP)), K),$$

$$C_{ap,aq} =$$
$$\mathbf{C}(\mathbf{S}, \mathbf{C}(\mathbf{Q}, \mathbf{M}(AP, BQ), \mathbf{M}(AP, BQ), \chi_S(AP), \chi_S(AQ)), K),$$

$$C_{bp,bq} =$$
$$\mathbf{C}(\mathbf{S}, \mathbf{C}(\mathbf{Q}, \mathbf{M})(AP, BQ), \mathbf{M}(AP, BQ), \chi_S(BP), \chi_S(BQ)), K),$$

$$C_{bq,bq} =$$
$$\mathbf{C}(\mathbf{S}, \mathbf{C}(\mathbf{Q}, \mathbf{M}(AP, BQ), \mathbf{M}(AP, BQ), \chi_S(BQ), \chi_S(BQ)), K).$$

The hypotheses we require can be formulated most simply if, instead of the two-termed relation $\mathbf{D}$ formerly used, we employ the three-termed relation $\mathbf{D}'$ which is easily defined as follows:

[D. 58] $\mathbf{D}'(x, y, z)$, if and only if $x\mathbf{D}y$ and $x\mathbf{D}z$ and $y \neq z$.

This three-termed relation can be used in the composition functor. Thus $\mathbf{c}(\mathbf{D}', x, y, z)$ will be the single object composed of the cells x, y and z when related by $\mathbf{D}'$.* Such an object can be called a *division triad*, x being called the first cell and y and z the two second cells of the triad. Accordingly, $\mathbf{C}(\mathbf{D}', X, Y, Z)$ will be the set of all division triads, in which the first cell is a member of X, one of the second cells belongs to Y and the other to Z.

---

* It will be noticed that the functors $\mathbf{c}(R, x, y)$ and $\mathbf{C}(R, X, Y)$ are multigrade, their degree depending upon the degree of R. If the latter is of degree n then the composition functor containing it will be of degree $n+1$.

The division triads which occur in a life belonging to a genetical system are divisible (in animals) into three mutually exclusive sub-sets. First, there are those which I call *pre-reduction* triads, in which the first cell is not a reduction cell and does not have a reduction cell standing in $\mathbf{D_{po}}$ to it. The second sub-set I shall call *reduction* triads, namely, those in which the first cell is a reduction cell. The third sub-set, called *post-reduction* triads, consists of those in which the first cell is a post-reduction cell, i.e. a cell to which a reduction cell stands in $\mathbf{D}$.* (In most plants there will also be post-post-reduction triads, i.e. those whose first cells have post-reduction cells standing in $\mathbf{D_{po}}$ to them.)

In addition to the general hypotheses given on p. 151 in connexion with sex systems we require the following hypotheses (E being the common environmental set):

[H. 49] $\mathbf{U}(\alpha\gamma, \beta\delta) \subset C_{ap,bq}.$

[H. 50]   Every pre-reduction triad which is a part of a member of $\mathbf{L}_E(\mathbf{U}(\alpha\gamma, \beta\delta))$ belongs to the set $\mathbf{C}(\mathbf{D}', C_{ap,bq}, C_{ap,bq}, C_{ap,bq}).$

[H. 51]   The set R of all reduction triads, which are parts of members of $\mathbf{L}_E(\mathbf{U}(\alpha\gamma, \beta\delta))$, falls into two mutually exclusive sub-sets R_1 and R_2 such that

$$R_1 \subset \mathbf{C}(\mathbf{D}', C_{ap,bq}, C_{ap,ap}, C_{bq,bq}),$$

$$R_2 \subset \mathbf{C}(\mathbf{D}', C_{ap,bq}, C_{ap,aq}, C_{bp,bq}),$$

and† $$D(R) = (1 - 2p) R_1 + 2p R_2.$$

[H. 52]   If P is the set of all post-reduction triads which are parts of members of $\mathbf{L}_E(\mathbf{U}(\alpha\gamma, \beta\delta))$, then P falls into four mutually

---

* Note that we have so far only defined 'reduction cell' for simple zygotic sex systems. In the present context therefore this phrase has the status of an undefined sign.

† Note that 'p' in this formula represents the recombination value (p. 120) and has nothing to do with the 'p' which appears as a sub-script to 'C'.

exclusive sub-sets P_1, P_2, P_3 and P_4 such that

$$P_1 = \mathbf{C}(\mathbf{D}', C_{ap,ap}, \alpha\gamma, \alpha\gamma),$$
$$P_2 = \mathbf{C}(\mathbf{D}', C_{bq,bq}, \beta\delta, \beta\delta),$$
$$P_3 = \mathbf{C}(\mathbf{D}', C_{ap,aq}, \alpha\gamma, \alpha\delta),$$
$$P_4 = \mathbf{C}(\mathbf{D}', C_{bp,bq}, \beta\gamma, \beta\delta).$$

[H. 53]   If $\mathbf{C}(\mathbf{D}', X, Y, Z)$ is any set of post-reduction triads, then $\mathbf{D}(Y \cup Z) = \frac{1}{2}Y + \frac{1}{2}Z$.

From H. 51 and H. 52 it will follow that

$$\mathbf{D}(P) = \tfrac{1}{2}(1 - 2p)\,P_1 + \tfrac{1}{2}(1 - 2p)\,P_2 + pP_3 + pP_4.$$

From this and H. 53 and with the help of the more general hypotheses mentioned it will follow that

$$\mathbf{D}(\mathbf{G}(\mathbf{L}_E(\mathbf{U}(\alpha\gamma, \beta\delta))))$$
$$= (\tfrac{1}{2}(1 - 2p) + \tfrac{1}{2}p)\,\alpha\gamma + \tfrac{1}{2}p\alpha\delta + \tfrac{1}{2}p\beta\gamma + (\tfrac{1}{2}(1 - 2p) + \tfrac{1}{2}p)\,\beta\delta$$
$$= \tfrac{1}{2}(1 - p)\,\alpha\gamma + \tfrac{1}{2}p\alpha\delta + \tfrac{1}{2}p\beta\gamma + \tfrac{1}{2}(1 - p)\,\beta\delta,$$

which is the theoretical gamete-set frequency required. By putting $a = b$ or $p = q$ or both in the subscripts of C, the other gamete-set frequencies for the Batesonian system are obtained. The generalization of hypotheses H. 49 to H. 53 to deal with Batesonian systems of order greater than 2 raises complications which will not be considered here, although it does not appear to involve the introduction of new functors (see Note 12, p. 211).

§ 4.   THE CLASSIFICATION OF GENETICAL SYSTEMS

If we now try to draw a rough map of the elements of genetics, in so far as they have been expounded here for illustrative purposes, it will be seen that zero level consists exclusively of mating descriptions. If the connexion between genetics and cytology had been fully worked out it would also include some generalizations of cytological observation records. Theoretical statements belonging to the other levels fall into five groups:

(1) the postulates governing the use of the undefined signs;

(2) the definitions formulated with the help of the undefined signs;

(3) embryological hypotheses, like H. 10 (p. 136);

(4) the hypotheses of first level giving gamete-set frequencies together with all those hypotheses of higher levels from which the former are derivable;

(5) finally, we have genetical hypotheses of a more general kind like conditions (α), (β) and (γ) (pp. 134–6) which embody the assumptions of the random union of gametes and the equi-productivity of sets with respect to $\mathbf{F}$, $\mathbf{L}$ and $\mathbf{U}$. In this group may also be included such cytological hypotheses as H. 32 (p. 151) and H. 42 (p. 155).

If we wish to axiomatize this part of genetics we should in the first instance treat all the statements which are not derivable from others in the system as postulates, and all the remaining ones would then be theorems of the system. But it might be found that the system could be simplified or otherwise improved by a different choice of postulates, so long as these yielded the required results. A set of postulates which had greater predictive power than another would obviously be preferable. But the choice of postulates would depend in part on the choice of undefined signs. In building up the pyramid of statements from zero level we have taken our undefined signs piecemeal as they have been required at each level. In this way we have adopted the following list of undefined signs: $\mathbf{F}_{X,Y,Z}$, $\mathbf{En}$, phenotype, $\mathbf{U}$, $\mathbf{B}(x)$, $\mathbf{G}_X$, $\mathbf{D}$, $\mathbf{P}$, reduction cell, $\mathbf{S}$, $\mathbf{Q}$ and $\mathbf{R}$.* In Note 14, p. 211, it is shown how a much smaller primitive vocabulary can be chosen with the help of which most of the above become definable.

In view of the fact, which was pointed out on p. 169, that we have three fundamental factors to deal with in genetical problems, namely, $\mathbf{N}(P)$, $\mathbf{K}(P)$ and $\mathbf{E}(P)$, for any phenotype P such that $\mathbf{H}(P) \neq \Lambda$, it will follow that there will be seven theoretically possible fundamental types of genetical system according to

---

* This suggests the question: What relation will be required in the composition functor in passing to the *next* level?

which factor (or factors) we suppose to vary and which one (or ones) we suppose to remain constant. (When I say, with reference to a given system, that the nuclear factor, for example, varies, I mean simply that there are at least two phenotypes P and Q such that $\mathbf{N}(P) \cap \mathbf{N}(Q) = \Lambda$. And when I say that the environmental factor remains constant, I mean simply that $\mathbf{E}(P) = \mathbf{E}(Q)$, and similarly for $\mathbf{K}(P)$ and $\mathbf{K}(Q)$.) In this way we obtain the following seven possible systems: (1) nuclear, (2) cytoplasmic, (3) environmental, (4) nucleo-cytoplasmic, (5) nucleo-environmental, (6) environmental-cytoplasmic, and (7) nucleo-cytoplasmic-environmental.

The familiar systems which have an allelic index and a partition, and which therefore exhibit the familiar mating descriptions, all belong to (1). These I call *regular* and *open* nuclear systems. *Open* but *irregular* nuclear systems would be those for which one or more of the hypotheses in our fifth category above (p. 173) do not hold. Concealed (as opposed to open) nuclear systems are certain systems belonging to possibilities (4) and (5). To (2) belong certain systems which have been studied in plants (see Note 18, p. 218). Of (6) we have an example in the environmental sex system described on p. 144. To (4) belong the zygotic sex systems and *Limnaea* with its two modes of shell-coiling. An imaginary example of (5) is worked out in Note 16, p. 215. It is isomorphic with the example there given of (4). Geneticists would not be interested in (3). Perhaps some natural or wild systems will exemplify (7).

As a prophylactic against dogmatism regarding the permanence of current theories in genetics it is well to remind ourselves of the recent history of physics and of the possibility that *every* hypothesis is capable of, and may some day require, revision. It is particularly useful to remember that even such an obvious and common-sense notion as that of the simultaneity of distant events was successfully subjected to drastic criticism by Einstein.

In order to end on a lighter note after so much rather heavy stuff, let me relate to you:

§ 5. THE PARABLE OF THE FOUR ISLANDS

Once upon a time there were four islands. They were called Adam and Eve Island, Mendel Island, Morgan Island and Opposite Island. They were too far apart, and their modes of water transport too primitive, to enable them to communicate. But at a remote epoch they had all been peopled from the same stock, and for that reason their languages closely resembled one another in certain basic features. Although primitive and indolent in many ways the inhabitants of all four islands were intellectually very advanced. They had all developed mathematics to a considerable extent. In all their scientific work they were as much interested in foundation problems as in the development and enlargement of their sciences. They had the lower functional calculus well developed and, curiously enough, they all used the same symbols for the formative signs, 'and', 'or', 'all', etc., on all the islands. Regarding their attainments in natural science, however, there were marked differences between them, especially in biology, which was much cultivated on them all.

On Adam and Eve Island the inhabitants naturally understood mating and had carried the investigation of hybridization as far as Mendel did. But like some of our modern scientists they had a horror of hypotheses. Moreover, they had no microscopes. The result was that, although they could formulate systems of mating descriptions—using something corresponding to my **F** functor to construct genetical equations—they knew nothing of gametes and made no attempt to frame explanatory hypotheses.

On Mendel Island, however, the situation was different. They had not only discovered genetical systems which they classified according to their allelic index and partition, but they had formulated first-level explanatory hypotheses in terms of gamete sets and sets of zygotes, after the manner of Mendel. Beyond that they were not able to go.

On Morgan Island genetics had been much further developed.

They had good microscopes and had formulated high-level hypotheses which covered both Mendelian and Batesonian systems.

One day a bottle, containing a concise axiomatization of the genetical theory of Mendel Island, was washed ashore on Adam and Eve Island. It was eagerly opened by the islanders and its contents carefully studied. They found that they could easily recognize the definitions of genetical systems and their classification according to allelic index and partition. The notation of Mendel Island for mating descriptions differed but little from their own; but the symbols corresponding to the functors **U, L, G** and **dlz** meant nothing to them. Nevertheless, owing to their grasp of the structure of their language, assisted by the use of common symbols for the formative signs, they were able to see how the mating descriptions followed from the first-level hypotheses and were able to use the Mendel Islanders' scheme for purposes of classification, calculation and prediction.

A somewhat similar event occurred on Mendel Island. One day they discovered a bottle from Morgan Island containing the genetical theory of that island in a compact axiomatic form. They had no difficulty in understanding all that part of the Morgan theory which corresponded with their own, but the rest was quite unintelligible to them. Nevertheless, they appreciated its structure, saw how their own hypotheses followed from its axioms and so were able to use it. They were particularly delighted to have a hypothesis, even a purely abstract one, from which they could derive mating descriptions of both Mendelian and Batesonian systems, the connexion between which had formerly completely baffled them.

On Opposite Island a curious situation prevailed. Their genetics was as far advanced as that of Morgan Island. In fact, by a most strange coincidence the theoretical genetics of these two islands resembled each other in every respect but one, and that a minor one. Wherever the word 'gene' occurred in the genetical statements of Morgan Island the word 'entelechy' occurred in the corresponding place in the genetical statements of Opposite Island, and wherever the word 'entelechy' occurred in the genetical statements of Opposite Island the word 'gene' occurred in the corresponding place in the genetical statements of Morgan Island. Consequently the two systems did not differ in structure, and whatever was predictable and testable on the one island was predictable and testable on the other. But when geneticists on Morgan Island talked of genes 'controlling this or that character' those of Opposite Island talked of entelechies 'controlling this or that character'. But the structure being the same in the two cases this made no difference whatever.*

* This suggests that the reason why those who have wished to use the word 'entelechy' in biology have been unsuccessful, is because they failed to use the word in statements having the right structure to provide fruitful predictions. It is not the words you use that is important but the structure of the statements in which they occur.

LECTURE V

§ 1. REQUIREMENTS OF A SCIENTIFIC LANGUAGE

One motive for searching for the basic functors of genetics, and for offering the foregoing analysis of its foundations, has been the wish to see whether it is possible to avoid certain expressions which have been sources of controversy and confusion during the short history of this subject. At the same time I have hoped that what I have done might provide a beginning for an eventual axiomatization of genetical theory.

In connexion with what I am about to say it is important to remember that geneticists use not one language, but many. There are the language of the laboratory, the language of the technical journals, the language of the general treatise and the language of the elementary text-book. With the first two I am not primarily concerned. They are used for communication between experts. The first especially is highly elliptical, but experts will understand one another in it, because they are able to make the necessary adjustments. But the use of an elliptical language in general treatises and text-books which are written by experts for non-experts will be a constant source of irritation and difficulty; and even experts, as we shall see, have been misled by it.

A good scientific language should be completely explicit and brief; it should contain no features which resist generalization and so create obstacles to further development; it should contain a minimum vocabulary of basic functors with the help of which the remaining ones can be defined; and these basic functors, if they are intelligible in the sense previously explained, should be as clear and free from ambiguity as possible. If they are abstract they are meaningless apart from the statements in which they occur and the place these latter occupy in the pyramid or map of genetical statements related by the consequence relation. For example, we can make no meaningful genetical statement about a gene unless it is a part of a chromosome, which in its turn is part of a nucleus, which again is part of a living cell and standing in the relation S to a cytoplasm, which cell again is part of a member of a phenotype developing in an environment. In other words, we deal only with sets of genes which are assumed to be defined relatively to certain other sets of genes, certain sets of chromosomes, a certain set of cytoplasms, a certain phenotype and a certain environmental set. Of these, what are observed in genetical experiments are the members of the phenotypes and environmental sets; and they are observed by means of sensible objects which stand in the relation OF to them, in the sense previously explained.

I think I can claim that my language goes some way towards satisfying these requirements. The conflicting claims of brevity and explicitness are reconciled by the use of functors which are fully explained when they are first introduced. As you have seen, some of them are abbreviations for expressions which occupy many lines when fully stated in English. It is not uncommon in the literature to find careless elliptical formulations excused on the ground that they provide a 'convenient shorthand'. But if this is done, as it usually is, without any provision being made for translating the shorthand into long hand, should occasion require it (and this is often a difficult thing to do), I would maintain that such shorthand cannot justly be called 'convenient'. All my statements can be expanded at once into English by reference to the explanations of the functors contained in them. I would also point out that the genetical equations which have been used are biological statements, not mathematical formulas, because they contain biological functors; just as chemical equations are chemical statements because they contain chemical functors.

Another feature of genetical books is a tendency to rely too much on diagrams. Diagrams are very useful devices, especially for teaching purposes. But the important thing to note about them is that they are not universal general statements and cannot completely take the place of such statements. The relation between mathematical equation and plotted curve is a particular instance of the general relation of statement to diagram, and the plotted curve does not enable us to dispense with the equation. A diagram is a particular object and cannot possibly represent all that a universal general statement asserts. Too much reliance on diagrams will therefore create obstacles to generalization.

§ 2. WORDS IN GENETICS BORROWED FROM EVERYDAY LANGUAGE

Among the expressions which have been responsible for controversy and misunderstanding in genetics are the following: (1) heredity, (2) hereditary or inherited character, (3) acquired character, (4) inheritance, (5) '...determines...' or '...is due to...', (6) identity.

It is, I think, a striking and significant fact that this list does not include a single technical term which has been deliberately introduced into genetics as it has developed, but consists exclusively of words taken, more or less uncritically, from the language of everyday life—words which have been in use in common-sense contexts long before genetics began. Professor L. Hogben quotes the late Professor Jennings as saying:

A burden of concepts and definitions has come down to us from pre-experimental days; the pouring of the new wine of experimental knowledge into these has resulted in confusion. And this confusion is worse confounded by the strange and strong propensity of workers in heredity to flout and deny and despise the observations of the workers in environmental action; the equally strange and strong propensity of students of environmental effects to flout and deny and despise the work on heritance. If one accepts the affirmative results of both sets, untroubled by their negations, untroubled by definitions that have come from the past, there results a simple, consistent, and useful body of knowledge, though with less pretentious claims than are set forth by either single set.*

I think I may claim therefore to have the support of at least one well-known geneticist when I say that these expressions

* *Genetic Principles in Medicine and Social Science* (1931), p. 34.

demand investigation from the point of view of their service-
ableness for modern genetics.* But, let me emphasize at the
outset, I am not saying that any of these expressions are meaningless in all contexts. Neither do I propose to lay down laws
for other people's use of language. I am concerned only to point
out some consequences of certain linguistic habits, and to show
how these consequences may be avoided if it is desired. Let me
also remind you of what I said in the beginning about the question
of a good correlation between the degree of precision of the
language we are using and the degree of precision demanded by
the occasion of its use. If we are told that a certain eminent man
is to give a lecture on heredity we shall know roughly what he
will be talking about and this will suffice. But it may well be
that, for formulating important biological generalizations and
hypotheses, 'heredity' is hopelessly abstract, vague and am-
biguous in all its uses.† If we apply to it the test of asking:
What is its extension? What is its degree? it is extremely difficult
to know what to answer. In any case we have now seen that it is
possible to express many genetical statements to a considerable
degree of precision, and even to offer a precise definition of
'genetics', without using this objectionable word at all. I therefore venture to suggest that a great gain in clarity could be
achieved, and a great improvement in biological writing generally could be made, if this word were banished from the vocabulary of scientific genetics entirely. At least we can ask of those
who insist upon using it that they should make clear in which
of its many senses they use it. It may well be that the effort
needed to do this, if conscientiously made, will convince them that
abandonment of the word would be the simpler course to take.

* For the views of W. Johannsen see Note 17, p. 217.
† For a list of some of the many so-called definitions of 'heredity' see my
Biological Principles (1948), pp. 384–5. To this collection we may add the
following specimen from p. 159 of the article by Johannsen quoted in Note 17:
'Heredity may then be defined as *the presence of identical genes in ancestors
and descendants*, or, as Morgan says in full accordance with this definition: "The
word heredity stands for those properties of the germ-cells that find their expression in the developing and developed organism."' This short passage illustrates
very well many of the points which have been discussed in these lectures.

§3. ENVIRONMENTAL RANGES

It is in connexion with the antithesis between heredity and environment that the word 'heredity' has done most damage. Professor Hogben has stated that 'genetical science has outgrown the false antithesis between heredity and environment productive of so much futile controversy in the past'. But what is true of genetical science is unhappily not true of the social sciences. The muddles which such futile controversies have engendered still persist in varying degrees in medical, legal and sociological literature. (See *postscript*, p. 357.)

It is plain that the use of the functor **dlz** and its derivative **Dlz** completely eliminates this antithesis because each functor is irreducibly three-termed. We cannot predict what phenotype a given zygote will develop into unless we know something about the environment in which it develops, and equally, knowing something about the environment will not suffice if we do not know enough about the zygote. When people use the word 'heredity' in such contexts, what they have in mind is the *sort* of zygote involved. They are thinking about some maximized set of zygotes; however, as we have seen, we cannot speak simply of a maximized set of zygotes, but only of a set which is maximized relatively to some phenotype and to some maximized environmental set.

If we consider a three-termed relation in physics, such as that involved in Ohm's law

$$C = \frac{E}{R},$$

we do not find physicists quarrelling about the relative importance of electromotive force and resistance, nor about how much of the current is 'due to' the one and how much to the other. Why is it then, when everything seems so plain, that in biology there has been so much controversy? One reason seems to be that, in discussions and expositions of these topics, one of the three terms in the matrix **Dlz**(Z, E, P) is frequently allowed to drop out, and the one most frequently dropped out is the middle term—the designation of the environmental set.

The reason why there is this tendency to drop all reference to the environmental set is easy to understand, but to make it quite plain certain technical terms are needed. Our previous definitions have already provided all that is necessary. We have (p. 130) already defined the P-environmental range of the set Z

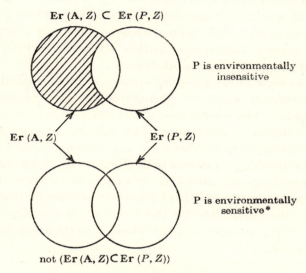

Er (A, Z) $\subset$ Er (P, Z)

P is environmentally
insensitive

Er (A, Z) Er (P, Z)

P is environmentally
sensitive*

not (**Er** $(A, Z)\subset$ **Er** (P, Z))

Diagram to illustrate environmental ranges

The circular areas represent environmental sets. The shaded area has no members. That part of the circle on the left in each pair which does not overlap the circle on the right represents those environments in which members of Z develop into adults but not into members of P.

* See explanation on p. 187.

of zygotes. We have denoted this set by **Er**(P, Z). In particular, the *adult* environmental range of a set Z of zygotes, i.e. **Er**(A, Z), using '**A**' to denote the set of adults, i.e. sexually mature lives, will be the set of all environments in which a member of Z will develop into an adult.

Now it is plain that if, for a given Z and P, the adult environmental range of Z is contained in the P-environmental range of Z, then it will never be necessary to worry much about the environment because, so long as we provide an environment in which members of Z attain the adult state, we shall also be providing one which will ensure the appearance of the phenotype P. It is also plain that when this is the case two other things may be expected: (1) it will be easy to overlook reference to the environment in constructing statements relating to such systems, and (2) it will be relatively easy to investigate such systems genetically, as compared with those systems in which the P-environmental range is only a small part of the adult environmental range of the sets of zygotes involved.

Now in most of the genetical systems so far investigated, at least in those in which the phenotypes are adult phenotypes, believe it will be correct to say that the adult environmental anges of the zygote sets concerned are included in the phenotype environmental ranges. There are exceptions of course, but generally speaking this seems to be the case. This is presumably because such systems are relatively easy to investigate, and the same circumstance, which has led to their selection for investigation, is also responsible for the fact that in describing such systems it is customary to omit reference to the environmental sets involved.

§ 4. VENN'S REQUIREMENT AND THE CONSTANT FACTOR PRINCIPLE

In connexion with this dropping out of any reference to the environmental sets and also with other omissions which will be discussed presently, I would draw attention to two important general methodological principles which, although most people would agree to them when they are stated in general terms, are nevertheless frequently forgotten in practice. The first I will call Venn's requirement because it is well stated in the following passage from a book* written by Venn, published in 1889:

We need hardly remind readers of Mill of the importance which he attaches to the enumeration of all the elements of the antecedent.

* *Empirical Logic.*

It forms the staple of his exposition of the causal relation. He criticises at considerable length the capricious way in which the popular estimate picks out some one circumstance, and regards this as the cause, or at least calls it so. For logical purposes the criticism is quite sound, but there is nevertheless some method in the seeming caprice. The great object of speech is to convey our meaning with the least trouble, and where anything can be reasonably taken for granted, we are naturally apt to omit the direct statement of it. If some of the antecedents can be thus taken for granted, we naturally incline to omit any reference to them. Moreover it must be remembered that the popular interest centres, not in speculation, but in practice. The reason why we look out for a cause is not to gratify any feeling of curiosity, at least not primarily, but because we want to produce some particular effect. Hence every element which can commonly be trusted to supply itself gives us no anxiety, and comes to slip out of our description of the producing circumstances.

Useful as it once was to insist upon the insufficiency of this popular makeshift for a true cause, it seems needless to dwell longer here upon the mere fact that accurate reasoning stands in need of something more than this. If we are to make sure of producing or inferring any particular effect, we must clearly make a point of requiring that all the elements of the antecedent are present, whatever may be the various names—such as condition, occasion, part-cause, etc.—which they may assume in the popular vocabulary.

This passage explains very well why it is that reference to the environmental sets involved is usually omitted in connexion with those genetical systems in which the adult environmental ranges of the zygote sets concerned are contained in the phenotype environmental ranges. For this is clearly a particular example of the omission to which Venn refers, and it can be excused in the way he suggests. At the same time, in so far as this practice continues to generate confusions—and, as we shall see, it is not only in connexion with environments that Venn's requirement is not satisfied—it can hardly be 'needless to dwell longer upon the mere fact that accurate reasoning stands in need of something more than this'. In spite of what Venn says, it still seems to be necessary to 'insist upon the insufficiency of this popular make-shift'. Now by the use of **Dlz** and by ensuring that such related expressions as $\mathbf{L}_E(\ )$, $\mathbf{G}_E(\ )$ and $\mathbf{F}_E(\ ,\ )$, are all carefully defined and all carry with them a reference to an environmental set, we succeed in having the best of both worlds: we achieve brevity and at the same time we satisfy Venn's requirement.*

Related to the foregoing is another point. When it is found that some factor can be omitted in formulating generalizations there is always a danger of slipping into the assumption that such factors can be omitted in fact and not only in expression. The following methodological principle bears on this point:

If, in a series of experiments, certain factors are constant, not necessarily in the sense of unchanging in time, but in the sense of being of the same kind in each experiment, then nothing can be asserted on the basis of those experiments about the role of such constant factors in the production of the observed result.†

This, which I shall call the *constant factor principle*, is also one to which most people would give their assent—indeed it is a commonplace of experimental procedure—and yet, as we shall see, it has more than once been forgotten in connexion with genetical problems. If we choose a system such that, for each of its zygote sets Z and each phenotype P, the adult environmental range of Z is included in the P-environmental range of Z, because then it is easy to investigate, and if we then omit reference to the environmental set because it is constant and common to all our experiments, we must obviously not slide into the assumption that the environments belonging to this set 'play no part' in the processes involved.

* For the sake of symbolical simplicity I have not provided '$\mathbf{U}$' with a subscript representing an environmental set. It usually occurs in such contexts as '$\mathbf{L}_E(\mathbf{U}(\ ,\ ))$'; and for animals, especially those in which fertilization is internal, this should suffice. Perhaps for some plants '$\mathbf{U}$' should have an independent subscript.

The tendency to forget the environment in formulating genetical statements is extremely powerful, even when one has recognized the danger. I have myself frequently forgotten it, only to be reminded of my omission by the occurrence of the subscript to $\mathbf{F}$, $\mathbf{L}$, etc. It is one of the many merits of a symbolic language (or one that is partly so) that it is able to do such services for us.

† For example, in a world in which nothing was opaque to light, and in which we had no means of varying the intensity of light, it would be impossible to discover the role of light in photosynthesis.

I hope it will not now be necessary to devote much time to the expressions 'hereditary characters' and 'acquired characters', although there are still differences of opinion regarding their use. Professor Hogben has said: 'Strictly speaking, it is meaningless to speak of hereditary characters.' Dr Julian Huxley, on p. 18 of his *Evolution: The Modern Synthesis*, writes: 'Characters as such are not and cannot be inherited.' But on p. 64 he says: 'Thus it may legitimately be argued that the majority of all inherited characters must rest on a Mendelian basis.' Also, these phrases continue to be used by many eminent geneticists, who would not agree that, in doing so, what they were saying was meaningless. I have already pointed out that theoretical genetics is not concerned with characters at all, but with phenotypes and still more with genotypes. To specify phenotypes, as we must do when we wish to *apply* genetics, it is necessary to *use* character words, but it is not necessary to *speak about* characters as we do when we classify them into hereditary and acquired ones, or when we use the absurd legal metaphor according to which characters are 'handed on' or 'transmitted' from one generation to another. It is, however, useful to classify *phenotypes* in the following way.

Let us say that a phenotype P is *environmentally insensitive* with respect to Z if and only if the adult environmental range of Z is included in its P-environmental range. This does *not* mean that a member of Z will develop in strong sulphuric acid. It means only what the definition says it means.*

Let us say also that P is *environmentally sensitive* with respect to Z if and only if there are members of the adult environmental range of Z which do *not* belong to the P-environmental range of Z. For example, the set of all red-haired human beings will be an environmentally insensitive phenotype relatively to the sets of zygotes from which they developed. But the set of all English men and women who exhibit a certain degree of sunburning will be an example of an environmentally sensitive phenotype, because it is quite possible for one member of a pair of identical

* See the diagram on p. 183.

twins to develop into an adult who is not sunburnt whilst his twin has developed into an adult who *is* sunburnt.

I think it is possible that this may be the distinction which forms the basis for the division of characters into hereditary and acquired, at least in some contexts. But as my language does not contain the expressions 'hereditary character' and 'acquired character' I am not called upon to say what they mean.

The words 'inherited' and 'inheritance' in other contexts are likewise easily dispensed with and are merely vestiges of the mistaken legal metaphor already alluded to. When someone asks: 'How is the phenotype P inherited?' or 'What is the mode of inheritance of P?' what is meant seems to be 'To what kind of genetical system does P belong? Is it Mendelian or Batesonian or mixed? What is its allelic index and partition? Or does P belong to some other kind of genetical system?'

§ 5. THE FORMULATION OF LAMARCKIAN HYPOTHESES

Although it is not possible in my language to ask the celebrated question: Are acquired characters inherited?—and this I claim to be a merit of the language—yet it is possible to formulate clearly hypotheses of a type which *might* be called Lamarckian. Some authors have maintained (e.g. Sir Ray Lankester) that even the formulation of such hypotheses involves a contradiction. But this is not so, provided we have a suitable language. Epidemics of Lamarckian controversy are a periodic occurrence in the history of biology. We are passing through one at the present day, complicated on this occasion by bitter political embroilments. Although it is not the business of methodology to take sides in such controversies, it *is* its business to try to analyse them.

A Lamarckian hypothesis would be one which asserts that there are mutually exclusive sets γ_1 and γ_2 of gametes, mutually exclusive sets E_1 and E_2 of environments, and phenotypes P_1 and P_2, satisfying the following conditions:

(1) P_2 is in some sense *superior* to P_1, in the sense, for example, that members of P_2 have greater economic value, such as greater

milk yield in cattle, or higher survival value in E_1, than those of P_1.

(2) $\mathbf{Dlz}(\mathbf{U}(\gamma_1, \gamma_1), E_1, P_1)$ and $\mathbf{Dlz}(\mathbf{U}(\gamma_1, \gamma_1), E_2, P_2)$.

(3)* $\mathbf{G}(\mathbf{L}_{E_1}(\mathbf{U}(\gamma_1, \gamma_1))) \subset \gamma_1$ and $\mathbf{G}(\mathbf{L}_{E_2}(\mathbf{U}(\gamma_1, \gamma_1))) \subset \gamma_2$.

(4) $\mathbf{Dlz}(\mathbf{U}(\gamma_2, \gamma_2), E_1, P_2)$.

(5) $\mathbf{G}(\mathbf{L}_{E_1}(\mathbf{U}(\gamma_2, \gamma_2))) \subset \gamma_2$.

Thus not only does $\mathbf{U}(\gamma_1, \gamma_1)$ yield P_2 in E_2 instead of P_1, but the gametes produced by a P_2 in an E_2 differ from those produced by a P_1 in an E_1 in such a way that, when zygotes are formed by union of members of this new set, they develop into members of P_2, even in environments belonging to E_1. Moreover, these members of P_2 go on producing such gametes in E_1. This, I think, is the possibility which Lamarckians believe actually happens.†

But this scheme can be extended. Let us enlarge our list of phenotypes to the sequence $P_1, P_2, \ldots, P_n$ such that for any P_i, P_j $(i, j = 1, 2, \ldots, n)$ if $i < j$ then P_j is superior in a certain respect to P_i, and let us similarly enlarge our collection of gamete sets to $\gamma_1, \gamma_2, \ldots, \gamma_n$. Then the above process could be continued as follows:

For any k such that $1 < k < n$,

(6) $\mathbf{Dlz}(\mathbf{U}(\gamma_k, \gamma_k), E_1, P_k)$ and $\mathbf{Dlz}(\mathbf{U}(\gamma_k, \gamma_k), E_2, P_{k+1})$ and $\mathbf{G}(\mathbf{L}_{E_2}(\mathbf{U}(\gamma_k, \gamma_k))) \subset \gamma_{k+1}$.

(7) $\mathbf{Dlz}(\mathbf{U}(\gamma_{k+1}, \gamma_{k+1}), E_1, P_{k+1})$, $\mathbf{G}(\mathbf{L}_{E_1}(\mathbf{U}(\gamma_{k+1}, \gamma_{k+1}))) \subset \gamma_{k+1}$.

In this way we should have what might be called *galloping evolution* or the Lamarckian's Dream.

But does anything of this sort happen? The orthodox answer among students of genetics is an emphatic No! But is orthodoxy always a virtue in natural science? Have not important advances frequently been made by people who have challenged the current orthodoxies? We are not really in a position to say that nothing

---

* I omit the subscript after G when it is the same as that after an immediately following L.

† As I am not acquainted with a Lamarckian I have not been able to test this hypothesis.

satisfying the Lamarckian hypothesis does or can happen. All we can say is that so far, when claims of this kind have been carefully tested experimentally, the results have not been such as to convince biologists. Neither can we confidently dismiss such claims merely on the basis of current genetical theory. Genetics is not a very old-established science, and, as the history of physics shows, even old-established theories sometimes require drastic revision. The fact that environmentally insensitive phenotypes have played such a large part in the building up of genetical theory should make us cautious. Perhaps if more environmentally sensitive phenotypes were studied the orthodox attitude would be different. Clearly, if someone claims to have actually found an instance satisfying the Lamarckian hypothesis, his claim can only be rejected after his experiments have been repeated. Until such experiments have been carried out discussion and vituperation on either side are useless and irrelevant. I hope this neutral attitude, which is the only one becoming a methodologist, especially an ignorant one, will not be interpreted as concealed propaganda. It is not intended to be.*

§ 6. CAUSAL LAWS IN GENETICS

I turn now to the examination of such expressions as '...determines...', or '...is due to...'. The chief objection to such expressions is that they once more commit us to trying to state with the help of a functor of degree 2 something that can usually

---

* The imaginary process depicted in the text is admittedly rather shocking. It is shocking because it violates the doctrine of the stability of genes. But this doctrine *may* be based too exclusively on experiments with environmentally insensitive phenotypes (in the sense explained in the text). Moreover, the stability of genes is not absolute even for orthodox genetics, otherwise there would be no evolution at all, except cytoplasmic evolution which itself is unorthodox. In any event the establishment of an instance of Lamarckism would in no sense involve the rejection of traditional genetics; it would merely involve a slight restriction on its generality. It is therefore difficult to understand why these discussions engender so much heat. The current controversy is complicated by the peculiarities of the Russian propaganda technique (which is referred to in Appendix C, p. 338) but the theoretical notions relating to genetics of recent Russian writers also seem to be rather woolly.

only be properly expressed by means of a functor of degree higher than 2. In other words these expressions will also lead to failure to satisfy Venn's requirement. What has already been said at some length about the functor **Dlz** is already an example of this. If someone says 'Sunburn is due to ultra-violet rays', he is speaking about a phenotype or about the Boolean sum of many phenotypes which are of the kind I have called environmentally sensitive. For this is a case where the adult environmental ranges of the zygote sets concerned are *not* contained in the sunburn environmental ranges. He is therefore in danger of forgetting that different people sunburn to different degrees with the same dosage of ultra-violet rays, and that correlated with this there may well be differences between the zygotes from which they have developed. This is an example of what Venn calls 'the capricious way in which the popular estimate picks out some one circumstance, and regards this as the cause, or at least calls it so'. In some contexts such rough-and-ready procedure will suffice; in others it is quite insufficient.

When the expression 'Z determines W' is used there seems to be a tendency to suppose that it means that the occurrence of a member of Z is a *sufficient* condition for the occurrence of a member of W. The following considerations illustrate this: In moths it is usually found that zygotes which contain a pair of chromosomes of the kind designated by X, Y develop, in any member of their adult environmental range, into females; and zygotes which contain a pair belonging to the set X, X develop, in such environments, into males. This is sometimes expressed by saying that X, X determines males and X, Y determines females. But then intersexes were discovered among moths of the genus *Lymantria*; that is to say, moths developed from both X, Y-containing zygotes and from X, X-containing zygotes which were *intermediate* between typical males and typical females. Referring to this Sinnott and Dunn write:

How can the occurrence of such individuals be reconciled with the theory that sex is determined at fertilization by the chance distribution of X and Y chromosomes to different gametes and different individuals? This theory provides for only two alternatives, that is, XX and XY, whereas in cases of intersexuality there appear to be several additional and intermediate possibilities.*

Now it seems clear that, only if the occurrence of X, Y is supposed to be a *sufficient*† condition for the development of females and of X, X for males, will there be any need for reconciliation of theory with observation, for otherwise there would be no conflict. Clearly the theory has been wrongly formulated. For when we recall that there are many parts in a zygote besides X and Y chromosomes, and when we remember that these zygotes must develop in an environment of some sort, we see that we have neglected Venn's requirement and that some of these neglected other factors may also be involved in the so-called 'determination of sex'. The use of the abbreviator Dlz and the composition functor will enable us to avoid all these difficulties. This may be illustrated by the following example provided by *Drosophila melanogaster*, where there are not two but six sexes according to the ratio of X-chromosomes to autosomes. If we use $2A$ as an abbreviation for

$$A_1, A_1, A_2, A_2, A_3, A_3,$$

and $3A$ as an abbreviation for

$$A_1, A_1, A_1, A_2, A_2, A_2, A_3, A_3, A_3,$$

where A_1, A_2 and A_3 are the three sets of autosomes for F and M in this animal, we can depict the composition of the zygotes and express the relevant embryological laws as follows (using 'K' to denote the Boolean sum of the sets of cytoplasms and 'E' the set of environments involved):

$$Dlz(C(S, C(Q, 2A, X, X, X), K), E, \text{super-female}),$$

$$Dlz(C(S, C(Q, 3A, X, X, X), K), E, \text{triploid female}),$$

$$Dlz(C(S, C(Q, 2A, X, X), K), E, \text{diploid female}),$$

---

* *Principles of Genetics* (1939), p. 259.
† See p. 153.

$$\mathbf{Dlz}(\mathbf{C}(\mathbf{S}, \mathbf{C}(\mathbf{Q}, 3A, \mathbf{X}, \mathbf{X}), K), E, \text{intersex}),$$

$$\mathbf{Dlz}(\mathbf{C}(\mathbf{S}, \mathbf{C}(\mathbf{Q}, 2A, \mathbf{X}, \mathbf{Y}), K), E, \text{male}),*$$

$$\mathbf{Dlz}(\mathbf{C}(\mathbf{S}, \mathbf{C}(\mathbf{Q}, 3A, \mathbf{X}, \mathbf{Y}), K), E, \text{super-male}).*$$

Let me give you an example of the horrible muddles which some authors get into in this connexion through the use of the phrase 'so-and-so determines so-and-so'. One well-known author I have in mind begins by saying that 'the genes controlling sex are carried in a special pair of chromosomes called "sex-chromosomes"', and that 'the remaining chromosomes, collectively known as "autosomes", are not directly concerned in actual sex-determination"'. He also speaks of the X-chromosomes as 'the actual agents deciding which sex shall develop'. Next he says that the genes 'carried in the X-chromosomes are female-determining, while others, in the autosomes, are male-determining', in spite of the fact that he has said that autosomes are *not* directly concerned in 'actual' sex-determination. Finally, he says that 'the sex-genes carried in the X-chromosomes act as the deciding elements in *sex-determination*, others equally responsible for the *development* of sex are carried in the autosomes'.

I hope you will agree with me, and not think I am being unduly fussy, when I say that this is very confusing for a student and that genetics has not got a language which is worthy of it. In this example the muddle is made rather worse by the use of such anthropomorphic phrases as 'controlling', 'deciding' and 'responsible', but the chief source of confusion is the inadequacy of the phrase 'determining' to do the work required of it.†

This is also an example of the violation of the constant factor principle. It is found by experiment that the corresponding pairs of maximized and mutually relativized autosome sets which are represented in sex systems and in genetical products

---

* 'Y' may be omitted.

† The distinction between 'sex-determination' and 'the development of sex' seems to indicate that the author is aware of the muddle, but the distinction is not discussed and it is not at all clear how it avoids the difficulty.

of such systems with other systems, although they may be mutually exclusive with respect to many other phenotypes, are nevertheless not mutually exclusive with respect to **F** and **M**. We may say therefore that with respect to sex they are genetically equivalent, so long as their *proportions* relatively to members of **X** remain constant. Accordingly, by the constant-factor principle, so long as this is the case we can say nothing about their role in the development of males and females. But the use of the composition functor serves to remind us of their presence and of the possibility that they may be involved in these processes.

The expressions 'determines' and 'due to', like 'the cause of', belong to the popular vocabulary. If we have a suitable notation for expressing embryological and genetical laws, such as **Dlz** and the genetical equations, there is no need to use these expressions in strict scientific contexts.*

§ 7. CYTOPLASMS IN GENETICS

I have several times remarked that there are three fundamental factors to be considered in any genetical problem for any phenotype P such that $\mathbf{H}(P) \neq \Lambda$, namely, $\mathbf{N}(P)$, $\mathbf{E}(P)$ and $\mathbf{K}(P)$. We have now seen the reasons why $\mathbf{E}(P)$ has sometimes been neglected by geneticists. Now we come to the reasons why $\mathbf{K}(P)$ has been neglected, and not only been neglected but also sometimes made the subject of uncomplimentary remarks.

The reasons why geneticists have neglected cytoplasms is very easy to understand—they have had no other alternative. For the vast majority of genetical systems so far studied are purely nuclear systems, and, as we have seen, if $P_1, P_2, ..., P_n$ are the phenotypes in a nuclear system such that for each P_i we have $\mathbf{H}(P_i) \neq \Lambda$, then if we take any two such phenotypes P_i

---

* A good example of the unscientific use of 'cause' is provided by the following passage from an embryological work: 'These results brought final confirmation of the view that the underlying of the dorsal ectoderm by the mesoderm is the full, perfect and sufficient cause for its determination for neural differentiation.' The author cannot possibly mean what he says because it clearly contradicts the doctrine of competence which is far from his intention.

and P_j such that $P_i \cap P_j = \Lambda$ we shall find $N(P_i) \cap N(P_j) = \Lambda$ but $K(P_i) = K(P_j)$. Consequently, by the constant-factor principle, such systems can teach us nothing about the role of the cytoplasms. They provide no basis for any sort of remarks about cytoplasms, complimentary or uncomplimentary.

Even in sex systems, although in addition to having $N_m \cap N_{m'} = \Lambda$ we also have $K_f \cap K_m = \Lambda$ (see p. 149), yet *each* zygote receives a contribution from a member of K_f and a member of K_m, so that, although the gametes can differ with respect to their cytoplasms, the zygotes of the system do not fall into two or more mutually exclusive sets with respect to their cytoplasms. Consequently such systems tell us absolutely nothing about the *separate* role of K_f and K_m.

These considerations seem to me to invalidate arguments of a certain type which we find very frequently in genetical books and which are exemplified by the following:

> The very common fact that the offspring of reciprocal crosses... are usually identical indicates that for most hereditary characters the influence of male and female gametes is equivalent; and since the nuclei of sperm and egg are equivalent, whereas their cytoplasmic contents differ (being practically absent in the sperm), this has served as a convincing argument that genetic similarities and hereditary variations are in general due to nuclear factors.

Quite apart from the fact that this passage contains such phrases as 'hereditary characters' and 'hereditary variations' and 'due to' which are not at all clear to me, I must confess that I find its argument very far from convincing. The cytoplasms of egg and sperm may differ as much as you please, but so long as each zygote receives a contribution from each, and so long as we are testing zygotes—not egg and sperm separately—then we can learn nothing about the role of the cytoplasm in the experiments concerned. All that reciprocal crossing teaches in this connexion is that it is a matter of indifference whether a zygote receives its contribution from K_f accompanied by a nucleus of kind Z (say) while it receives its contribution from K_m accompanied by a nucleus of kind W, *or* whether it receives its member of $\mathbf{K}_f$ accompanied by a W and its member of $\mathbf{K}_m$ accompanied by a Z.

Here then is another example of the violation of the constant-factor principle: because in nuclear systems the cytoplasmic sets concerned are all identical, we are not at all entitled to say that cytoplasms 'play no part' in genetical processes.*

To these remarks about cytoplasms the following may be added. Not only is there in the overwhelming majority of genetical systems so far investigated only one maximized set of cytoplasms involved (the nucleo-cytoplasmic system furnished by the pond snail *Limnaea* being one of the very few exceptions), but we should expect this to be so even for larger taxonomic groups, which do not constitute genetical systems at all because breeding within them is impossible. The reason for this is as follows: development, we may say, has a magnifying effect in the following sense. If we throw a circle of light on to a screen by means of a projection lantern and disturb it in any way by placing an opaque object in the beam, the nearer the object is to the lantern the greater will be the blackened area on the screen. Something analogous happens in development; the effect of any departure from normal development on the adult will, in general and allowing for such exceptions as are presented by the regulative eggs, be the greater the earlier the departure from normal takes place. Now we have embryological generalizations of observation records which suggest the hypothesis that the cytoplasmic organization of the zygote is very important in the early differentiation process. The nuclei of the early blastomeres, however, are not believed to differ with respect to the developmental processes at this stage. In consequence of this it is not to be expected that there will be great differences between the cytoplasms, even in zygotes belonging to different species or even to different genera. Because lives so closely related in the taxonomic system do not, in general, differ in their early develop-

---

* Corresponding remarks of course apply, in relation to such systems, to other parts of cells described by cytologists, e.g. to centromeres and parts of chromosomes which are not believed to have genes as parts.

ment. On the other hand, with wider taxonomic separation we should expect cytoplasmic differences. But these could not be investigated by present genetical methods on account of the absence of interbreeding. It seems clear then that cytoplasms, no less than those genes which are operative in early development, must be conservative factors. Any great deviation from normal in cytoplasmic organization would tend to wreck development completely. *Limnaea* provides an exception because a change from right coiling to left coiling of the shell does *not* involve wreckage of the whole developmental process.

The question remains: 'Is this conservative cytoplasmic organization of zygotes wholly formed anew in each female reduction cell, or does a foundation for it persist by successive duplications over the divisions which separate each zygote from the reduction cells to which it stands in $\mathbf{D}_{po}$?' To this question, which is a very difficult one, we cannot yet claim to give an answer supported by experiment.*

§ 8. IDENTITY IN GENETICS

Regarding confusions connected with the use of 'identity' (which I have included in my black list) the following remarks may here be added to what has already been said. When once we have recognized the distinction between individuals and sets of individuals we should not be in any difficulty about the distinction between identity of individuals and identity of sets. The set X is identical with the set Y if and only if every member of X is a member of Y and every member of Y is a member of X (see Statement 3 in Note 2, p. 201). By contrast, identity between individuals can have two meanings. We may mean strict identity, as when we say Paris is identical with the capital of France (in which case we are speaking about one individual object, not about two), or we may mean identity *in certain respects*. In the latter case we do not mean that the individual *objects* are identical in the strict sense, but that the *respects* are identical in that sense or are

* See Note 18, p. 218.

indistinguishable. This can be expressed from the extensional or set-theoretical standpoint as follows (to give first a simple illustration). Suppose X is the set of all black objects, Y the set of all objects made of iron and Z the set of all objects which weigh 2 lb. Then to say that my kettle a and my poker b are identical with respect to, or relatively to, X, Y and Z is simply to say that $a \in X$ and $b \in X$, $a \in Y$ and $b \in Y$ and $a \in Z$ and $b \in Z$. To say simply that two objects x and y are identical can only mean (if we do not mean strict identity) that there is *some* (at least one) X such that $x \in X$ and $y \in X$. When we say that x and y are identical twins we mean (in addition to asserting that they are twins) either (1) that there is a natural number n greater than zero, and certain specifiable sets $X_1, X_2, ..., X_n$ such that x and y are both of them members of each of these n sets, and that n is greater than the corresponding number for non-identical twins; or (2) that there is a zygote u and environments v and w such that $v \neq w$ and $\mathbf{dlz}(u, v, x)$ and $\mathbf{dlz}(u, w, y)$. That is to say that the zygote from which x developed is strictly identical with that from which y developed. One is a definition on zero level and the other on level 1 of our genetical analysis.

Often the relativization which is necessary in order to make quite clear what is meant in asserting an identity is not a simple matter of enumerating the sets with respect to which there is common membership, but is much more complicated. I have already explained that we can say that two zygotes x and y are *developmentally* identical if there is a zygote set X, an environmental set Y and a phenotype P such that $\mathbf{Dlz}(X, Y, P)$ and x and y both belong to X. This is developmental identity with respect to Y and P, although x and y do not themselves belong to Y and P.

Correspondingly, *genetical* identity (between individual objects) will involve reference to mating descriptions, some phenotype and some environmental set. Thus we can say that two lives are genetically identical with respect to a phenotype P if they both belong to $\mathbf{H}(P)$ or if there is a phenotype Q and both lives belong to $\mathbf{Ht}(P, Q)$. Here there is an implicit relativization to an

environmental set, namely, $\mathbf{E}(P)$, and an implicit reference to
a mating description, through the definition of $\mathbf{H}(P)$ or that of
$\mathbf{Ht}(P, Q)$. With the same reservations we can say that two
zygotes are genetically identical with respect to P if they both
belong to a set X of zygotes which is developmentally homo-
geneous with respect to $\mathbf{E}(P)$ and to $\mathbf{H}(P)$ or $\mathbf{Ht}(P, Q)$. Similarly,
two gametes will be genetically identical with respect to P if
they both belong to $\mathbf{Gm}(P)$. And so on for members of sets of
nuclei, $\mathbf{N}(P)$, sets of cytoplasms $\mathbf{K}(P)$, sets of chromosomes
$\chi_S(P)$ and sets of genes $\Gamma_S(P)$. But identity between individuals
seems to be of less importance than identity between sets,
because in genetical literature, when the notion of identity is
used, it is usually sets that are being referred to (see end of
Note 8, p. 209).

§ 9. CONCLUSION OF PART II

In attempting a brief summary of this part of my lectures let
me remind you that I have been concerned primarily not with
the subject-matter of genetics but with its language. I have
shown that it is possible to construct a genetical language which
is more analytical than those commonly in use and is consequently more explicit. It enables us to attain a considerable
degree of precision and to avoid completely certain expressions
which have been troublesome in the past. If I have sometimes used more symbols than may have seemed to be necessary,
this is because I have wanted my constructions to be useful
for methodological analysis (and for that purpose they must
be genuine biological statements, rather than mathematical
formulas accompanied by biological explanations), and also
because I have wanted to satisfy Venn's requirement. I do not
at all wish to deny that for many purposes of rapid calculation
it is often possible to work satisfactorily with *ad hoc* symbols.
But it is very useful for careful formulations to have precisely
defined sets, such as $\mathbf{H}(P)$, $\mathbf{N}(P)$, etc., as functions of any phenotype P. This language has made it possible not only to offer

analytical definitions of intuitive notions in common use, but also some new ones, such as allelic index, environmental range, environmentally sensitive phenotype, etc. A considerable part has been played by the Boolean operations on sets, especially addition and multiplication, and use has been made of their laws. With their help we have been able to construct the combined algebra. This has been possible on account of the purely extensional procedure which was explained in the earlier lectures and which has been consistently adhered to. I strongly believe that if biologists would make themselves acquainted with the elements of the theory of sets they would find it very useful.

I have shown that the language here developed has a comparatively slender minimum vocabulary and provides hints for a possible future axiomatization of genetical theory. It enables us not only to argue but to calculate, not only to differ but to see precisely where and how we differ. If I have seemed too fussy over details, or if I have confined myself to topics which geneticists have long left behind (as my ignorance compels me to do), I would remind you that we are laying the foundations of a new science of genetical methodology and we must not grudge the effort needed to make them secure.*

* The reader must not suppose that what is offered here claims to be in any sense complete. I have done most of the spade-work that is needed as far as the foundations are concerned and I believe I have overcome most of the difficulties connected with that. But I do not at all claim that my formulations of these foundations are the best possible ones. A beginning has been made, that is all. The present formulation (all its predecessors having been rejected) is the last of many attempts, so many in fact that I have long lost count of the number. It is therefore the product of a great deal of hard work, not a casually composed or hastily constructed scheme. But there is plenty of scope for discussion about the suitability of some of the basic definitions, and there is an enormous amount of working out and elaboration to be done. Moreover, little has been done from the purely cytological aspect and its precise connexion with the genetical remains to be analysed. But this can only properly be done by experts who have some understanding of the results of the Boole-Frege movement. This first attempt at a methodological analysis of genetics will have fulfilled more than its original purpose if it stimulates some geneticist into an attempt to axiomatize the subject.

NOTES TO PART II

Note 1 (p. 99). See J. B. S. Haldane, art. 'Heredity', *Encyclopedia Britannica* (ed. 14), vol. II, p. 485. Regarding other uses of the word 'genotype', for reasons which will be clear from what was said in Part I, I do not find such statements as the following very illuminating:

(i) 'While the chromosomes contain the 'something' which we identify with the genotype they themselves cannot be directly identified with it.'

(ii) 'Genotype: the kind or type of the hereditary properties of an individual organism.'

For a further discussion of this difficult topic see p. 167.

Note 2 (p. 97). The following note on the Boolean operations and their laws will supplement the brief explanations given in the text.

Inclusion. A set X is said to be included in a set Y (written $X \subset Y$) if and only if every member of X is a member of Y. The *complement* of a set X (written $\overline{X}$) is the set of all objects in the universe of discourse which do not belong to X. Thus we have

$$X = \overline{\overline{X}}.$$

(The universe of discourse of a theory is the set of all objects which are regarded as individuals (as opposed to sets) in that theory.)

The *Null* set (Λ) for a given universe of discourse is the set which has no members. Its complement (V) is the universe of discourse itself. For any sets X, Y and Z the following hold:

(1)　$X \subset X.$　　　(2)　$\Lambda \subset X$ and $X \subset V.$

(3)　If $X \subset Y$ and $Y \subset X$ then $X = Y.$

(4)　If $X \subset Y$ and $Y \subset Z$ then $X \subset Z.$

Boolean *Sum* and *Product*. The Boolean sum of X and Y (written $X \cup Y$) is the set of all objects which belong to X or to

Y or to both. The Boolean product of X and Y (written $X \cap Y$) is the set of all objects which belong both to X and to Y:

$(5a)$ $\quad X \cap X = X.$

$(5b)$ $\quad X \cup X = X.$

$(6a)$ $\quad X \cap Y = Y \cap X.$

$(6b)$ $\quad X \cup Y = Y \cup X.$

$(7a)$ $\quad X \cap (Y \cap Z) = (X \cap Y) \cap Z.$

$(7b)$ $\quad X \cup (Y \cup Z) = (X \cup Y) \cup Z.$

$(8a)$ $\quad X \cap (Y \cup Z) = (X \cap Y) \cup (X \cap Z).$

$(8b)$ $\quad X \cup (Y \cap Z) = (X \cup Y) \cap (X \cup Z).$

$(9a)$ $\quad \Lambda \cap X = \Lambda.$

$(9b)$ $\quad \Lambda \cup X = X.$

$(10a)$ $\quad V \cap X = X.$

$(10b)$ $\quad V \cup X = V.$

$(11a)$ $\quad X \cap \bar{X} = \Lambda.$

$(11b)$ $\quad X \cup \bar{X} = V.$

$(12a)$ $\quad \overline{X \cap Y} = \bar{X} \cup \bar{Y}.$

$(12b)$ $\quad \overline{X \cup Y} = \bar{X} \cap \bar{Y}.$

In spite of the fact that Boolean algebra was invented over 100 years ago, two recent writers have found it desirable to remark that

...few people are aware that there is a consequential algebra of classes. This is not surprising, as the full importance of this algebra has been recognized only very recently, even by professional mathematicians. (G. Birkhoff and S. MacLane, *A Survey of Modern Algebra*, 1947.)

As the sequel will show, Boolean algebra is very useful in genetics.

Readers interested in the application of other algebraical methods to genetical problems are referred to the following:

L. Hogben, 'A matrix notation for Mendelian populations', *Proc. Roy. Soc. Edinb.* (1933), vol. LIII, pp. 8–25.

I. M. H. Etherington, 'On the non-associative combinations', *Proc. Roy. Soc. Edinb.* (1939), vol. LIX, pp. 153–62; 'Genetic algebras', *Proc. Roy. Soc. Edinb.* (1939), vol. LIX, pp. 242–58; 'Non-associative algebra and the symbolism of genetics', *Proc. Roy. Soc. Edinb.* (1941), vol. LXI, pp. 24–42.

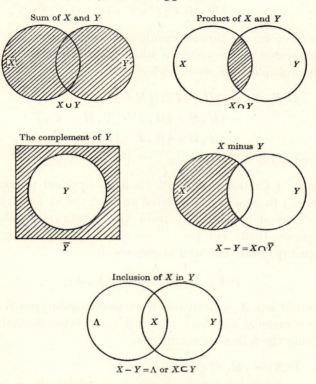

Boolean operations on sets illustrated by sets of points.

In each of the four upper diagrams the set referred to is indicated by shading.

In the bottom diagram the area marked 'Λ' is supposed to have no members. X thus reduces to $X \cap Y$.

Note 3 (p. 101). No biological example is given in the text of the use of the combined Cartesian product. By way of a simple example the following is offered. Suppose $X \times Y$ is a set of throws of *two* unbiased coins thrown *successively*, members of

X being those thrown first, and members of Y those thrown second. Then using 'H' to denote the set of throws of heads and 'T' for that of tails we should have

$$D(X \times Y) = (\tfrac{1}{2}H + \tfrac{1}{2}T) \mathbin{\dot{\times}} (\tfrac{1}{2}H + \tfrac{1}{2}T),$$
$$= \tfrac{1}{4}H \times H + \tfrac{1}{4}H \times T + \tfrac{1}{4}T \times H + \tfrac{1}{4}T \times T.$$

But if the coins are thrown simultaneously, or supposing we are not interested in the order in which they fall, then combined simple multiplication would suffice:

$$D(X, Y) = (\tfrac{1}{2}H + \tfrac{1}{2}T) \mathbin{;} (\tfrac{1}{2}H + \tfrac{1}{2}T)$$
$$= \tfrac{1}{4}H, H + \tfrac{1}{4}H, T + \tfrac{1}{4}T, H + \tfrac{1}{4}T, T$$
$$= \tfrac{1}{4}H, H + \tfrac{1}{2}H, T + \tfrac{1}{4}T, T$$

(because $H, T = T, H$).

The use of Cartesian multiplication (as opposed to combined Cartesian) in genetics is referred to in Note 11 (p. 210). The term 'Cartesian' is taken from C. Kuratowski's *Topologie* (Warszawa, 1933), vol. I.

Note 4 (p. 105). The well-known result

$$D(\mathbf{F}_E(X, X)) = D(\mathbf{F}_E^2(X, X))$$

for certain sets X, is derivable if we have phenotypes P and Q, positive rational numbers p and q and environmental set E satisfying the following conditions:

(1) $D(X) = p\mathbf{H}(P) + q\mathbf{H}(Q)$,

(2) $p + q = 1$,

(3) $\mathbf{H}(P) \cup \mathbf{H}(Q) \cup \mathbf{Ht}(P, Q)$ is a genetical system of allelic index (2) and $E = \mathbf{E}(P) = \mathbf{E}(Q)$,

(4) $\mathbf{H}(P) \cup \mathbf{H}(Q) \cup \mathbf{Ht}(P, Q)$ is equiproductive with respect to $\mathbf{F}_E$, (see p. 106), and mating is random within X,

and if we have

D. 4, D. 11, D. 12 and T. 8 of combined algebra.

The assumption of random mating has played a great part in modern discussions within the theory of evolution. In this connexion the following considerations may be of interest.

First I must explain what I mean by the *ecological trumpet* of a life x. Consider a worm-like organism x living on a flat plane. At any given moment which intersects the whole time-extent of x (which I call the complete life x) it must be somewhere within a circle with the place of birth or hatching, $\mathbf{B}(x)$, of x as its centre and having a radius dependent upon the locomotor capacities of x from birth (or hatching) onwards. It cannot exceed a distance which would be reached if x had exerted its locomotory powers to the utmost and in a straight line from birth (or hatching) onwards. Now consider the locus of all space-time points falling on or within all such circles. If we wish to represent this locus in a space-time diagram we can do so as follows:

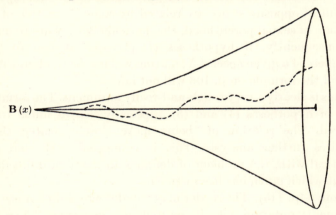

This locus I call the ecological trumpet of x. The straight line represents the place of birth (or hatching) of x throughout the time-extent of x, and the dotted line represents x itself in its meanderings within its trumpet. For the sake of simplicity I have assumed that the magnitude of the trumpet depends only on the unaided efforts of x itself. If x is picked up by a bird and dropped alive at a distance which it could not otherwise have reached its trumpet would have been larger.

Now consider the following hypotheses:

(1) The more likely two lives x and y of the same species X but of opposite sexes are to meet, the more likely they are to mate.

(2) The more the ecological trumpets of two lives, x and y, intersect, the more likely x and y are to meet.

(3) The nearer the birth (or hatching) places of two lives, x and y, are to one another, the more their ecological trumpets will intersect.

(4) The closer two lives x and y are related by some derivative of the relation $\mathbf{Ps}$ of sexual parenthood (e.g. $\breve{\mathbf{Ps}} \mid \mathbf{Ps}$, $\breve{\mathbf{Ps}} \mid \mathbf{Ps}^2$, $\breve{\mathbf{Ps}}^2 \mid \mathbf{Ps}$, $\breve{\mathbf{Ps}}^2 \mid \mathbf{Ps}^2$, etc.),* the nearer their places of birth or hatching will be.

From (1)–(4) it will follow that

(5) The closer two lives x and y belonging to the same species X, but of opposite sexes, are related by some derivative of the relation of sexual parenthood, the more likely they are to mate.

Consequently, if hypotheses (1)–(4) are satisfied for the members of a given species X, mating will not be random within X and the formula on p. 106 will not hold for X.

This is clearly a very rough-and-ready argument. The formulation of hypotheses (4) and (5), especially, leaves much to be desired. The relation of 'being more closely related than' requires further analysis. This is connected with, but not identical with, the problem of defining an index of inbreeding, about which much has been written.

Note 5 (p. 115). The reader may wonder why I do not use the customary notation AA, Aa, aa to denote genotypes. There are various reasons. The chief reason is that I am seeking the maximum generalization possible. The above expressions are perfectly satisfactory, no doubt, when we are dealing with some particular example; but in general we see that genotype designations must be relativized to a phenotype and an environmental set. Moreover, although the above notation suffices so long as

* For the stroke sign in $\breve{\mathbf{Ps}} \mid \mathbf{Ps}$ see Part III, Note 1, p. 320. For the cup sign $\cup$ see Appendix B, p. 222.

the allelic index is (2), it does not lend itself to the general case of allelic index (n), with $n > 2$. Finally, it is not at *all* times clear exactly what 'AA', etc., denote (see text, p. 165).

Note that the genetical equation

$$D(\mathbf{F}_X^2(\mathbf{H}(P), \mathbf{H}(Q))) = \tfrac{3}{4}P + \tfrac{1}{4}Q \tag{1}$$

takes the place of such schemata as

$$
\begin{array}{c}
P \times Q \\
| \\
P(Q) \times P(Q) \\
| \\
\end{array} \tag{2}
$$

$$\tfrac{1}{4}P \qquad \tfrac{1}{2}P(Q) \qquad \tfrac{1}{4}Q$$

The reasons for preferring (1) to (2) in some contexts are: (*a*) that (1) is a statement, whereas (2) is a diagram; (*b*) that (1) is completely explicit and can stand alone if the definitions for D, $\mathbf{F}_X$ and H have been formulated; (*c*) that (1) occupies one line and (2) occupies four; (*d*) that (1) distinguishes explicitly between phenotype designations and genotype designations and does not use the former in places where only the latter are appropriate; (*e*) that (1) contains an explicit reference to the environmental set; and (*f*) that (1) can be used for the purpose of calculation.

Note 6 (p. 124). There are systems of allelic index (2) (2) which are not *visibly* genetical products of two systems each of allelic index (2). Consider, for example, S($\mathbf{W}, \mathbf{R}, \mathbf{P}, \mathbf{S}$), where $\mathbf{W}$ is the set of all fowls with Walnut combs, $\mathbf{R}$ the set of all those with Rose combs, $\mathbf{P}$ that of all those with Pea and $\mathbf{S}$ that of all those with Single combs. It is found that $\mathbf{W}$ contains one homozygous, two singly heterozygous and one doubly heterozygous genotype, $\mathbf{R}$ and $\mathbf{P}$ each contain one homo- and one singly heterozygous genotype, and $\mathbf{S}$ only contains one homozygous genotype. The partition is therefore (4, 2, 2, 1). This system is isomorphic with the system S($\mathbf{Y}, \mathbf{G}$) $\times$ S($\mathbf{R}, \mathbf{W}$) described in the text. We can therefore say that S($\mathbf{W}, \mathbf{R}, \mathbf{P}, \mathbf{S}$) has allelic index (2) (2) not because it is the product of two systems each of allelic index (2), but because it is isomorphic with such a system. We could of course construct the embryological hypothesis that we have four phenotypes P_1, P_2, Q_1 and Q_2, each specified by reference to a distinct developmental process and such that

$$S(\mathbf{W}, \mathbf{R}, \mathbf{P}, \mathbf{S}) = S(P_1, P_2) \times S(Q_1, Q_2),$$

each factor system being of allelic index (2) and

$$P_1 Q_1 = \mathbf{W}, \quad P_1 Q_2 = \mathbf{R}, \quad P_2 Q_1 = \mathbf{P} \quad \text{and} \quad P_2 Q_2 = \mathbf{S}.$$

Note 7 (p. 142). Quite generally we can say that a genetical system S with environmental set E is of order m, if and only if there are m systems of order 1:

$$S_1 = \mathbf{L}_E\left(\mathbf{U}\left(\sum_1^{n_1} \alpha_{1i}, \sum_1^{n_1} \alpha_{1i}\right)\right),$$

$$S_2 = \mathbf{L}_E\left(\mathbf{U}\left(\sum_1^{n_2} \alpha_{2i}, \sum_1^{n_2} \alpha_{2i}\right)\right),$$

$$\vdots$$

$$S_m = \mathbf{L}_E\left(\mathbf{U}\left(\sum_1^{n_m} \alpha_{mi}, \sum_1^{n_m} \alpha_{mi}\right)\right),$$

and
$$S = \mathbf{L}_E\left(\mathbf{U}\left(\prod_{j=1}^m \sum_{i=1}^{n_j} \alpha_{ji}, \prod_{j=1}^m \sum_{i=1}^{n_j} \alpha_{ji}\right)\right),$$

the summation and multiplication being Boolean.*

The allelic index of S will be a distribution of $n_1, n_2, \ldots n_m$, among k pairs of brackets, k being the number of linkage groups.

Note 8 (p. 125). The notion of environment as here conceived may be explained with the help of the Minkowski cone-diagram. If $y = \mathbf{en}(z)$† then y will be the sum (in the sense defined on p. 64 of my *Axiomatic Method in Biology*) of the set of all places which are neither before nor after the beginning of z in time (but excluding that beginning itself) and from which it is possible for a physical signal to reach some part of the time-extent of z. Its magnitude will therefore depend on the time-length of z, and

---

* For Batesonian systems of order greater than 2 it is necessary to use Cartesian multiplication (see Note 11, p. 210). With mixed systems it would be Boolean between some factors, Cartesian between others, if the order is greater than 3.

† See p. 127.

the velocity of light. The following postulates governing the relation **En** are here adopted:

[P. 1] If x**En**y and z**En**y, then $x = z$.

[P. 2] If $y =$ **en**(z), then **B**$(z) \neq$ **E**(z). (Here '**E**(z)' denotes the end of z.)

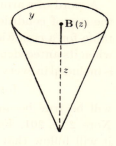

[P. 3] If $y =$ **en**(z), then **B**(z) and y have no parts in common.

[P. 4] If **en**$(z) =$ **en**(w), then $z = w$.

[P. 5] If $y =$ **en**(z) and $x =$ **en**(w), then z is part of w if and only if y is part of x.

With the definition of **dlz** given in the text and the postulates for **En** given here, the following will be theorems:

(1) $(x)(y)(z)(w)$ (if **dlz**(x, y, z) and **dlz**(x, y, w) then $z = w$).

(2) $(x)(y)(z)(w)$ (if **dlz**(x, y, z) and **dlz**(x, w, z) then $y = w$).

In current biological writing individuals and sets are not clearly distinguished, and language appropriate to the former is frequently used when the latter are intended. For example, we read in a work on genetics that

if a zygote receives the same gene from each germ-cell, the individual produced from it is said to be homozygous for that gene.

Since a zygote cannot possibly receive the same individual gene from each gamete it is obvious that a certain *set* of genes is intended (see text, p. 199, and Note 7, Part I, p. 63).

In the following passage it is not so obvious which is intended:

A number of such changes may sometimes occur in the same gene and so form a series of multiple allelomorphs.

(When geneticists speak of multiple allelomorphs they are referring (usually) to a genetical system of allelic index (n) where $n > 2$.)

Note 9 (p. 129). Notice that we do not have

(z) (if $z \in P$ then $(\exists x)(\exists y)($**dlz**(x, y, z) and $x \in Z$ and $y \in E))$.

This is in case members of P may arise in other ways, from zygote sets of kinds other than Z and in environments other than those belonging to E. If it is desired to exclude this possibility, then the above clause must be added.

A word of warning should be uttered here in connexion with the use of conditionals in definitions. Reference to the truth-table for a conditional statement (p. 35) shows that it is true when its antecedent is false. It is for this reason that the null set is included in every set, for, whatever set X may be, the statement

$$\text{for all } x, \text{ if } x \in \Lambda \text{ then } x \in X$$

will be true because '$x \in \Lambda$' is false. Consequently $\Lambda \subset X$, see Note 2, p. 201. For the same reason with our definition D. 29 it will follow that $\mathbf{Dlz}(\Lambda, E, P)$ and $\mathbf{Dlz}(Z, \Lambda, P)$ whatever sets Z, E and P may be. It is for this reason also that such definitions as D. 32 are dangerous. It is always possible to add to the set α in this definition terms which would make the antecedent of the conditional which is implicit in this definition false and would thus still satisfy the definition. The set α would thus become unduly large and would contain all manner of objects (e.g. some which were not gametes at all) which are not wanted in the set $\mathbf{Gm}(P)$.

Note 10 (p. 136). By way of an example of a genetical system for which condition (β) holds but condition (α) does *not* hold, consider a system of allelic index (2)

$$S = \mathbf{L}_E(\mathbf{U}(\alpha \cup \beta, \alpha \cup \beta)),$$

and suppose every member of $\mathbf{U}(\alpha, \alpha)$ and every member of $\mathbf{U}(\alpha, \beta)$ produces *two* lives of the same time-length in members of E, but every member of $\mathbf{U}(\beta, \beta)$ produces only *one*. Then putting

$$A' = \mathbf{L}_E(\mathbf{U}(\alpha, \alpha)), \quad A'' = \mathbf{L}_E(\mathbf{U}(\alpha, \beta)), \quad B' = \mathbf{L}_E(\mathbf{U}(\beta, \beta)),$$

we should have

$$D(\mathbf{F}_E(A'', A'')) = \tfrac{2}{7}A' + \tfrac{4}{7}A'' + \tfrac{1}{7}B'$$

and

$$D(\mathbf{F}_E(B', A'')) = \tfrac{1}{3}B' + \tfrac{2}{3}A''$$

in place of the customary frequencies when condition (α) holds.

Note 11 (p. 142). In Batesonian systems of order greater than 2 the order in which the factors are written down becomes significant. Thus if S is of order 3 and $S = S_1 \times S_2 \times S_3$, and if the recombination value for S_1 and $S_2 = p$, that for S_1 and $S_3 = q$ and that for S_2 and $S_3 = r$, it is found that $q \leqslant p + r$. It is then said that S_2 is 'between' S_1 and S_3. On level 1 the order between the terms in each gamete-set product can be depicted and preserved by the use of *Cartesian* multiplication (see p. 101) instead of Boolean. Thus if the system is of allelic index $(2, 2, 2)$ and $(\alpha \cup \beta)$, $(\gamma \cup \delta)$ and $(\eta \cup \theta)$ are the Boolean sums of the gamete sets of S_1, S_2 and S_3 respectively, we can describe the system on level 1 by

$$S = \mathbf{L}_E(\mathbf{U}((\alpha \cup \beta) \times (\gamma \cup \delta) \times (\eta \cup \theta), (\alpha \cup \beta) \times (\gamma \cup \delta) \times (\eta \cup \theta))).$$

Note 12 (p. 172). In this connexion see H. Geiringer, (1) 'On the probability theory of linkage in Mendelian heredity', *Ann. Math. Statist.* (1944), vol. xv, pp. 25–57; (2) 'Further remarks on linkage theory in Mendelian heredity. On the definition of distance in the theory of the gene', *Ann. Math. Statist.* (1945), vol. xvi, pp. 390–8.

Note 13 (p. 149). The genetical product of a sex system with a genetical system of allelic index (2) is easily obtained.* Suppose for example

$$S_1 = \mathbf{L}_E(\mathbf{U}(\mathbf{f}, (\mathbf{m} \cup \mathbf{m}'))) = \mathbf{F} \cup \mathbf{M},$$

Then
$$S_2 = \mathbf{L}_E(\mathbf{U}(\alpha \cup \beta, \alpha \cup \beta)) = P' \cup P'' \cup Q'.$$

$$S_1 \times S_2 = \mathbf{L}_E(\mathbf{U}((\alpha \cup \beta) \cap \mathbf{f}, (\alpha \cup \beta) \cap (\mathbf{m} \cup \mathbf{m}')))$$
$$= \mathbf{L}_E(\mathbf{U}(\alpha \mathbf{f}, \alpha \mathbf{m} \cup \beta \mathbf{f}, \alpha \mathbf{m} \cup \alpha \mathbf{f}, \alpha \mathbf{m}' \cup \beta \mathbf{f}, \alpha \mathbf{m}' \cup \beta \mathbf{f}, \beta \mathbf{m} \cup \beta \mathbf{f}, \beta \mathbf{m}'))$$
$$= P' \mathbf{F} \cup P'' \mathbf{F} \cup P' \mathbf{M} \cup P'' \mathbf{M} \cup Q' \mathbf{F} \cup Q' \mathbf{M}.$$

If we now put $\alpha \mathbf{m}' = \beta \mathbf{m}' = \mathbf{m}'$, the above becomes

$$S_1 \times S_2 = \mathbf{L}_E(\mathbf{U}((\alpha \cup \beta) \cap \mathbf{f}, (\alpha \cup \beta) \cap (\mathbf{m} \cup \mathbf{m}')))$$
$$= \mathbf{L}_E(\mathbf{U}(\alpha \mathbf{f}, \alpha \mathbf{m} \cup \beta \mathbf{f}, \alpha \mathbf{m} \cup \beta \mathbf{f}, \beta \mathbf{m} \cup \alpha \mathbf{f}, \mathbf{m}' \cup \beta \mathbf{f}, \mathbf{m}'))$$
$$= P' \mathbf{F} \cup P'' \mathbf{F} \cup Q' \mathbf{F} \cup P' \mathbf{M} \cup Q' \mathbf{M},$$

which is a system exhibiting one of the forms of sex linkage.

Note 14 (p. 41). In my *Technique of Theory Construction* (1939), a beginning was made towards constructing (for the purpose of illustrating the thesis of that book) a biological theory on the basis of only three undefined signs: '**P**' (denoting the relation *part of*), '**T**' (denoting the relation of precedence in time) and '**cell**' (denoting the set of all cells). If to this modest

---

* For the notation P', P'', etc., see p. 118.

set of primitives we add 'En' (as explained in the text), we can define a great many of the genetical functors that have here been used. The definability relations between these functors is shown on the accompanying chart. But if we substitute the 'S' of Part II for 'cell' the latter becomes definable.* If we add the 'Q' and 'R' of the text the resulting set, P, T, En, S, Q and R, provides a very powerful minimum vocabulary. Whether 'phenotype' is definable on this basis (or is perhaps not necessary), and whether 'En' is definable with the help of 'P' and 'T', are questions about which I have not yet reached a decision.

I will now give some definitions (which are not given in the text) in support of the claims made in the chart. $B(x)$ is explained in the text; '$E(x)$' denotes the corresponding last time-slice of x. Both of these are defined in the monograph mentioned above. The relation F ('xFy' meaning that x is one of the cells which have fused to form the cell y) is also defined (together with D) in the monograph. The following are defined below (some of them appear in the text as undefined signs for reasons which were there explained):

(1) $u(x, y) = the$ cell z such that xFz and yFz and $x \neq y$ and there is no cell w such that wFx or wFy. (This functor thus denotes the zygote formed by the union of x with y. The last clause is added to exclude endosperm cells in flowering plants.)

(2) $U(X, Y) = $ the set of all cells z such that for some x and some y, $x \in X$ and $y \in Y$ and $z = u(x, y)$.†

(3) $dlz(x, y, z)$ if, and only if, for some u and some $v, x = u(u, v)$, $B(x) = B(z)$ and $y = en(z)$. (A more general relation, not confining x to the set of zygotes, could also be defined.)

---

* I have since discovered that it is possible to define 'cell' by means of 'P' and 'T'. This is an example of a reduction of a biological sign to physical ones (in the narrow sense of 'physical').

† Professor Quine has kindly drawn my attention to the fact that, for technical reasons, it would be more correct to define '$U(X, Y)$' as follows:

$U(Z) = $ the set of all cells z, such that for some X, some Y, some x and some y, $Z = X$, Y and $x \in X$ and $y \in Y$ and $z = u(x, y)$.

The same applies to '$F_{X, Y, Z}(W, U)$'. But as I have never had occasion to use a single dummy name in the brackets of these functors I have allowed the above definitions to stand.

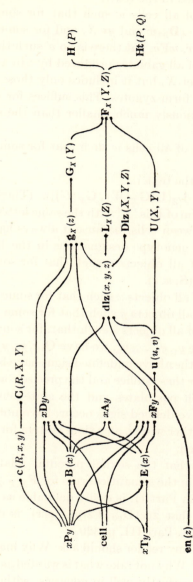

Chart showing the definability relations between some biological functors and abbreviators

Where a line runs from one functor or abbreviator and ends with a dot at another, this indicates that the former is used in the definition of the latter. The functor 'A' is discussed in Part III. **Dlz** is an abbreviator, the remaining signs are functors.

(**Dlz**(X, Y, Z) is defined in the text.)

(4) $\mathbf{\dot{g}}_X(z) =$ the set of all cells w such that for some x and some y, **dlz**(x, y, z) and $x\mathbf{D}_{\text{po}}w$ and $y \in X$, and for some u, $u\mathbf{P}w$ and $u\mathbf{P}z$, and for some v, $w\mathbf{F}v$, but there is no v' such that $v'\mathbf{F}w$. (Thus $\mathbf{\dot{g}}_X(z)$ is the set of all gametes produced by z in a member of the environmental set X, but it includes only those gametes which actually fuse to form zygotes. This suffices for genetical purposes, but it is obviously much smaller than the set of all cytologist's gametes.)

(5) $\mathbf{G}_X(Y) =$ the set of all cells w such that for some z, $z \in Y$ and $w \in \mathbf{\dot{g}}_X(z)$.

($\mathbf{L}_X(Z)$ is defined in the text.)

(6) $\mathbf{F}_{X, Y, Z}(W, U) = \mathbf{L}_Z(\mathbf{U}(\mathbf{G}_X(W), \mathbf{G}_Y(U)))$. (There should be no danger of confusion of this '**F**' with the same letter used for the fusion relation between cells, because it always has at least one subscript and two genotype designations in the brackets.)

(7) **cell** = the set of all objects x such that for some u and some v, $u\mathbf{S}v$ and $x = \mathbf{c}(\mathbf{S}, u, v)$.

(8) **nuc** = the set of all objects x such that for some y, $x\mathbf{S}y$.

(9) **cyt** = the set of all objects y such that for some x, $x\mathbf{S}y$.

(10) **chr** = the set of all objects x such that, for some natural number $n > 0$ and some $y_1, y_2, ..., y_n$, we have $\mathbf{Q}(x, y_1, y_2, ..., y_n)$.

Some postulates for the above undefined signs have been given in the text; but how far these suffice and the precise consequence relations between such postulates and the statements in the text, in which the above-defined signs occur, have not yet been fully worked out. In other words, an axiom system for them has not yet been established.

(It may be added that the sexual parental relation (**Ps**), which was mentioned in the semantical rule for $\mathbf{F}_{X, Y, Z}$ but does not otherwise appear in Part II, is easily definable as the set of all couples x, y such that $\mathbf{z}(x)\,\mathbf{D}_{\text{po}}\,|\,\mathbf{F}\mathbf{z}(y)$. '$\mathbf{z}(x)$' is defined on p. 127, and '$|$' in Note 1, Part III, p. 320.)

Note 15 (p. 152). If any reader should ask: Why make all this fuss about definitions? Why not take what is wanted as undefined signs? We get along perfectly well in genetics, without definitions, so why worry? My answer would be this: It is a question of interest. I am interested in reducing the number of unanalysed ideas in genetics. I want to discover the minimum set of undefined signs which will suffice for genetics. Unanalysed notions are a nuisance in so far as you do not know what they commit you to. If you can analyse them and express the result in a definition with the help of a satisfactory set of undefined signs, then you *do* know what they commit you to. (Incidentally, the story of the **X**- and **Y**-chromosomes illustrates this point to perfection.) This is part (but only part) of the use of definitions and of the aim of methodological analysis. To realize such aims we must construct a language which will differ in some respects from one which suffices for other purposes. With reference to what was said in Part I (p. 8) about the resemblance between language and dress, we may say that using a language which is suitable for methodological analysis for situations in which an untamed language suffices is like playing tennis in evening dress; and using an untamed language for methodological analysis is like attending a state ball in tennis kit. In neither case does this mean that one equipment is superior to the other in any absolute sense. Each is appropriate to its own purpose. If you are not interested in methodological analysis you need not concern yourself with the problem of whether your language is suitable for it, just as you need not provide yourself with evening dress if you are not interested in state balls and similar functions.

Note 16 (p. 174). Concealed genetical systems:

A. Nucleo-cytoplasmic:

Phenotypes (included in the monoecious species *Limnaea peregra*):*

> **D** snails with dextrally coiled shells,
> **S** snails with sinistrally coiled shells,
> Δ snails producing female gametes of kind δ,
> Σ snails producing female gametes of kind σ,
> $$(\mathbf{D}\cup\mathbf{S})\cap(\Delta\cup\Sigma) = \mathbf{D}\Delta\cup\mathbf{S}\Delta\cup\mathbf{D}\Sigma\cup\mathbf{S}\Sigma.$$

* See Boycott, Diver, Garstang and Turner, *Phil. Trans. Roy. Soc.* (1930), B, vol. ccxix, pp. 51–131.

Common maximized environmental set: **E**.

Gamete-sets: Male **d∪s**,

Female $(\mathbf{d}\cup\mathbf{s})\cap(\delta\cup\sigma) = \mathbf{d}\delta\cup\mathbf{s}\delta\cup\mathbf{d}\sigma\cup\mathbf{s}\sigma.$

(Members of sets **d** and **s** are distinguished by their nuclei, those of sets δ and σ by their cytoplasms.)

Genotypes: $\mathbf{L_E}(\mathbf{U}(\mathbf{d}\cup\mathbf{s}\,,(\mathbf{d}\cup\mathbf{s})\cap(\delta\cup\sigma)))$

$= \mathbf{L_E}(\mathbf{U}(\mathbf{d},\mathbf{d}\delta\cup\mathbf{s},\mathbf{d}\delta\cup\mathbf{s},\mathbf{s}\delta\cup\mathbf{d},\mathbf{d}\sigma\cup\mathbf{d},\mathbf{s}\sigma\cup\mathbf{s},\mathbf{s}\sigma)).$

Embryological laws:

$\mathbf{Dlz}(\mathbf{U}(\mathbf{d}\,,\mathbf{d}\delta),\mathbf{E},\mathbf{D}\Delta),$	$\mathbf{Dlz}(\mathbf{U}(\mathbf{d}\,,\mathbf{d}\sigma),\mathbf{E},\mathbf{S}\Delta),$
$\mathbf{Dlz}(\mathbf{U}(\mathbf{s}\,,\mathbf{d}\delta),\mathbf{E},\mathbf{D}\Delta),$	$\mathbf{Dlz}(\mathbf{U}(\mathbf{d}\,,\mathbf{s}\sigma),\mathbf{E},\mathbf{S}\Delta),$
$\mathbf{Dlz}(\mathbf{U}(\mathbf{s}\,,\mathbf{s}\delta),\mathbf{E},\mathbf{D}\Sigma),$	$\mathbf{Dlz}(\mathbf{U}(\mathbf{s}\,,\mathbf{s}\sigma),\mathbf{E},\mathbf{S}\Sigma).$

Gamete-set frequencies:

$$\left.\begin{array}{l}\mathbf{G}(\mathbf{L_E}(\mathbf{U}(\mathbf{d}\,,\mathbf{d}\delta)))\\ \mathbf{G}(\mathbf{L_E}(\mathbf{U}(\mathbf{d}\,,\mathbf{d}\sigma)))\end{array}\right\} \subset \quad \begin{array}{cc}\text{Female} & \text{Male}\\ \mathbf{d}\delta & \mathbf{d}\end{array}$$

$$\mathbf{D}(\mathbf{G}(\mathbf{L_E}(\mathbf{U}(\mathbf{s}\,,\mathbf{d}\delta)))) = \mathbf{D}(\mathbf{G}(\mathbf{L_E}(\mathbf{U}(\mathbf{d}\,,\mathbf{s}\sigma)))) = \tfrac{1}{2}\mathbf{s}\delta + \tfrac{1}{2}\mathbf{d}\delta \ \tfrac{1}{2}\mathbf{d}+\tfrac{1}{2}\mathbf{s}$$

$$\left.\begin{array}{l}\mathbf{G}(\mathbf{L_E}(\mathbf{U}(\mathbf{s}\,,\mathbf{s}\delta)))\\ \mathbf{G}(\mathbf{L_E}(\mathbf{U}(\mathbf{s}\,,\mathbf{s}\sigma)))\end{array}\right\} \subset \qquad \mathbf{s}\sigma \qquad \mathbf{s}$$

Some mating descriptions:

$$\mathbf{F_E}(\mathbf{L_E}(\mathbf{U}(\mathbf{d}\,,\mathbf{d}\delta))\,,\ \mathbf{L_E}(\mathbf{U}(\mathbf{s}\,,\mathbf{s}\sigma)))\subset\mathbf{L_E}(\mathbf{U}(\mathbf{d}\delta\,,\mathbf{s}))$$

or $\mathbf{L_E}(\mathbf{U}(\mathbf{d}\,,\mathbf{s}\sigma))$ (according to which parent is male),

$$\mathbf{D}(\mathbf{F_E}(\mathbf{L_E}(\mathbf{U}(\mathbf{d}\,,\mathbf{s}\delta))\,,\ \mathbf{L_E}(\mathbf{U}(\mathbf{d}\,,\mathbf{s}\delta))))$$

$$= \tfrac{1}{4}\mathbf{L_E}(\mathbf{U}(\mathbf{d}\,,\mathbf{d}\delta)) + \tfrac{1}{2}\mathbf{L_E}(\mathbf{U}(\mathbf{d}\,,\mathbf{s}\delta)) + \tfrac{1}{4}\mathbf{L_E}(\mathbf{U}(\mathbf{s}\,,\mathbf{s}\delta)),$$

$$\mathbf{F_E}(\mathbf{L_E}(\mathbf{U}(\mathbf{s}\,,\mathbf{s}\delta))\,,\ \mathbf{L_E}(\mathbf{U}(\mathbf{d}\,,\mathbf{s}\delta)))\subset\mathbf{L_E}(\mathbf{U}(\mathbf{s}\,,\mathbf{s}\sigma)).$$

B. Nucleo-environmental (imaginary example):

Phenotypes:

G, green butterflies; Y, yellow butterflies; P, butterflies which lay their eggs on food plant occurring in environment E_1.

Q, butterflies which lay their eggs on food plant occurring in environment E_2.

$$G\cap Y = P\cap Q = E_1\cap E_2 = \Lambda,$$

$$(G\cup Y)\cap(P\cup Q) = GP\cup YP\cup GQ\cup YQ.$$

Put $E = E_1 \cup E_2$.

Gamete sets: $p \cup q$.

Embryological laws:

$$\mathbf{Dlz}(\mathbf{U}(p,p), E_1, PG), \quad \mathbf{Dlz}(\mathbf{U}(p,p), E_2, PY),$$
$$\mathbf{Dlz}(\mathbf{U}(p,q), E_1, PG), \quad \mathbf{Dlz}(\mathbf{U}(p,q), E_2, PY),$$
$$\mathbf{Dlz}(\mathbf{U}(q,q), E_1, QG), \quad \mathbf{Dlz}(\mathbf{U}(q,q), E_2, QY).$$

Gamete-set frequencies:

$$\mathbf{G}(\mathbf{L}_E(\mathbf{U}(p,p))) \subset p, \quad \mathbf{D}(\mathbf{G}(\mathbf{L}_E(\mathbf{U}(p,q)))) = \tfrac{1}{2}p + \tfrac{1}{2}q,$$
$$\mathbf{G}(\mathbf{L}_E(\mathbf{U}(q,q))) \subset q.$$

Some mating descriptions:

$$\mathbf{F}_E(\mathbf{L}_{E_1}(\mathbf{U}(p,p)), \mathbf{L}_{E_2}(\mathbf{U}(q,q))) \subset \mathbf{L}_{E_1}(\mathbf{U}(p,q))$$

(if $\mathbf{L}_{E_1}(\mathbf{U}(p,p))$ is female),

$$\mathbf{D}(\mathbf{F}_E(\mathbf{L}_{E_1}(\mathbf{U}(p,q)), \mathbf{L}_{E_1}(\mathbf{U}(p,q))))$$
$$= \tfrac{1}{4}\mathbf{L}_{E_1}(\mathbf{U}(p,p)) + \tfrac{1}{2}\mathbf{L}_{E_1}(\mathbf{U}(p,q)) + \tfrac{1}{4}\mathbf{L}_{E_1}(\mathbf{U}(q,q)),$$

$$\mathbf{F}_E(\mathbf{L}_{E_1}(\mathbf{U}(q,q)), \mathbf{L}_{E_1}(\mathbf{U}(q,q))) \subset \mathbf{L}_{E_2}(\mathbf{U}(q,q)),$$
$$\mathbf{F}_E(\mathbf{L}_{E_1}(\mathbf{U}(q,q)), \mathbf{L}_{E_1}(\mathbf{U}(p,p))) \subset \mathbf{L}_{E_2}(\mathbf{U}(p,q)).$$

Note 17 (p. 181). That W. Johannsen was aware of the linguistic difficulties of genetics is well illustrated by the following extracts from his paper 'The genotype conception of heredity' in *Amer. Nat.* (1911), vol. XLV, pp. 129–59:

Biology has evidently borrowed the terms 'heredity' and 'inheritance' from everyday language, in which the meaning of these words is the '*transmission*' of money or things, rights or duties—or even ideas and knowledge—from one person to another or to some others: the 'heirs' or 'inheritors' (p. 129).

The view of natural inheritance as realized by an act of transmission, viz. the transmission of the parent's (or ancestor's) *personal qualities* to the progeny, is the most naïve and oldest conception of heredity. We find it clearly developed in Hippocrates (p. 129).

But no profound insight into the biological problem of heredity can be gained on this basis, for the transmission-conception of heredity represents exactly the reverse of the real facts (p. 130).

It is a well-established fact that language is not only our servant, when we wish to express—or even conceal—our thoughts, but that it may also be our master, overpowering us by means of the notions attached to current words. This fact is the reason why it is desirable to create a new terminology in all cases where new or revised conceptions are being developed. Old terms are mostly compromised by their application in antiquated or erroneous theories and systems, from which they carry splinters of inadequate ideas, not always harmless to the developing insight (p. 132).

Note 18 (p. 174). See P. and G. Michaelis, 'Über die Konstanz des Zytoplasmons bei *Epilobium*' in *Planta, Arch. wiss. Bot.* (1948), Bd. xxxv, Heft 5/6, S. 467–512.

This paper is summarized as follows:

Überblickt man nun nochmals die hier an mehr als 100 Rückkreuzungslinien festgestellten Beobachtungen, so kann kein Zweifel darüber bestehen, dass ausserhalb des Zellkernes, im Protoplasma, noch weitere Erbträger lokalisiert sein müssen. Nachdem eine mütterliche Übertragung bestimmter Reaktionsnormen wenigstens in einem Falle über mindestens 24 Generationen, in zahlreichen anderen Fällen über mehr als 10 Generationen (vgl. Tabelle 1, S. 470) bewiesen ist, ist die Berechtigung gegeben, als Symbol für diese plasmatischen Erbträger den Begriff 'Plasmon' (v. Wettstein) zu verwenden. Durch die Versuche ist weiterhin das Vorkommen zahlreicher verschiedener Plasmone bei *Epilobium* belegt. Gleichzeitig konnten berechtigte Gründe dafür angeführt werden, dass auch in solchen Fällen das Plasmon von Bedeutung ist, in denen der Nachweis von Plasmonunterschieden bisher misslang. An dem Vorhandensein und an der Bedeutung der Plasmavererbung kann kein Zweifel mehr bestehen.

See also *The Elements of Genetics*, by C. D. Darlington and K. Mather (1949), Chapter 9.

Experiments on sea-urchin eggs in which nuclei from distinct species are exchanged do not bear on the point raised in the text (p. 197), because the cytoplasm of the egg is already fully elaborated in the presence of a nucleus of its own species. Even if such experiments could be performed on the primary oocyte they would not be decisive.

APPENDIX B

SOME LINGUISTIC AIDS TO THE
STUDY OF EVOLUTION

The progress of the art of rational discovery, depends in part on the art of characteristic (*ars characteristica*). The reason why people usually seek demonstrations only in numbers and lines and things represented by these is none other than that there are not, outside numbers, convenient characters corresponding to the notions. (Leibniz.)

It was not until 131 years after the death of Leibniz that Boole's first work was published; and then another thirty-two years were to pass before Frege published his *Begriffschrift*. To-day, 234 years after Leibniz's death, it is high time we began to make use of the work of these men and their successors in order to 'seek demonstrations' in biology. This appendix will show how a beginning can be made in relation to evolutionary problems.*

What is set forth in this appendix began with an attempt to reconcile two seemingly conflicting features of evolution and classification. In the first place we have Darwin's emphasis on the *gradualness* of evolution. He estimated that it required some 1000 generations to pass from one variety to another, and some 10,000 generations to pass from one species to another, and correspondingly greater numbers for the larger taxonomic categories. But when I came to reflect upon the matter it seemed to me that one must pass from one taxonomic category (small or large) into another in *one* generation, in the sense that there must be at least two organisms, x and y, such that x is parent of y, and x belongs to one category, say a species or genus, and y to

---

* In saying this I am not at all forgetting the splendid work that has been done by Professors Fisher, Haldane and S. Wright in seeking demonstrations in relation to evolutionary problems with the help of traditional mathematics. I am only urging that this work should be extended to all aspects of these problems with the help of non-traditional mathematics.

another distinct from the first. How is this to be reconciled with Darwin's 10,000 generations?

A second point is this. The taxonomic system is usually depicted as a system of taxonomic categories or sets such that, if we take any two of them, either the one is wholly contained in the other, or they have no members in common. Thus the Carnivora and the Ungulata are both contained in the Mammalia, but the Carnivora and the Ungulata have no member in common. But if we consider the taxonomic sets in their time-extent and in connexion with the notion of gradualness of evolution, must there not be overlapping of some sort? At the present day the Amphibia and the Reptilia have no members in common, but will not evolutionary considerations force us to assume that at some time in the past they had members in common? This leads to the problem: What exactly do the systems of branching lines represent which we sometimes find in biological books under the name 'phylogenetic trees'?

That was my starting-point. But as the work progressed I found that I was creating a postulate system analogous to those we find in geometry. And just as in geometry we have different geometries according to the way we make our choice of postulates, so we shall have different theories of evolution according to our choice of evolutionary postulates. Our problem is ultimately to find at least one set of postulates which is consistent with all the data we possess about evolutionary processes. No attempt to find such a set will be made here, only a few postulates will be proposed for the purpose of illustration and discussion.

In setting about this task I have found it necessary to develop a special branch of set theory which I call the theory of the joining of sets by one-one relations with finite fields. To begin with we must therefore forget about evolution and concentrate on these preliminaries. Their relevance to evolution will become clear later.

First I must explain what I mean by a one-one relation with a finite field. Consider the accompanying list of ordered couples of natural numbers. Let us call this set the relation K. The fact that the couple 1, 2 belongs to this set can be expressed by writing $1K2$ which may be read ' 1 stands in K to 2'. The set of single numbers, 1, 2, 3, 4, 5, 6, 7 and 8, is called the *field* of K (written $C(K)$). It will be noticed that each member of the field stands in K to *one* other member of the field at most, and each member of the field has at most *one* other member of the field standing in K to it. For this reason K is called a one-one relation (written $K \in 1 \to 1$). This is also true of the next set of couples which we can call L and which is a sub-set of K. But there is an important difference between K and L which is expressed by saying that K has *one and only one first* and *one and only one last* term. The first term or beginner of K (written $B(K)$) is that member of its field which has no term standing in K to it, and the last term is that member of its field which stands in K to nothing (written $B(\breve{K})$; see below). L has four beginners and four enders.

1, 2
2, 3
3, 4
4, 5
5, 6
6, 7
7, 8

1, 2
3, 4
5, 6
7, 8

K has a third feature which is very important in the sequel. Owing to the fact that its field is finite it is possible to pass from

Table to illustrate the powers of K, K_{po} and K_*

K^0	1, 1	2, 2	3, 3	4, 4	5, 5	6, 6	7, 7	8, 8
K	1, 2	2, 3	3, 4	4, 5	5, 6	6, 7	7, 8	
K^2	1, 3	2, 4	3, 5	4, 6	5, 7	6, 8		
K^3	1, 4	2, 5	3, 6	4, 7	5, 8			
K^4	1, 5	2, 6	3, 7	4, 8				
K^5	1, 6	2, 7	3, 8					
K^6	1, 7	2, 8						
K^7	1, 8							

$$K_{po} = K \cup K^2 \cup K^3 \cup K^4 \cup K^5 \cup K^6 \cup K^7$$
$$K_* = K^0 \cup K \cup K^2 \cup K^3 \cup K^4 \cup K^5 \cup K^6 \cup K^7$$

the first term to all the remaining members of the field by a succession of K-steps—from 1 to 2, from 2 to 3, and so on. This is expressed by saying that 1 stands in K_{po} to every member of the field but itself. K_{po} is the relation of standing in some *power* of K to something. K itself is the first power of K, 1 stands in the second power of K (K^2) to 3, and so does 2 to 4. 1 stands in the third power of K (K^3) to 4, in the fourth (K^4) to 5 and so on. K_{po} is the Boolean sum of all the powers of K (excluding K^0). If we call identity in the field of K the zero power of K (writing it K^0) and add this to K_{po} we have a new relation called K_*. These notions are illustrated by the accompanying table.

We can also represent K by means of an arrow figure as follows: $1 \rightarrow 2 \rightarrow 3 \rightarrow 4 \rightarrow 5 \rightarrow 6 \rightarrow 7 \rightarrow 8$,

in which pairs belonging to K are connected by arrows. If we write down the pairs in reverse order,

$$8 \rightarrow 7 \rightarrow 6 \rightarrow 5 \rightarrow 4 \rightarrow 3 \rightarrow 2 \rightarrow 1,$$

we obtain another set of pairs called the converse of K (written $\breve{K}$). A term x is said to stand in $\breve{K}$ to a term y if yKx. It will be noticed that the last term of K is identical with the first of its converse and is therefore denoted by $B(\breve{K})$.

Another feature of our relation K is that no term stands in K to itself. For that reason K is said to be *irreflexive*. Moreover, it will be noticed that, when a term stands in K to another, the latter never stands in K to the former. For that reason K is said to be *asymmetrical*. Finally, if a term stands in K to a second and this in turn stands in K to a third term, then the first does not stand in K to the third. If it did, K would not be one-one. This is expressed by saying that K is *intransitive*. K_{po}, on the other hand, is transitive.

I have now explained what I mean by a one-one relation which is such that its first term stands in some power of the relation to its last term. As we shall frequently have occasion to speak about such relations it will be very desirable to have a name for them. In the present context I shall call them *lines*. As we shall not need to use the word in any other sense there will be no risk of ambiguity. The formal definition may be written:

[D. 1] $R \in$ line if and only if $R \in 1 \rightarrow 1$ & $B(R)\,R_{po}\,B(\breve{R})$.*

* Within the theory of shared and unshared names 'line' and '$1 \rightarrow 1$' would not be shared names but abbreviators. This applies to many of the defined signs in this appendix.

By way of an example of a relation which does *not* satisfy D. 1, although it is

Now I can explain what is meant by saying that a relation of this kind, a line, *joins* one set *to* another. I shall say that a line R joins a set X to a set Y if and only if the first term of R belongs to $X - Y$ and the last term of R belongs to $Y - X$. ($X - Y$ is another way of writing $X \cap \overline{Y}$, see Note 2, p. 201.) This I shall write $J(R, X, Y)$.

[D. 2] $J(R, X, Y)$ if and only if

$$B(R) \in X - Y \ \& \ B(\breve{R}) \in Y - X \ \& \ R \in \text{line}.$$

Thus, to go back to our example, suppose A is the set of all natural numbers less than 4, and B is the set of all natural numbers greater than 3, then K joins A to B, because its first term is less than 4 but not greater than 3 and its last term is greater than 3 and so not less than 4. The following are some consequences of the definitions:

[T. 1]   If $J(R, X, Y)$, then not $(X \subset Y) \ \& \ \text{not} \ (Y \subset X)$.

[T. 1.11]   If $J(R, X, Y)$, then $X - Y \neq \Lambda \ \& \ Y - X \neq \Lambda$.

[T. 1.12]   Not $J(R, X, X)$.

[T. 1.2]   If $J(R, X, Y)$, then $X \neq \Lambda \ \& \ X \neq V \ \& \ Y \neq \Lambda \ \& \ Y \neq V$.

[T. 1.3]   If $J(R, X, Y)$, then not $J(R, Y, X)$.

[T. 1.4] $J(R, X, Y)$ if and only if $J(\breve{R}, Y, X)$.

[T. 1.5] $J(R, X, Y)$ if and only if $J(R, X - Y, Y - X)$.

(T. 1.5 follows because $(X - Y) - (Y - X) = X - Y$ and $(Y - X) - (X - Y) = Y - X$.)

I shall say that a line R joins a set X to a set Y *directly* if and only if R joins X to Y and every member of the field of R belongs to X or to Y or to both. Thus

[D. 3] $Jd(R, X, Y)$ if and only if $J(R, X, Y) \ \& \ C(R) \subset X \cup Y$.

one-one and has a first and last term, consider the relation R defined as the relation in which an integer x (positive or negative but excluding zero) stands to an integer y (satisfying the same condition) when $y = x + 1$. Then the first term of R ($+1$) does not stand in R_{po} to the last term (-1).

I now pass to another notion, namely, the set of all R-steps *from* a set X *to* a set Y. I denote this set by $S(R, X, Y)$. I shall say that a couple x, y is an R-step from X to Y if and only if x stands in R to y and belongs to X and y belongs to Y.

[D. 4] $x, y \in S(R, X, Y)$ if and only if xRy & $x \in X$ & $y \in Y$.

In particular, $S(R, X, \overline{X})$ will be the set of all R-steps *out of* X and $S(R, \overline{Y}, Y)$ will be the set of all R-steps *into* Y.

The following are some consequences of these definitions:

[T. 2]   If $Jd(R, X - Y, Y - X)$, then $C(R) \cap ((X \cap Y) \cup (\overline{X} \cap \overline{Y})) = \Lambda$.

[T. 2.1]   If $Jd(R, X, Y)$ & $C(R) \cap X \cap Y = \Lambda$, then
$$Jd(R, X - Y, Y - X).$$

[T. 2.2]   If $Jd(R, X, Y)$ & $X \cap Y = \Lambda$, then $Jd(R, X - Y, Y - X)$.

[T. 3]   If $J(R, X, Y)$, then $S(R, X, \overline{X}) \neq \Lambda$ & $S(R, \overline{Y}, Y) \neq \Lambda$.

[T. 3.022] $S(R, X, \overline{X}) \cap S(R, \overline{Y}, Y) \subset S(R, X, Y)$.

[T. 3.032]   If $C(R) \cap X \cap Y = \Lambda$, then
$$S(R, X, Y) = S(R, X - Y, Y - X).$$

[T. 3.033]   If $C(R) \cap X \cap Y = \Lambda$, then
$$S(R, X, \overline{X}) \subset S(R, X - Y, \overline{X}) \text{ & } S(R, \overline{Y}, Y) \subset S(R, \overline{Y}, Y - X).$$

[T. 3.034]   If $C(R) \subset X \cup Y$, then
$$S(R, X, \overline{X}) \subset S(R, X, Y - X) \text{ & } S(R, \overline{Y}, Y) \subset S(R, X - Y, Y).$$

[T. 3.035]   If $C(R) \subset X \cup Y$ & $C(R) \cap X \cap Y = \Lambda$, then
$$S(R, X, Y) = S(R, X, \overline{X}) = S(R, \overline{Y}, Y) = S(R, X - Y, Y - X).$$

[T. 3.22]   If $Jd(R, X, Y)$ and $S(R, X - Y, Y - X) = \Lambda$, then
$$X \cap Y \neq \Lambda.$$

[T. 3.32]   If $Jd(R, X - Y, Y - X)$, then
$$S(R, X, \overline{X}) = S(R, \overline{Y}, Y) = S(R, X - Y, Y - X).$$

A set X is said to be *closed with respect to* a relation R if and only if, whenever we have a term x standing in R to a term y

which belongs to X, then x also belongs to X. In *Principia Mathematica* the set of terms which stand in R to members of X is denoted by $R``X$. Consequently closure with respect to $R$ can be expressed briefly by writing $R``X \subset X$.

A set Y will be said to be closed with respect to the *converse* of R if and only if, whenever we have a term x standing in R to a term y and belonging to Y, then y also belongs to Y. With the notation explained above this can be expressed by writing $\breve{R}``Y \subset Y$.

If X is closed with respect to R, then when once we are out of X by an R-step there is no returning by an R-step, and if Y is closed with respect to the converse of R, then when once we are in Y by an R-step there is no R-step out of Y. The condition of closure thus has the effect of ensuring uniqueness of steps in or out of a given set with respect to a given relation. This is expressed in the following statements, in which $Nc(\ )$ denotes the cardinal number of the set whose designation occurs in the brackets:

[T. 4]   If $J(R, X, Y)$ & $R``X \subset X$ & $\breve{R}``Y \subset Y$, then
$$Nc(S(R, X, \overline{X})) = Nc(S(R, \overline{Y}, Y)) = 1.$$

[T. 4.01]   If $R``X \subset X$, then $S(R, \overline{X}, X) = \Lambda$.

[T. 4.02]   If $\breve{R}``Y \subset Y$, then $S(R, Y, \overline{Y}) = \Lambda$.

I shall say that the couple x, y belongs to the *sum* of two lines R and S, or that x stands in $R + S$ to y, if and only if the last term of R is identical with the first term of S and x stands in R to y or in S to y.

[D. 5] $xR + Sy$ if and only if
$$R \in \text{line} \ \& \ S \in \text{line} \ \& \ B(\breve{R}) = B(S) \ \& \ xRy \text{ or } xSy.$$

Using $D(R)$ to denote the set of all terms which stand in R to something and $\mathrm{C}(R)$ for the set of all terms which have something standing in R to them, with corresponding designations for S, we can express the following consequences:

[T. 5]   If $D(R) \cap D(S) = \mathrm{C}(R) \cap \mathrm{C}(S) = \Lambda$, then $R + S \in 1 \rightarrow 1$.

[T. 5.11] $(R \breve{+} S) = \breve{S} + \breve{R}.$

[T. 5.12] If $R \epsilon$ line & $S \epsilon$ line & $B(\breve{R}) = B(S)$, then
$$B(R) = B(R + S) \,\&\, B(\breve{S}) = B(R \breve{+} S).$$

[T. 5.13] If $R \epsilon$ line & $S \epsilon$ line & $B(R) \neq B(\breve{S})$, then $R + S \neq S + R.$

[T. 5.14] If R, S and $Q \epsilon$ line, then $(R + S) + Q = R + (S + Q).$

[T. 5.15] If $J(R, X, Y) \,\&\, J(S, Y, Z) \,\&\, X \cap Z = \Lambda \,\&\, B(\breve{R}) = B(S)$, then $J(R + S, X, Z).$

The reader will be beginning to wonder when, if at all, we shall ever reach the theory of evolution. Soon I shall provide a bridge which connects this abstract set theory with the doctrine of evolution. But it will not be without interest, I hope, first to inquire a little into the variety of ways in which two sets can be joined by relations of the kind I have called lines.*

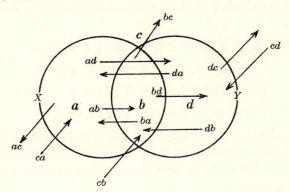

Consider two sets X and Y, and let us denote $X - Y$ by a, $X \cap Y$ by b, $Y - X$ by d and $\overline{X} \cap \overline{Y}$ by c. Let us also denote the set of all ordered couples whose first term belongs to $X - Y$ and whose second term belongs to $Y - X$ by ad, and their converses by da. Then ad will be the set of shortest possible lines which join X to Y. In the same way we can define the sets ab, ac; ba, bc, bd; and da, db, dc. Each of the four sub-sets of the universe

---

* The reader who is not interested in this problem should turn to p. 231.

of discourse has *three* sets of couples leading *out* of it, and their converses leading *into* it. Let us assign capital letters to these sets of sets of couples as follows:

$$A = ab, ac, ad; \quad B = ba, bc, bd; \quad C = ca, cb, cd; \quad D = da, db, dc.$$

A contains all (see top of p. 229) the three possible sets of initial couples for lines joining *X* to *Y*, and also the single set of terminal couples *ad*, since these are both terminal and initial. *B*, *C* and *D* have no set of initial couples. But *A*, *B* and *C* each have one set of terminal couples. *D* has no terminal couple.

By successive additions of couples chosen from the above sets, lines of great variety and infinite in number can be constructed, because additional couples can always be added and at each step there is always a choice of a couple from three possible sets. Addition can be expressed thus:

$$ab + bc = abc,$$
and
$$ab + bc + cd = abcd.$$

abc would be the set of all lines formed by adding a member of *bc* to one of *ab*; and *abcd* would be the set of all lines which are sums of three couples from *ab*, *bc* and *cd* respectively. Members of this set would join *X* to *Y*.

If we suppose all these couples to be sub-relations of some one relation *R*, then, if the following conditions are imposed on *R*, they will have the effect of limiting certain of the possible ways in which *X* can be joined to *Y*.

(1) If $R``X \subset X$ and $R``Y \subset Y$, we eliminate the couples *ba*, *ca* and *da* and also the couples *bc* and *db*. This has the effect of ensuring one-way traffic only from *X* to *Y*. It leaves only three sets of lines, *ad*, *abd* and *acd*.

(2) If $C(R) \subset X \cup Y$, we eliminate the couples *ac*, *bc* and *dc* and also *ca*, *cb*, *cd*, i.e. we eliminate the whole block *C* and its three sets of converses. This has the effect of confining traffic between *X* and *Y* to those sets themselves. It leaves couples belonging to the sets *ab*, *ad* and *da*, *db*. It therefore does not forbid oscillation backwards and forwards between *X* and *Y*.

(3) If we impose the condition expressed by

for all u and v, if uRv & $u \in X$ then $v \in \overline{Y}$,

we eliminate all couples belonging to ab, bd and ad. This only leaves the route by way of c. Thus conditions (2) and (3) are mutually exclusive. If (2) holds we can say that the lines join X to Y directly, if (3) holds we can say that they join X to Y indirectly.

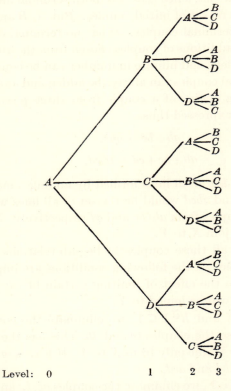

Level: 0   1   2   3

(4) If we impose the condition $C(R) \cap X \cap Y = \Lambda$, we eliminate the couples belonging to the sets ab, cb, db and to ba, bc and bd, thus the whole block B and its converses. This leaves the direct route ad open and also the route by way of c.

Let us say that a line which is composed of the sum of n

couples has length n, and let us consider now the number of possible ways in which X can be joined to Y by lines of a given length. In what follows I shall consider only those lines which are composed of couples of the above kinds, i.e. couples which lead out of one subset into another. Purely internal couples, like aa, bb, etc., will be ignored. Since A has all the sets of initial couples and these end only in members of b, c and d, any couple belonging to a set in A can only be followed by one of a set in B, C and D. In the same way we can say that B can only be followed by A, C and D; C only by A, B and D; and D only by A, B and C. Lines of increasing length thus have their terms in sets belonging to sets forming an infinite $1 \to 3$ hierarchy* formed of A, B, C and D, and having A as the single member of its zero level; B, C, D constituting its first level; A, C, D, and A, B, D, and A, B, C its second level and so on.

Now if, in an infinite $1 \to k$ hierarchy, each term belongs to one and only one of $k+1$ sets $X_1, X_2, ..., X_{k+1}$, and the immediate successors of each term belong to the sets to which that term does *not* belong, and if there are m terms belonging to a given set in level n, then there will be $k^n - m$ belonging to that set in level $n+1$.

Suppose the single member of level 0 belongs to the set X_i so that for $n = 0$ we have $m = 1$, then for *any* of the other sets X_j $(i \neq j)$ we shall have, for $n = 0$, $m = 0$ and in succeeding levels the values of m will be as shown in the following table:

n	X_i m	X_j m
0	1	0
1	$k^0 - 1$	$k^0 - 0$
2	$k - 0$	$k - 1$
3	$k^2 - k$	$k^2 - k + 1$
4	$k^3 - k^2 + k$	$k^3 - k^2 + k - 1$
⋮		
n	$k^{n-1} - k^{n-2} + ... - k$ (n odd)	$k^{n-1} - k^{n-2} + ... - k + 1$ (n odd)
n	$k^{n-1} - k^{n-2} + ... + k$ (n even)	$k^{n-1} - k^{n-2} + ... + k - 1$ (n even)

Taking X_i first, if we put

$$s = k^{n-1} - k^{n-2} + ... - k,$$

* See my *Axiomatic Method in Biology*, pp. 42–7.

then $$sk = k^n - k^{n-1} + \ldots - k^2,$$

and $$sk + s = k^n - k,$$

so $$s = \frac{k(k^{n-1} - 1)}{k+1} \quad \text{(for } n \text{ odd)},$$

similarly $$s = \frac{k(k^{n-1} + 1)}{k+1} \quad \text{(for } n \text{ even)}.$$

These formulas give the number of X_i in the nth level. In the same way, for X_j we obtain

$$s = k^{n-1} - k^{n-2} + \ldots - k + 1$$

$$= \frac{k^n + 1}{k+1} \quad \text{(for } n \text{ odd)};$$

and $$s = k^{n-1} - k^{n-2} + \ldots + k - 1$$

$$= \frac{k^n - 1}{k+1} \quad \text{(for } n \text{ even)}.$$

These give the number of X_j in the nth level.

Returning now to our hierarchy of A, B, C and D, it will be seen that $k = 3$ and that A corresponds to X_i and each of B, C and D corresponds to X_j.

Let us denote by $N_A(n)$ the number of A's in the nth level of the hierarchy, and by $N_B(n)$, $N_C(n)$ and $N_D(n)$ the corresponding numbers for B, C and D.

Let us use $N_{ad}(n)$ to denote the number of distinct kinds of line of length n which end in a member of ad. And let $N_{bd}(n)$ and $N_{cd}(n)$ have corresponding definitions for bd and cd. Then we shall have
$$N_{ad}(n) = N_A(n-1), \text{ etc.,}$$

and $$N_A(n-1) + N_B(n-1) + N_C(n-1) + N_D(n-1) = 3^{n-1},$$

so $$N_{ad}(n) + N_{bd}(n) + N_{cd}(n) = 3^{n-1} - N_D(n-1).$$

If we now denote the total number of lines of length n and ending in ad or bd or cd by $N(n)$, it will be seen that

$$N(n) = N_{ad}(n) + N_{bd}(n) + N_{cd}(n)$$

$$= 3^{n-1} - N_D(n-1);$$

but $$N_D(n+1) = 3^n - N_D(n),$$

so $$N_D(n) = 3^{n-1} - N_D(n-1),$$

and $$N(n) = N_D(n).$$

Applying the formula for X_j we obtain

$$N(n) = \tfrac{1}{4}(3^n + 1) \quad \text{(for } n \text{ odd)}$$
$$= \tfrac{1}{4}(3^n - 1) \quad \text{(for } n \text{ even),}$$

or, combining these into one formula,

$$N(n) = \tfrac{1}{4}(3^n + (-1)^{n-1}).$$

When the condition $C(R) \subset X \cup Y$ or the condition

$$C(R) \cap X \cap Y = \Lambda$$

is imposed the hierarchy reduces to a $1 \to 2$ hierarchy, because B is eliminated by the one condition and C by the other. Consequently we have

$$N(n) = \tfrac{1}{3}(2^n + (-1)^{n-1}).$$

The following table shows the values of these functions for values of n from 1 to 10:

	$N(n)$	
n	$1 \to 3$	$1 \to 2$
1	1	1
2	2	1
3	7	3
4	20	5
5	61	11
6	182	21
7	547	43
8	1,640	85
9	4,921	171
10	14,762	341

Thus X can be joined to Y by lines composed of the sum of only ten couples in 14,762 ways, exclusive of those which contain couples aa, bb, etc., which do not step out of one of the four sub-sets a, b, c and d.

So far we have been using a language which contains no word or other sign which is in any way characteristic of biology. I have spoken of sets in general, but not of sets of organisms or lives. What I have said about sets in general applies, however, to *any* sets and hence to sets of lives. To this bare skeleton of a language as it has so far been explained I now propose to add, one at a time, only three signs which belong to biology, in order to see how much can be said on this very meagre basis.

The first bridge to biology is provided by the *parental relation*. I denote this relation (in the present context) by '**P**', and by it I mean the set of all couples x, y such that x is parent of y. This relation is very complicated. An organism may have one or two parents, and in the former case the relation may be sexual or asexual. But in what I am about to say these complications fortunately will not arise. I shall make *one and only one* assumption about the relation **P**, namely, that $\mathbf{P}_{po}$ is irreflexive, in other words, that no organism is its own ancestor. I think it will be agreed that this is a very innocent and safe assumption, and one in which all biologists will concur. I call this assumption the first postulate of the parental relation P.P. 1. Thus:

P.P. 1   For all x, not $(x\mathbf{P}_{po}x)$.

I now proceed to define, with the help of **P**, a set of relations which is very useful in the theory of evolution. I call it the set of **P**-lines. I shall say that a relation R is a **P**-line, if and only if R is a line (in the sense already defined) and R is included in **P**. By saying that a relation R is included in **P** I mean that every R-couple is also a **P**-couple. That is to say, whenever we have a couple x, y such that xRy, we also have x is parent to y.

[D. 6] $R \in \mathbf{P}\text{-line} \equiv (R \in \text{line} \,\&\, R \subset \mathbf{P})$.

By way of a concrete example of a **P**-line we can consider the succession of historical persons beginning with Henry VII, the founder of the royal house of Tudor, and ending with George I of Hanover, and passing in the following order through Margaret (daughter of Henry VII), James V of Scotland (her son), Mary Stuart (his daughter), James I of England (her son), Elizabeth (his daughter), Sophia (her daughter and mother of George I). Each of these intermediate terms has one parent in the set and is parent of one member of the set. This relation is thus one-one, its first term stands in some power of the relation to its last and it is included in **P**. It is therefore a **P**-line. Incidentally it *joins* (in the sense defined) the set of Tudors to the set of Hanoverians, because Henry VII is a Tudor but not a Hanoverian, and George belongs to the house of Hanover but not to the Tudors.

The following are some consequences of the definition of **P**-line and our single postulate regarding **P**.

[T. 6.01]   **P** is asymmetrical.

$$(x)\,(y)\,(\text{if } x\mathbf{P}y \text{ then not } (y\mathbf{P}x)) \quad \text{(by P.P. 1)}.$$

[T. 6.011]   If R is any **P**-line, its first and its last terms are not identical.

$$(R)\,(\text{If } R\epsilon\,\mathbf{P}\text{-line then } B(R) \neq B(\breve{R})) \quad \text{(by D. 6, P.P. 1)}.$$

[T. 6.02]   If R is any **P**-line, then R_{po} is included in $\mathbf{P}_{po}$.

$$(R)\,(\text{If } R\epsilon\,\mathbf{P}\text{-line then } R_{po} \subset \mathbf{P}_{po}) \quad \text{(by D. 6)}.$$

[T. 6.03]   If R and S are any **P**-lines such that the last term of R is identical with the first of S, then the first term of R is identical with the first of $R+S$, and the last term of S is identical with the last of $R+S$.

$$(R)\,(S)\,(\text{If } R\epsilon\,\mathbf{P}\text{-line } \& \ S\epsilon\,\mathbf{P}\text{-line } \& \ B(\breve{R}) = B(S)$$

then $\quad B(R) = B(R+S)\ \& \ B(\breve{S}) = B(R \breve{+} S)) \quad$ (by D. 5, D. 6).

[T. 6.2]   If R and S are any **P**-lines such that the last term of R is identical with the first of S, then the last term of S is not identical with the first of R.

$$(R)\,(S)\,(\text{If } R\epsilon\,\mathbf{P}\text{-line } \& \ S\epsilon\,\mathbf{P}\text{-line } \& \ B(\breve{R}) = B(S)$$

then $\qquad\qquad B(\breve{S}) \neq B(R)) \quad$ (by D. 6, P.P. 1).

[T. 6.21]   If R and S are any **P**-lines such that the last term of R is identical with the first of S, then $R+S$ is one-one.

$$(R)\,(S)\,(\text{If } R\epsilon\,\mathbf{P}\text{-line } \& \ S\epsilon\,\mathbf{P}\text{-line } \& \ B(\breve{R}) = B(S)$$

then $\qquad R + S \epsilon\, 1 \to 1)$ $\quad$ (by D. 5, D. 6, P.P. 1).

[T. 6.22] $\quad$ If R and S are any **P**-lines, then $R + S$ is included in **P**.

$\qquad (R)\,(S)$ (If $R \epsilon$ **P**-line & $S \epsilon$ **P**-line then $R + S \subset$ **P**)

(by D. 5, D. 6).

[T. 6.23] $\quad$ If R and S are any **P**-lines such that the last term of R is identical with the first of S, then the first term of $R + S$ stands in some power of $R + S$ to the last term of $R + S$.

$\qquad (R)\,(S)$ (If $R \epsilon$ **P**-line & $S \epsilon$ **P**-line & $B(\check{R}) = B(S)$

then $\qquad B(R + S)\,(R + S)_{\mathrm{po}}\,B(R \overset{\smile}{+} S))$ $\quad$ (by D. 6, T. 6.03).

From the last three statements it follows that

[T. 6.24] $\quad$ If R and S are any two **P**-lines such that the last term of R is identical with the first of S, then $R + S$ is a **P**-line.

$\qquad (R)\,(S)$ (If $R \epsilon$ **P**-line & $S \epsilon$ **P**-line & $B(\check{R}) = B(S)$

$\qquad\qquad\qquad\qquad\qquad$ then $R + S \epsilon$ **P**-line).

By way of illustration of the method of derivation I give the derivation ot T. 6.01 in full (references preceded by *P.M.* refer to the numbered statements of *Principia Mathematica*):

Omitting the universal quantifiers we have:*

$\quad$ (1) $\quad x \mathbf{P} y \,.\, y \mathbf{P} x \,.\, \supset .\, x \mathbf{P}_{\mathrm{po}} y \,.\, y \mathbf{P}_{\mathrm{po}} x$ $\quad$ (by *P.M.* 91.502).

$\quad$ (2) $\quad x \mathbf{P}_{\mathrm{po}} y \,.\, y \mathbf{P}_{\mathrm{po}} x \,.\, \supset .\, x \mathbf{P}_{\mathrm{po}} x$ $\quad$ (by *P.M.* 91.56).

$\quad$ (3) $\quad$ not $(x \mathbf{P}_{\mathrm{po}} x) \supset$ not $(x \mathbf{P}_{\mathrm{po}} y \,.\, y \mathbf{P}_{\mathrm{po}} x)$ (by *P.M.* 2.16 and (2)).

$\quad$ (4) $\quad$ not $(x \mathbf{P}_{\mathrm{po}} y \,.\, y \mathbf{P}_{\mathrm{po}} x) \,.\, \supset .\,$ not $(x \mathbf{P} y \,.\, y \mathbf{P} x)$ (by *P.M.* 2.16 and (1)).

$\quad$ (5) $\quad$ not $(x \mathbf{P}_{\mathrm{po}} x) \,.\, \supset .\,$ not $(x \mathbf{P} y \,.\, y \mathbf{P} x)$ (by $\quad$ *P.M.* 3.33 $\quad$ and $\quad$ (3) and (4)).

---

* For the use of dots in the following statements see my *Axiomatic Method in Biology*, pp. 20 and 49. A dot between two adjacent matrices is functioning as the sign of conjunction and is therefore to be read 'and'. One or more dots immediately before or after the conditional sign function as brackets and their scope extends to the end of the statement or until a greater number of dots is reached.

(6)   not $(x\mathbf{P}_{\mathrm{po}}x)$. $\supset$ .not $(x\mathbf{P}y)$ or not $(y\mathbf{P}x)$ (by $P.M.$ 3.13 and (5)).

(7)   not $(x\mathbf{P}_{\mathrm{po}}x)$. $\supset$: $x\mathbf{P}y \supset$ not $(y\mathbf{P}x)$ (by $P.M.$ 1.01 and (6)).

(8) $x\mathbf{P}y$. $\supset$ .not $(y\mathbf{P}x)$ (by $P.M.$ 9.12 and (7) and P.P. 1).

(9) $(x)(y)(x\mathbf{P}y$. $\supset$ .not $(y\mathbf{P}x))$.

I now make a further addition to our biological vocabulary. I introduce the notion of a *taxonomic set*. By a taxonomic set I simply mean any set occurring in the taxonomic system of animals and plants. Thus a species, a genus, a family, an order, etc., will all be taxonomic sets. So will a sub-species, a sub-genus, etc. I denote the set of all taxonomic sets by '**ts**'.

This being another undefined sign of the system, it must be introduced by means of postulates. I adopt, to begin with, the following three postulates, which I call evolutionary postulates, E.P. 1, E.P. 2 and E.P. 3.

[E.P. 1]   If X and Y are any taxonomic sets, and a **P**-line joins X to Y, then for every member u of Y there is a **P**-line S such that the first term of S belongs to $X - Y$ and the last term of S is identical with u.

$$(X)(Y)(X \in \mathbf{ts} \& Y \in \mathbf{ts} \& (\exists R)(R \in \mathbf{P}\text{-line} \& J(R, X, Y))$$
$$. \supset (u)(u \in Y \supset (\exists S)(S \in \mathbf{P}\text{-line} \& B(S) \in X - Y \& B(\breve{S}) = u))).$$

This seems a fairly safe assumption to make. It does not seem likely to arouse much controversy, but we cannot judge it until we have worked out its consequences. The next one is a little more complicated:

[E.P. 2]   If X, Y and Z are any taxonomic sets such that a **P**-line joins X to Y, and a **P**-line joins Y to Z, then *every* **P**-line which joins $X - Y$ to $Z - Y$ is the sum of a **P**-line which joins X to Y and a **P**-line which joins Y to Z.

$$(X)(Y)(Z)(X \in \mathbf{ts} . Y \in \mathbf{ts} . Z \in \mathbf{ts} . (\exists R)(\exists S)(R \in \mathbf{P}\text{-}$$
$$\text{line} . J(R, X, Y) . J(S, Y, Z)) . \supset . (Q)(Q \in \mathbf{P}\text{-line} . J(Q, X - Y,$$
$$Z - Y) . \supset . (\exists P)(\exists T)(P \in \mathbf{P}\text{-line} . T \in \mathbf{P}\text{-line} . J(P, X, Y) .$$
$$J(T, Y, Z) . Q = P + T))).$$

The effect of this postulate is this: when we have $X - Y$ joined to Y by a **P**-line, and $Y - Z$ joined to Z by a **P**-line, this postulate excludes the possibility of stray **P**-lines reaching Z from $X - Z$ without having some members of their fields in Y. It excludes the skipping of Y when passing from $X - Z$ to Z along **P**-lines. This postulate is perhaps more debatable than the others. We can only judge it by what it commits us to. The third evolutionary postulate is very simple:

[E.P. 3] If X, Y and Z are any taxonomic sets such that a **P**-line joins X to Y, and a **P**-line joins Y to Z, then X and Z have no members in common.

$$(X)(Y)(Z)(X \in \textbf{ts} . Y \in \textbf{ts} . Z \in \textbf{ts} . (\exists R)(\exists S)(R \in \textbf{P}\text{-line} . S \in \textbf{P-line} . J(R, X, Y) . J(S, Y, Z)) \supset X \cap Z = \Lambda).$$

In working out the consequences of these postulates in order to see what they commit us to, it will be convenient to introduce certain new expressions by way of definition. This simply means that we use these new expressions as abbreviations for frequently recurring combinations of expressions constructed exclusively with the help of the primitive or undefined signs. They therefore introduce nothing new into the system. At the same time to facilitate reading I accompany these new signs with a verbal expression, but it is important not to be misled by the latter. Nothing must be read into it, so to speak, which is not in the definition. For example, the first definition is as follows:

[D. 7] I shall say that a taxonomic set X stands in an evolutionary relation to a taxonomic set Y, if and only if there is a **P**-line joining X to Y. I denote this relation by '**E**' and write $\mathbf{E}(X, Y)$.

$$\mathbf{E}(X, Y) \equiv (\exists R)(R \in \textbf{P}\text{-line} \mathbin{\&} X \in \textbf{ts} \mathbin{\&} Y \in \textbf{ts} \mathbin{\&} J(R, X, Y)).$$

Now it is open to anyone to say: 'That is not what I mean by being in an evolutionary relation.' But that would not be to the point. I am not saying what anybody means by being in an evolutionary relation. All I have done is to announce that

I shall use '$E(X, Y)$' as an abbreviation for 'some **P**-line joins taxonomic set X to taxonomic set Y' (i.e. at least one **P**-line does so), and I shall also sometimes read this expression as 'X stands in an evolutionary relation to Y'. But this last phrase does not belong to the system at all. Corresponding remarks apply to the subsequent definitions. But before we introduce further definitions we must look at some of the consequences of D. 7 and our three evolutionary postulates.

[T. 7.11]   If X is included in Y or Y in X, we do not have $E(X, Y)$ or $E(Y, X)$.

$$(X)(Y)((X \subset Y \text{ or } Y \subset X) \supset (\text{not } (E(X, Y)) \,\&\, \text{not } (E(Y, X))))$$

(by D. 7, T. 1).

[T. 7.12]   For no X can we have $E(X, X)$.

$$(X)(\text{not}(E(X, X)))   \text{(by T. 7.11)}.$$

[T. 7.121]   If $E(X, Y)$ then X is not closed with respect to the converse of **P**.

$$(X)(Y) \,(\text{If } E(X, Y) \text{ then not } (\breve{\mathbf{P}}``X \subset X))$$

(by D. 7, T. 3, D. 4, D. 6).

[T. 7.2]   If $E(X, Y)$, then there is a **P**-line joining X to every sub-set of $Y - X$ which is not null.

$$(X)(Y)(Z)((E(X, Y) \,\&\, Z \neq \Lambda \,\&\, Z \subset Y - X) \supset (\exists R)$$
$$(R \in \mathbf{P}\text{-line} \,\&\, J(R, X, Z)))   \text{(by D. 7, E.P. 1)}.$$

[T. 7.21]   If $E(X, Y)$, then X stands in an evolutionary relation to every taxonomic set which is included in $Y - X$.

$$(X)(Y)(Z)((E(X, Y) \,\&\, Z \in \mathbf{ts} \,\&\, Z \neq \Lambda \,\&\, Z \subset Y - X)$$
$$\supset E(X, Z))   \text{(by D. 7, T. 7.2)}.$$

[T. 7.22]   If $E(X, Y)$ and $E(Y, Z)$, then X and Z have no members in common.

$$(X)(Y)(Z)((E(X, Y) \,\&\, E(Y, Z)) \supset X \cap Z = \Lambda)$$

(by D. 7, E.P. 3).

[T. 7.23]   The relation **E** is transitive.

$$(X)(Y)(Z)((\mathbf{E}(X, Y) \& \mathbf{E}(Y, Z)) \supset \mathbf{E}(X, Z))$$

(by D. 7, D. 2, E.P. 1, T. 6.24, T. 7.22, T. 6.03, D. 6).

[T. 7.24]   The relation **E** is asymmetrical.

$(X)(Y)$ (If $\mathbf{E}(X, Y)$ then not $\mathbf{E}(Y, X)$)   (by T. 7.12, T. 7.23).

[T. 7.3]   If $\mathbf{E}(X, Y)$ and $\mathbf{E}(Y, Z)$ then, belonging to the field of every **P**-line which joins X to Z, there are members of Y which do not belong to X or to Z.

$$(X)(Y)(Z)(\mathbf{E}(X, Y) \& \mathbf{E}(Y, Z) \supset (R)((R \in \text{P-line} \& J(R, X, Z))$$
$$\supset C(R) \cap Y - (X \cup Z) \neq \Lambda)).$$

This follows from D. 7, D. 5, D. 2 and E.P. 2.

[T. 7.31]   If $\mathbf{E}(X, Y)$ and $\mathbf{E}(Y, Z)$, then no **P**-line joins X to Z directly.

$$(X)(Y)(Z)(\mathbf{E}(X, Y) \& \mathbf{E}(Y, Z)$$
$$\supset \text{not } (\exists Q)(Q \in \text{P-line} \& Jd(Q, X, Z))).$$

This follows from D. 7, D. 3 and T. 7.3.

I shall say that evolution is non-oscillatory between X and Y, if and only if X stands in an evolutionary relation to Y, and, if R is *any* **P**-line which joins X to Y, then X is closed with respect to R and Y is closed with respect to the converse of R. This is written $\mathbf{NO}(X, Y)$.

[D. 8] $\mathbf{NO}(X, Y) \equiv (\mathbf{E}(X, Y) \& ((R)(R \in \text{P-line} \& J(R, X, Y))$
$$\supset (R``X \subset X \& \breve{R}``Y \subset Y))).$$

[T. 8.11]   If evolution is non-oscillatory between X and Y and R is any **P**-line which joins X to Y, then there is one and only one R-step out of X and one and only one R-step into Y and there is no R-step into X and no R-step out of Y.

$$(X)(Y)(R)((\mathbf{NO}(X, Y) \& R \in \text{P-line}) \supset (Nc(S(R, X, \overline{X}))$$
$$= Nc(S(R, \overline{Y}, Y)) = 1 \& S(R, \overline{X}, X) = S(R, Y, \overline{Y}) = \Lambda)).$$

This follows from D. 8, T. 4, T. 4.01 and T. 4.02. That **NO** is irreflexive and asymmetrical follows from D. 8 and T. 7.12 and T. 7.24. But with our three evolutionary postulates it does not follow that **NO** is transitive.

(If we wish to have the transitivity of **NO** in our system it will be necessary to add the following to our evolutionary postulates:

If X, Y and Z are any three taxonomic sets such that a **P**-line joins X to Y and a **P**-line joins Y to Z, then no **P**-line joining X to $Y - Z$ has any member of its field belonging to Z, and no **P**-line joining $Y - X$ to Z has any member of its field belonging to X.)

I shall say that evolution is *direct* from X to Y, if and only if X stands in an evolutionary relation to Y and every **P**-line which joins X to Y joins X to Y directly. This is written: $\mathbf{Ed}(X, Y)$.

[D. 9] $\mathbf{Ed}(X, Y) \equiv (\mathbf{E}(X, Y) \,\&\, (R)\,((R \in \mathbf{P}\text{-line} \,\&\, J(R, X, Y))$
$$\supset Jd(R, X, Y))).$$

[T. 9.1]   If $\mathbf{E}(X, Y)$ and $\mathbf{E}(Y, Z)$, then not $(\mathbf{Ed}(X, Z))$.

This follows from D. 9 and T. 7.31.

From the last statement and D. 9 it will follow that **Ed** is intransitive. That it is irreflexive and asymmetrical follows from D. 9 and the corresponding statements concerning **E**.

I now define gradual evolution. I say that evolution is direct and gradual from X to Y, if and only if it is direct and if, for every **P**-line R which joins X to Y, there is no R-step from $X - Y$ to $Y - X$. This is written $\mathbf{Gd}(X\ Y)$.

[D. 10] $\mathbf{Gd}(X, Y) \equiv (\mathbf{Ed}(X, Y) \,\&\, (R)\,((R \in \mathbf{P}\text{-line} \,\&\, J(R, X, Y))$
$$\supset S(R, X - Y, Y - X) = \Lambda)).$$

Finally, I shall say that evolution is non-gradual from X to Y, if and only if X stands in a direct evolutionary relation to Y and, for every **P**-line R which joins X to Y, every R-step from X to Y is a step from $X - Y$ to $Y - X$. This is written $\mathbf{NG}(X, Y)$.

[D. 11] $\mathbf{NG}(X, Y) \equiv (\mathbf{Ed}(X, Y) \,\&\, (R)\,((R \in \mathbf{P}\text{-line} \,\&\, J(R, X, Y))$
$$\supset (S(R, X, Y) \subset S(R, X - Y, Y - X)))).$$

It will follow that both of these relations are irreflexive, asymmetrical and intransitive. Each excludes the other although neither is the complement of the other; hence they do not exclude other possibilities.

It will follow from D. 10, D. 9 and T. 3.22 that, if evolution from X to Y is direct and gradual in the above sense, then X and Y must have members in common. But it does not follow, if we have $\mathbf{NG}(X, Y)$, that X and Y do not have members in common. It will, however, follow that, if X stands in a direct evolutionary relation to Y, and X and Y have no member in common, then evolution from X to Y is non-gradual.

So much, for the present, for gradualness, at least in one sense of the word. I turn now to the problem of what is involved if we allow two taxonomic sets, neither of which is included in the other (and this must be so if they stand in an evolutionary relation to one another), to have members in common. For this purpose I make one more addition to our primitive biological vocabulary. I use 'tu' to denote the set of all *taxonomic units*, and by a taxonomic unit I mean simply any set which is specified by reference to only one taxonomic diagnostic character. For example, the set of all animals which have a parasphenoid bone would constitute a taxonomic unit, and so would the set of all animals having a metanephric kidney, and so would the set of all plants having two cotyledons, and so on.

Now it is customary to define each taxonomic set by reference to a number of such taxonomic units, namely, as their Boolean *product*. The Amphibia, for example, are usually defined as the Boolean product of some eight or nine such taxonomic units. Moreover they are defined in such a way that two taxonomic sets are always mutually exclusive, unless one is contained in the other; consequently it will be impossible for evolution from one such set to another to be direct and gradual, since this requires that they should have members in common. But this difficulty is easily overcome if we define each taxonomic set, not as the Boolean product, but as the Boolean *sum* of the taxonomic units. But this, as it stands, would perhaps make our taxonomic sets too big. Some further condition might be imposed in order to avoid this. How this can be done will be seen if it is noticed that every taxonomic set is contained in a taxonomic set which is closed with respect to the converse of the parental relation. For the set of all lives is itself closed in this sense and every taxonomic set is included in it.* Moreover, since there is only a finite number of taxonomic sets there must be a *smallest* taxonomic set in which any given one is included and which is closed with respect to the converse of the parental relation. I therefore state, as the first taxonomic postulate:

[T.P. 1]   To every taxonomic set X there is a smallest taxonomic set Y, which is closed with respect to the converse of the parental relation and in which X is included.

With this in mind we can formulate a second taxonomic postulate:

[T.P. 2]   If X is any taxonomic set and Y is the smallest taxonomic set satisfying T.P. 1 in which X is included, then there are n $(n > 1)$ taxonomic units $X_1, X_2, ..., X_n$ such that X is identical with the Boolean sum of all members of these n units which belong to Y, i.e. $X = \sum_1^n Y \cap X_i$ (for each $i = 1, 2, ..., n$).

If we agree to proceed in this way we can at once distinguish two important sub-sets of any given taxonomic set X. These I call the *core* of X (written $\mathbf{C}(X)$) and the *fringe* of X (written $\mathbf{F}(X)$). By the core of X I mean what is ordinarily identified with X itself, namely, the Boolean product of all the taxonomic units involved in the definition of X. Thus if $X_1, X_2, ..., X_n$ are the defining taxonomic units of X we can say:

[D. 12] $\mathbf{C}(X) = \prod_1^n X_i.$

---

* For example, Pisces is not closed with respect to the converse of **P** because **P**-lines are believed to join Pisces to Amphibia; but Chordata is closed with respect to converse **P**. This involves the assumption that in future Chordata will give rise only to Chordata and this hypothesis is based on the doctrine that a very great departure from the typical, *early* in development, is lethal in its consequences. For that reason it might be better to formulate the statement in the text in such a way as to confine it to the *adult* members of the taxonomic sets concerned.

By the fringe of X I mean those members of X which do *not* belong to the core of X. Thus:

[D. 13] $\mathbf{F}(X) = X - \mathbf{C}(X)$.

Point-set diagram of core and fringe

$$n = 4 \quad X = X_1 \cup X_2 \cup X_3 \cup X_4$$
$$\mathbf{C}(X) = X_1 \cap X_2 \cap X_3 \cap X_4$$

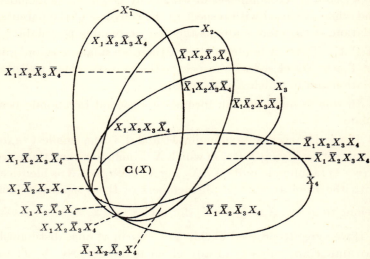

(Juxtaposition of set-designations indicates Boolean product)

This distinction between the core and the fringe of a taxonomic set not only enables us to understand the problem of the overlapping of taxonomic sets, but it also, I think, illuminates the distinction which systematists make between 'good' and 'bad' species. If a systematist lives during a period of time which intersects only the core of a species he will call it a good one, but if this period of time intersects the fringe to any large extent he will call that species a bad one. The core corresponds to times of stability and the fringe to times of instability of a taxonomic set, but of course there is nothing to prevent members of both core and fringe being contemporary with one another.

In this connexion I will point out in passing the rather curious fact that in what has been said so far it has not been necessary to make any explicit reference to precedence in time. This is because we have taken **P** as a primitive notion and the irreflexivity of $\mathbf{P}_{po}$ as a postulate. It would have been possible to adopt precedence in time as a primitive notion and with its help, together with certain other biological functors, we could have introduced **P** by definition. The part played by precedence in time in our system would then have been explicit. (For example, the present system could be incorporated into the system discussed in Note 14, p. 211. Then it would be necessary to use '**Ps**' for the '**P**' of the present system in order not to conflict with the '**P**' which denotes 'part of'.)

It is now necessary to introduce a fourth evolutionary postulate. In formulating this postulate I omit, for the sake of simplicity, all reference to the smallest taxonomic sets which are closed with respect to the converse of **P** which are mentioned in T.P. 1 and T.P. 2. It must be understood that the X_i's and Y_i's referred to are the members of taxonomic units which belong to such smallest taxonomic sets:

[E.P. 4]   If a taxonomic set X stands in a direct evolutionary relation to a taxonomic set Y (i.e. if $\mathbf{Ed}(X, Y)$), then there is a set of n X_i's and a set of n Y_i's (with $n > 1$ and $i = 1, 2, ..., n$) such that X is identical with the Boolean sum of the X_i's and Y is identical with the Boolean sum of the Y_i's, and the X_i's and Y_i's can be put into one-one correspondence with one another in such a way that the members of each couple of taxonomic units under this correspondence are mutually exclusive. We shall assume that corresponding couples share the same subscript, so that we shall have

$$X_1 \cap Y_1 = \Lambda, \quad X_2 \cap Y_2 = \Lambda,$$

and so on.

Roughly speaking we may say that evolution is here conceived as a process of replacement of each X_i by a Y_i with which it has no member in common. For example, in passing along a **P**-line from the core of the Amphibia to the core of the Reptilia we begin with terms which have a mesonephric kidney but not a metanephric kidney in the adult and end with terms which have a metanephric kidney in the adult but no mesonephric kidney.

Transition zone between X and Y

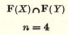

$$n = 4$$

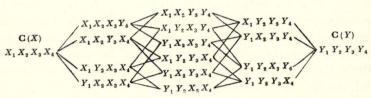

If oscillations are excluded, the number of paths from $C(X)$ to $C(Y)$ in the general case by successive single replacements is equal to $n!$. The number of sub-sets of the transition zone, having exactly r X_i's (or exactly r Y_i's) is equal to $\binom{n}{r}$.

From D. 12 and D. 13 it will follow that, for any taxonomic set X,

[T. 13.11] $C(X) \cap F(X) = \Lambda$.

[T. 13.12] $C(X) \cup F(X) = X$.

From these definitions and E.P. 4 it will follow that, for any taxonomic sets X and Y,

[T. 13.21]   If $\mathbf{Ed}(X, Y)$, then $C(X) \cap C(Y) = \Lambda$.

[T. 13.22]   If $\mathbf{Ed}(X, Y)$, then $C(X) \cap F(Y) = \Lambda$.

Let us call the common part of the fringe of a taxonomic set X and the fringe of a taxonomic set Y the *transition zone* between X and Y, denoting it by $T(X, Y)$, thus:

[D. 14] $T(X, Y) = F(X) \cap F(Y)$.

Then we shall have, for any taxonomic sets X, Y and Z,

[T. 14.1] $T(X, Y) = T(Y, X)$.

[T. 14.11]   If $\mathbf{Ed}(X, Y)$, then $\mathbf{T}(X, Y) = X \cap Y$.

[T. 14.12]   If $\mathbf{Ed}(X, Y)$ and $\mathbf{T}(X, Y) = \Lambda$, then $\mathbf{NG}(X, Y)$.

[T. 14.13]   If $\mathbf{E}(X, Y)$ and $\mathbf{E}(Y, Z)$, then $\mathbf{T}(X, Z) = \Lambda$ (by E.P. 3 and D. 7).

[T. 14.14]   If $\mathbf{Gd}(X, Y)$, then $\mathbf{T}(X, Y) \neq \Lambda$.

We can now sum up the position reached regarding the problem mentioned at the outset. If evolution from X to Y is gradual and direct in the sense defined, then X and Y must have members in common, and this common part will consist of those members of the fringe of X which also belong to the fringe of Y. We can also now formulate the factors upon which the *degree* of gradualness depends. Let me first explain what I mean by a *replacement*. I shall say that a couple x, y is a replacement relatively to X and Y, if and only if $x \mathbf{P} y$ and if y belongs to a sub-set of the transition zone between X and Y, which has at least *one more* Y_i than that to which x belongs, or y belongs to the core of Y and x to the transition zone. For example, any member of the set of couples $S(\mathbf{P}, X_1 X_2 X_3 Y_4, X_1 X_2 Y_3 Y_4)$ will be a replacement.

Now we can see that the degree of gradualness of evolution between X and Y will depend upon

(1) how many replacements are needed to pass from the core of X to the core of Y (i.e. upon n in E.P. 4);

(2) the frequency with which replacements occur in each $\mathbf{P}$-line joining X to Y;

(3) whether the members of a replacement couple can differ with respect to more than one taxonomic unit, e.g. whether, for example, such replacements as $S(\mathbf{P}, X_1 X_2 X_3 Y_4, X_1 Y_2 Y_3 Y_4)$ occur (supposing $n = 4$);

(4) whether evolution from X to Y is oscillatory or not.*

Now that we have distinguished core and fringe it will be seen that we can define a more strict kind of non-oscillatory evolution than that defined at first. We have said that evolution is

* The arithmetical considerations on pp. 226–31 are relevant here.

non-oscillatory from X to Y, if X is closed with respect to every **P**-line joining X to Y and if Y is closed with respect to the converse of every such **P**-line. A much more drastic requirement would be that every taxonomic *unit* in the transition zone between X and Y should be closed in a corresponding way, so that for each X_i and Y_i, when once we have left X_i, there is no return, and, when once we have entered Y_i, there is no escape by any **P**-line which joins X_i to Y_i.

It will also be seen that, although the passage from one taxonomic set to another must take place in a single **P**-step, nevertheless the passage from $C(X)$ to $C(Y)$ may require 10,000 generations as Darwin estimated, on account of the infrequency of replacements in the **P**-lines joining them.* This I take to be in accord with modern beliefs about the rarity of mutations. It seems obvious that the occurrence of oscillations would very much slow down the process.

So far we have been working with a very meagre biological vocabulary. You may think it is a vocabulary with which we can hardly expect to express anything of importance about evolution. There are many things to be said about evolution which cannot be expressed with these slender means. But I am deliberately pursuing what I believe to be an important principle of method, namely, to introduce our undefined notions one at a time in order to see how much can be done with them before we introduce another. Corresponding remarks apply also to the postulates. Moreover, I would point out that, although what I have said may not seem very exciting and has left many evolutionary problems untouched, nevertheless I have been able to give a tolerably precise formulation to some fundamental postulates which are basic in any theory of evolution and regarding which current theories must take *some* attitude, even although that attitude may never be made explicit. What I have tried to do is to drag some of these issues into the light by formulating them explicitly.

---

* Not because, as Darwin seems to have supposed, it required a vast number of *imperceptible* steps.

But in spite of the meagreness of our present vocabulary we have still by no means come to the end of what can be done with it.

In biological books we sometimes find diagrams of what are called *phylogenetic trees*. These diagrams consist of systems of branching lines which usually begin at the top or bottom of the page with a single line, the branches of which do not join again. What do these lines represent? What happens at the branching? Let us see whether answers to these questions can be formulated with the help of the parental relation.

Pedigrees and barriers of pedigrees

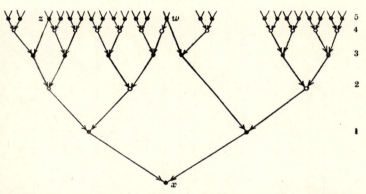

Diagram of part of the pedigree of x to illustrate barriers. The horizontal rows of terms marked 1, 3 and 5 on the right-hand side of the diagram are barriers of the pedigree, but those marked 2 and 4 are not, because there is a P-line beginning with w and ending in x which has no term in 2, and there is a P-line beginning with z and ending in x which has no term in 4, and there is a P-line beginning with w and ending in x which has no term in 4.

First I must explain what I mean by the *pedigree* of a member of a taxonomic set and by a *barrier* of such a pedigree. I shall say that a set X is the pedigree of a member y of some taxonomic set if and only if X consists of y together with all the ancestors of y.

[D. 15] $X = \mathbf{Ped}(y) \equiv (\exists Y)\,(Y \in \mathbf{ts}\ \&\ y \in Y\ \&\ (x)\,(x \in X \equiv x\mathbf{P}_{*}y)).$

I shall say that a set Z is a barrier of a pedigree X if and only if the following conditions are satisfied:

(1) there is a y such that $X = \mathbf{Ped}(y)$;

(2) Z is not null and is included in X;

(3) there are ancestors of members of Z which do not belong to Z;

(4) there are descendants of members of Z which belong to X but not to Z;

(5) if R is any **P**-line whose first term belongs to the ancestors of members of Z but not to Z and whose last term is y, then the field of R contains at least one member of Z.

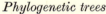

Phylogenetic trees

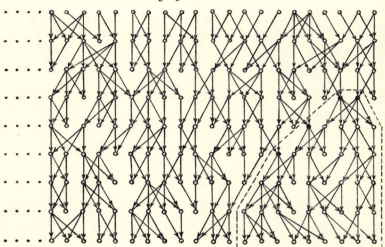

Diagram to illustrate the beginner set (Y) of a phylogenetic tree X. The members of X are enclosed by the dotted line. Members of Y are represented by the black dots. The time-direction runs from the top to the bottom of the page.

[D. 16] $\quad Z \in \mathbf{Bar}(X) \equiv (\exists y)\,(X = \mathbf{Ped}(y) . Z \neq \Lambda . Z \subset X$

$\qquad . (\mathbf{P}_{po}\text{``}Z) - Z \neq \Lambda . (\breve{\mathbf{P}}_{po}\text{``}Z) \cap X \cap \bar{Z} \neq \Lambda . (R)\,((R \in \mathbf{P}\text{-line}$

$\qquad . B(R) \in (\mathbf{P}_{po}\text{``}Z) - Z . B(\breve{R}) = y) \supset C(R) \cap Z \neq \Lambda)).*$

* In D. 16 dots are used instead of '&'.

Roughly speaking a barrier of a pedigree is a sub-set Z of the pedigree such that it is not possible to pass along a **P**-line from one side to the other without passing through a member of Z.

With the help of the notion of a barrier of a pedigree we can now define *phylogenetic tree*. I shall say that a set X is a phylogenetic tree with beginner set Y if and only if the following conditions are satisfied:

(1) X consists of Y together with all the descendants of members of Y;

(2) no parent of a member of Y belongs to X;

(3) if y is any member of Y, then there is an x and a z such that $x\mathbf{P}y$ and $x\mathbf{P}z$ and z does not belong to X;

(4) there is at least one member x of $X - Y$ such that Y is a barrier of the pedigree of x;

(5) if x is any member of $X - Y$, then there is a sub-set Z of Y which is a barrier of the pedigree of x.

[D. 17] $\mathbf{Ph}(X, Y) \equiv (X = \mathbf{\breve{P}_*}``Y . (\mathbf{P}``Y) \cap X = \Lambda$

$. (y) ((y \in Y) \supset (\exists x) (\exists z) (x\mathbf{P}y . x\mathbf{P}z . z \in \bar{X})) . (\exists x) (x \in X - Y$

$. Y \in \mathbf{Bar}(\mathbf{Ped}(x))) . (x) ((x \in X - Y) \supset (\exists Z) (Z \subset Y$

$. Z \in \mathbf{Bar}(\mathbf{Ped}(x)))))$.*

It follows from this definition that, if X is a phylogenetic tree with beginner set Y, and Z is a phylogenetic tree with beginner set Y, then X is identical with Z. This is immediately evident from the definition. But it also follows that if X is a phylogenetic tree with beginner set Y, and X is a phylogenetic tree with beginner set Z, then Y is identical with Z. In consequence of this, it follows that the relation between X and Y when X is a phylogenetic tree with beginner set Y is a one-one relation. We can therefore speak of *the* beginner set of X:

[D. 18] $Y = \mathbf{Bg}(X) \equiv \mathbf{Ph}(X, Y)$.

Branching is now easily defined. I shall say that a phylogenetic tree Z *branches into* a phylogenetic tree W, if and only if

* In D.17 dots are used instead of '&'.

the beginner set of W is included in Z minus the beginner set of Z:

[D. 19] $\mathbf{Br}(Z, W) \equiv \mathbf{Bg}(W) \subset Z - \mathbf{Bg}(Z).$*

The following are some consequences of the foregoing definitions, including some already mentioned:

[T. 16.1]   If X is a barrier of the pedigree of x and R is any **P**-line whose first term belongs to the set Y consisting of those ancestors of members of X which do not belong to X and whose last term is x, and if Z is the set of all descendants of members of X which do not belong to X, then $J(R, Y, Z)$ but not $Jd(R, Y, Z)$.

[T. 17.1]   If $\mathbf{Ph}(X, Y)$ and $\mathbf{Ph}(Z, Y)$, then $X = Z$.

[T. 17.2]   If $\mathbf{Ph}(X, Y)$ and $\mathbf{Ph}(X, Z)$, then $Y = Z$.†

[T. 17.3]   If $\mathbf{Ph}(X, Y)$, then, if x and y are any members of Y, x stands in $\mathbf{P}_{po} \mid \breve{\mathbf{P}}_{po}$ to y (see Note 1, p. 320).

[T. 17.4]   If $\mathbf{Ph}(X, Y)$ and Z is any taxonomic set which is closed with respect to the converse of **P** and Y is included in it, then X is included in it.

[T. 19.1]   The relation of branching between phylogenetic trees is irreflexive, asymmetrical and transitive.

This brings me to the end of my tether for the moment. The next step will be to introduce postulates connecting phylogenetic trees with taxonomic sets, especially postulates concerning how the cores of taxonomic sets and their fringes are related to branching. This is a difficult problem requiring much expert knowledge. When we have done this and have exhausted the possibilities of the three undefined signs **P**, **ts** and **tu**, it will then be necessary to add further undefined signs to the system—

---

* D. 17 and D. 19 are an improvement on the corresponding definitions (which are defective), 2.7.1 and 2.7.4, given in my *Axiomatic Method in Biology*. Fortunately the latter definitions were merely suggestions and were not used in later sections of that book.

† For the derivation of this theorem see the note at the end of this Appendix.

those belonging to genetics, embryology and ecology. Some hints towards accomplishing this task have been given in Part II.*

The method I have been following is called the method of postulates or the axiomatic method. After what has been said in Part I, it should hardly be necessary to point out that postulates are not to be regarded as dogmas but as tentative formulations which are to be rejected if their consequences are not in agreement with experience. I hope what I have said has been sufficient to illustrate the applicability and utility of this procedure in relation to biological problems and to show that it is possible, in the words of Leibniz, to 'seek demonstrations' in such biological contexts.†

Note. The following gives the derivation of T. 17.2:

If $\mathbf{Ph}(X, Y)$ and $\mathbf{Ph}(X, Z)$ then $Y = Z$.

It depends only on the following three immediate consequences of D. 17:

(i)   if $\mathbf{Ph}(X, Y)$, then $X = \breve{\mathbf{P}}_*``Y$,

(ii) if $\mathbf{Ph}(X, Z)$, then $X = \breve{\mathbf{P}}_*``Z$,

(iii) if $\mathbf{Ph}(X, Y)$, then $(\mathbf{P}``Y) \cap X = \Lambda$.

It follows from (i) that

(1) (y) (if $y \in Y$ then $y \in X$).

* The following are some problems which are not discussed in the text but which may interest the reader: Let us say that a taxonomic set Z is of *convergent origin*, or belongs to the set **CO**, if and only if there exist taxonomic sets X and Y such that $\mathbf{E}(X, Z)$ and $\mathbf{E}(Y, Z)$ but not $\mathbf{E}(X, Y)$, not $\mathbf{E}(Y, X)$, not $X \subset Y$ and not $Y \subset X$. Problem 1: Can either of the following two statements be derived from the postulates and definitions of the present system: (i) $\mathbf{CO} \neq \Lambda$, (ii) $\mathbf{CO} = \Lambda$? Problem 2: Which of these two statements is to be preferred in the light of existing evolutionary data? Problem 3: What additions to, or other alterations in, our existing postulates must be made in order that the preferred statement should be derivable? Problem 1 only demands skill in the art of deriving consequences from statements. Problem 2 requires an expert knowledge of evolutionary data, i.e. of observation records by which evolutionary hypotheses can be tested. Problem 3 requires skill in the art of theory construction.

† The reader will notice that, in this Appendix, I have made use of two sets of sets, **ts** and **tu**. As these are undefined signs it is difficult to see how they can be regarded as abbreviators after the manner of **Dlz**. There may be some way of treating them as abbreviators; but at the moment I do not see exactly how this is to be done.

And it follows from (ii) that

(2) (y) (if $y \epsilon X$ and $y \epsilon \bar{Z}$ then $(\exists z)$ $(z \epsilon Z$ and $zP_{po}y))$.

From (1) and (2), with the help of principles (3) and (6) in Part I, pp. 37, 38, we obtain

(3) (y) (if $y \epsilon Y$ then: if $y \epsilon \bar{Z}$ then $(\exists z)$ $(z \epsilon Z$ and $zP_{po}y))$.

From (ii) with the help of $P.M.$ 91.57 we obtain

(4) if $(\exists z)$ $(z \epsilon Z$ and $zP_{po}y)$ then $(\exists u)$ $(uPy$ and $u \epsilon X)$.

And from (iii) we get

(5) if $(\exists u)$ $(uPy$ and $u \epsilon X)$ then $y \epsilon \bar{Y}$.

From (3), (4) and (5), by principle (6) on p. 38, we obtain

(6) (y) (if $y \epsilon Y$ then: if $y \epsilon \bar{Z}$ then $y \epsilon \bar{Y})$.

From (6) by transposition we get

(7) (y) (if $y \epsilon Y$ then: if $y \epsilon Y$ then $y \epsilon Z)$.

From which it follows that

(8) (y) (if $y \epsilon Y$ then $y \epsilon Z)$.

Hence

(9) $Y \subset Z$.

By an exactly analogous procedure we obtain

(10) $Z \subset Y$.

Consequently, from (9) and (10) we have

(11) $Y = Z$.

PART III

METHODOLOGICAL PROBLEMS IN NEUROLOGY AND RELATED SCIENCES

Nay, I'll ne'er believe a madman till I see his brains.

Twelfth Night, IV, ii.

LECTURE VI

NEUROLOGICAL AND RELATED STATEMENTS

I propose now to leave genetics and to turn the Boole-Frege searchlight upon statements of a totally different kind. This third part of my lectures originated in a study of some utterances of neurologists which have puzzled me. In addition to formulating ordinary physiological statements, some neurologists permit themselves to construct statements which contain a mixture of both physiological and what are commonly called psychological words, and it is sometimes very difficult to decide what precisely is being asserted by such statements, or whether they can be regarded as belonging to neurology at all.

But when I came to reflect upon such matters I soon found myself becoming involved in wider and wider topics, some of which have already been touched upon in Part I. In Part II these fell into the background—we were able to use a homogeneous language—but here it will be necessary to take note of them again.

Connected with these methodological problems of neurology are also certain problems regarding a discrepancy between the training of medical students and the practice of medicine, a discrepancy which has puzzled me for a long time and about which I should like to say something. For this discrepancy is also a result of the lack of relations between the different departments of knowledge.

When, in what follows, I use the phrase 'physical sciences', I must be understood to include not only physics and chemistry but also biology, and I shall use the phrase 'physical objects' to cover all objects whose designations occur in the theoretical statements of these sciences.

Now neurologists, and also students of animal behaviour, are divisible into two great classes: First there are those who explicitly hold that the language of neurology and of behaviour theory should be strictly physiological, that it should be a purely physical language which speaks exclusively about physical objects, scrupulously avoiding all words characteristic of psychology and sociology. A second group does not accept this restriction but freely mingles in its physiological statements words which are foreign to the physical sciences. This class has two sub-sets. Members of one sub-set are more or less aware that they are using a mixed language, and that this procedure may have unfortunate consequences; but they consider that its advantages outweigh any possible dangers of confusion. The second sub-set includes those who do not seem to be aware that they are using a mixed language at all. Anyone who uses language uncritically—as we all do until we begin to reflect about it —will belong to this sub-set because the natural languages are themselves mixtures.

The discussion of these problems usually takes place in a context which presupposes the traditional body-mind dualism. It is easy to say: Neurologists deal with bodies and psychologists with minds, and so long as they each attend to their own business and do not mix their languages all will be well. But apart from the fact that people often find it difficult to confine their attention in this way, and apart from other objections, this attitude offers no answer to the interesting methodological questions: (i) How do you know what belongs to the language of neurology and what belongs to that of psychology? and (ii) Why must they not be mixed? or (iii) Assuming that there is no objection in principle to their mixture, what are the rules governing the mixing? These are genuine methodological problems to which we may reasonably hope to find answers. The metaphysical issues involved will not be discussed.*

It is common enough to find authors deploring the body-mind dualism and yet at the same time continuing to use a language which inevitably commits them to it. If we wish to avoid this

---

* What do I mean by 'metaphysical issues'? I mean any attempt to say what anything 'really is in itself' as opposed to the construction of explanatory hypotheses which are testable (as explained in Part I) by means of observation records.

result we must devise or find a language which carries with it no such commitments; that is to say, we must find a *pre-dualistic language*. In attempting to follow this latter course I must not be supposed to be condemning the use of the notions of body and mind, but merely to be seeking for an alternative starting-point which may be useful in setting old problems in a somewhat new light and in enabling us to see under what conditions these notions may be significantly used. My procedure is simply an attempt to rediscover the obvious, which has become buried under layers of unacknowledged or unexamined assumptions, in the belief that, in the words of Whitehead, 'almost any idea which jogs you out of your current abstractions may be better than nothing'.

Attempts to understand the use of the words 'body' and 'mind' have been befuddled by the way in which judgements of value have been mixed up with them. Some people have been impressed with the vast superiority of bodies over minds, others with the no less vast superiority of minds over bodies (and if we had sufficient patience we might come finally to see how, in suitable contexts, both views are significant and acceptable); and as these topics have usually been approached from the point of view of the alleged *entities* which these words are supposed to name, the question of how the words function in various scientific uses, which surely is the prior question, has not been sufficiently considered. That is to say, these problems are more often discussed from a naïve, metaphysical, rather than from a linguistic or methodological, point of view.

The view I shall take is simply this: that the notions of body and mind are both reached by abstraction from something more concrete. For these more concrete objects we have the convenient and familiar word *persons*. Let us speak, then, in the first instance of persons.* But even the notion of person is abstract in the sense that every person is a member of some *community* of persons, upon which the *kind* of person he is, and

---

* The body-mind dualism cannot be satisfactorily dealt with simply by accepting one abstractum and ignoring the other.

even his continued existence, *as* a person, depends. That is to say, in specifying the environments of persons it is necessary to use words belonging to sociology, especially that branch of it which is chiefly concerned with the study of *small* communities, such as families. I shall maintain later that the branch of sociology in question is identical with, or contains as a large part, that branch of applied science which is more commonly known as medical psychology. To make this clearer let me try to explain what I mean by a family. This will, at the same time, provide illustrations of interesting methodological problems which arise in such contexts and of ways of dealing with them.

First, let us use '**Ps**' to denote the relation of sexual parenthood, so that 'x**Ps**y' reads: 'x is sexual parent of y'. And let us use '**R**' to denote the relation between two persons which is commonly expressed by saying that they both live under the same roof. I assume that this relation is symmetrical and transitive, so that it gives rise to abstractive classes, that is to say, sets of persons such that each includes all the persons living under any one roof and no one else. Such sets would not suffice to define families, because without the parental relation they would only constitute communities of the institutional type. Next I define a three-termed relation **f** as follows: I shall say that three persons x, y and z stand in **f** to one another, if and only if x and y are distinct, x**Ps**z and y**Ps**z and x**R**y and y**R**z. With the help of this relation we could formulate general statements of the form

$$(x)\,(y)\,(z)\,(\text{if } \mathbf{f}(x,y,z) \,\&\, x\epsilon\, X \,\&\, y\epsilon\, Y \text{ then } z\epsilon\, Z). \qquad (1)$$

Superficially this has the same form as

$$(x)\,(y)\,(z)\,(\text{if } \mathbf{dlz}(x,y,z) \,\&\, x\epsilon\, X \,\&\, y\epsilon\, Y \text{ then } z\epsilon\, Z). \qquad (2)$$

And just as we used $\mathbf{Dlz}(X, Y, Z)$ as an abbreviation for (2), so we could use $\mathbf{F}(X, Y, Z)$ as an abbreviation for (1). For example, if G is the set of all German-speaking persons the statement

$$\mathbf{F}(G, G, G) \qquad (3)$$

would assert that all children who live under the same roof with their German-speaking parents are themselves German-speaking.

But this example shows that the resemblance between (1) and (2) is deceptive, for (1) does not satisfy Venn's requirement. A child may be a cretin or so intellectually feeble as to be incapable of learning any language at all. Moreover, there is nothing to fix the time-length of z in (1), so that z might be too young to speak a language. It might also be pointed out that some parents have very little to do with their children but hand them over to the companionship of a foreign nurse who does not speak the language of her employer. This objection can easily be met by providing for it in the specification of the parental sets X and Y. The former difficulties are not so easily dealt with. To overcome them we must make use of the functor **dlz**, because the set of all German-speaking people is a phenotype, no less than is the set of all peas with yellow cotyledons. We also require the notion of what I shall call *normal zygotic range* which is, so to speak, an inverse of the notion of adult environmental range. Assuming that we know what we mean by the set N of normal persons, at least as far as learning languages is concerned, then, by the normal zygotic range of an environmental set E, I shall mean the set of all zygotes x, such that if x develops in an environment belonging to E it develops into a normal person. By the G-zygotic range of E, I shall mean the set of all zygotes x, such that if x develops in a member of E it develops into a German-speaking person. Now if the normal zygotic range of E is contained in its G-zygotic range and if u develops in v into z, and u belongs to the normal zygotic range of E and v belongs to E, it will follow that z belongs to G.

Now what the statement (3) is intended to express is that, if the parents of any child z are German-speaking, they will provide an environment for z which is of the kind E. It is also tacitly assumed that the normal zygotic range of this E is contained in its G-zygotic range. What must now be added to the antecedent is the further information that the child z develops from a zygote belonging to the normal zygotic range of E. Let us use W to denote the set of all lives developing from members of this range. Then the statement (3) becomes

$$(x)\,(y)\,(z)\ (\text{if } \mathbf{f}(x,y,z)\ \&\ x\,\epsilon\,G\ \&\ y\,\epsilon\,G\ \&\ z\,\epsilon\,W \text{ then } z\,\epsilon\,G),$$

or
$$\mathbf{F}(G,G,W,G).$$

Thus, in genetics the tendency is to study phenotypes P such that the adult environmental range of a set Z of zygotes is co tained in its P-environmental range, because we are interest in zygote analysis, whereas in sociology we frequently have do with phenotypes P such that the normal zygotic range set E of environments is contained in its P-zygotic ra because we are interested in the analysis of environments.

A serious objection to the three-termed relation $\mathbf{f}$ is the that it only mentions one child, and so provides no mea expressing the effects of one child on another. This is als obstacle to its use as a basis for defining 'family'. It woul better, therefore, to define a multigrade relation—a relatio degree $n+2$, where n is the number of children. Thus we define $\mathbf{f'}$ as follows:

$\mathbf{f'}(x,y,z_1,z_2,\ldots,z_n)$ if and only if $x \neq y\ \&\ x\mathbf{P}\mathbf{s}z_1\ \&\ y\mathbf{P}\mathbf{s}z_1\ \&$
$\quad x\mathbf{P}\mathbf{s}z_2\ \&\ y\mathbf{P}\mathbf{s}z_2\ \&\ \ldots\ \&\ x\mathbf{P}\mathbf{s}z_n\ \&\ y\mathbf{P}\mathbf{s}z_n\ \&\ x\mathbf{R}y\ \&\ y\mathbf{R}z_1\ \&$
$\quad z_1\mathbf{R}z_2\ \&\ \ldots\ \&\ z_{n-1}\mathbf{R}z_n.$

With this, together with the form of the composition fu which is appropriate to individuals, as opposed to sets c dividuals, we can define 'family'. I use '$\mathbf{c}(R,x,y)$' to de *the* object consisting of x in relation R to y (see p. 146). $\mathbf{c}(\mathbf{f'},x,y,z_1,z_2,\ldots,z_n)$ will be a family if and only if

$$\mathbf{f'}(x,y,z_1,z_2,\ldots,z_n).$$

This, of course, does not cover *all* varieties of families. It not provide for maiden aunts, aged grandparents or lod These varieties would require separate definition. I have de one common type of family for purposes of illustration. T are also other ways of defining this type.* Which definition is adopted will depend upon how the definition is to be used in a theory of families. I would also mention in passing that the other composition functor can be used to denote sets of families. Thus $C(f', G_1, G_2, ..., G_{n+2})$ would denote the set of all families in which there were n children all of whom together with their parents speak German. With the help of such expressions as these we can briefly formulate laws belonging to the pathology of families.

In connexion with the fact that persons are parts of families I would point out the importance of beginning the analysis of anything with *big units* in order that nothing important is omitted, and of course families themselves are parts of still larger communities. In treating persons under the notion of body we are thus being exceedingly abstract, and it is then quite easy to lose sight of this fact and, indeed, difficult even to be aware of it at all. But this is the only way in which we can treat them so long as we confine ourselves to the physical sciences, since these sciences do not provide a vocabulary for speaking about them in any other way.

But physical objects, persons and communities are not the only objects we have to consider (or, if it is preferred, physical object-words, person-words and community-words are not the only words we have to consider). We must recall what was said in Part I about sensible objects. Let us approach this question from a somewhat wider angle. Consider the following statements, which are all of types familiar to everyone:

   (i) You get a fine view of the sea from this window;

  (ii) If you listen carefully you get a sound of running water;

 (iii) If you stroke this you get a feel of velvet;

 (iv) You get a lovely smell of lavender in this garden;

  (v) When you swallow this you get a taste of vinegar.

From these five statements we can distil a matrix containing

---

* We could, for example, treat families by means of finite sequences in the sense defined by Tarski in his 'Der Wahrheitsbegriff in den formalisierten Sprachen' *Studia Philosophica*, Leopoli, 1935, p. 287. This would have many advantages.

a functor of degree four, namely,

x gets y which is of z under circumstance w.

It is easy to see how the relations, **S** (see below) and **OF** in P
can be defined with the help of this matrix. **S** is the relati
which x stands to y when for some z and some w—x gets y wl
is of z under circumstance w. And **OF** is the relation in wl
y stands to z when for some x and some w—x gets y which i
z under circumstance w. When, therefore, we use **S** and **OF** al
there is a tacit reference to two other terms.

Now the objects, whose names can be significantly substitu
for 'x' in the matrix (M), form what is called the *first domain*
the relation expressed by (M), those whose names can be su
stituted for 'y' constitute the second domain, those whose names
can be substituted for 'z' form the third and those whose names
can be substituted for 'w' the fourth or last domain of this
relation. This provides a nice non-committal terminology which
permits us to talk about things without treading upon people's
ontological and epistemological pet corns, and for that reason is
to be preferred. But as it is unfamiliar and technical I shall
continue (under protest) to use ordinary phrases. I shall call the
values of 'x' *persons* and the values of 'y' *sensible objects*. The
values of 'z' may be persons or physical objects. For some values
of 'w', x and z may be identical (you can sometimes get a fine
view of yourself in a mirror). It seems clear to me that y and z
can never be identical, although some persons apparently do
not agree with me about this. But, if y and z are always identical,
then when I bathe in the sea I must bathe in the view I get of it
from this window, and when a blind man bathes with me he
also must bathe in the view I get of it from this window. And
when I drink running water I must also drink the sound I get of
it. But to say such things seems to me to be a plain misuse of
language. Some persons appear to wish to abolish y altogether.
But I can only report that I get views and sounds and feels, etc.,
of things from time to time and other persons tell me they do the
same. The values of 'w' are complexes of persons and physical

objects. It is important to note that they frequently include *actions* on the part of *x* (e.g. *x* strokes this, *x* swallows this, etc.).

Now let us consider a *day*. By a day in this context I mean the totality of what a person *gets* from waking up one morning to sinking into dreamless sleep at night. This is the sense of 'day' involved when someone asks: 'What sort of a day have you had?' and you reply 'Fine!' or 'Much as usual', or something of that sort. But this question and answer are concerned with an aspect of a day about which it will not be necessary for me to speak here, namely, the running commentary of approval or disapproval which is usually an ingredient of a day.

If we consider two days which are near together in the succession of days of the same person, the feature which most impresses us is their massive similarity. Even if we are on holiday on our second day, and are refreshed by a change of scene, there is still the same pervasive possibility of recognition. Although the houses, persons, mountains, etc., are all so different, yet they are still recognizable *as* houses, persons, mountains, etc. If we ignore the differences and consider only the resemblances in a succession of days we can discern certain elements which we can call *routines*. Thus putting on one's clothes in the morning, having breakfast, or going out to post a letter are examples of routines. Each routine has a terminus, like fastening the last button, swallowing the last mouthful or dropping the letter into the letter-box. These are routines of doing, each terminus is the completion of an act. But we can also have routines of knowing, such as dissecting an animal to demonstrate the course of a nerve, or looking up a word in a dictionary. Here the routine terminates in an observation.

But houses, persons and mountains are not ingredients of days as I am using the latter word. The ingredients of days are the looks, feels, sounds, etc., which are **OF** such objects. Consider the terminus of posting a letter a little more closely. It will have been preceded by the looks of the houses and of the road and by the sounds of my shoes on the pavement. It will include the red cylindrical look of the letter-box which swells visibly as

I approach the box. There is also the black rectangular look of the slit into which I drop the letter, the absence of resistance as I push it in, and the soft rustling sound when the letter drops.

When we have come to an end of describing the looks, feels, and sounds of the letter-box, we are next led to reflect on the status of the letter-box itself and the relation of the sensible objects to it. It is clear that, although we commonly speak of seeing, feeling and perhaps hearing the letter-box, this is only an abbreviated way of saying that we see a look, feel a feel and hear a sound which is **OF** a letter-box. The physical letter-box itself is not and cannot be seen, felt or heard in the *same* sense.*
Nevertheless, most people believe, when they post a letter, that they are in the presence of something, a physical object, which is distinct from the feels and sounds, if not the looks, which are **OF** it, and which persists long enough at least to guard their letter, another physical object, until the postman comes to collect it. Physical objects thus belong to what I have called the converse domain of **OF**. And the same is true of persons. We also believe that, when we are living through a routine of doing, we are actually moving ourselves and other objects belonging to the converse domain of **OF**.

But, if we do not see, hear or feel the letter-box, but only looks, sounds, feels, etc., which we suppose to be **OF** it, the question may be asked how we distinguish times when such sensible objects really are **OF** a letter-box from times when, although they seem to be genuine letter-box looks, yet we believe there to be no letter-box present for them to stand in **OF** to. The only answer open to us seems to be that we distinguish two such instances by the *routines* in which the sensible objects occur. If they occur as elements in a terminus of a typical letter-posting routine, we assume that we are dealing with a letter-box and

---

* The reason why we use the same word 'hearing' (for example) both in 'hearing a sound' and in 'hearing a bell' seems to be partly because in practical affairs we are usually more concerned with the bell than with the sound, and still more because, until we come to reflect about such matters, we do not distinguish between objects belonging to the converse domain of **OF** and the objects which are **OF** them, especially in the case of visual sensible objects.

we entrust our letter to it. Our hypothesis will, for most practical purposes, be confirmed to a very high degree if we subsequently receive an answer to our letter. But if we become aware of a sensible object, of the kind normally associated with letter-boxes, in a routine in which such objects do not ordinarily occur (e.g. during a visit to a theatre), we are suspicious and seek (and usually find) a different explanation of what we have seen or heard. Thus perceptual judgements of this kind (to which our scientific observation records belong) are always hypotheses based upon experienced routines. We say that perception is veridical when such hypotheses are confirmed and illusory when they are falsified. In this case also it is important to begin with big units. We do not decide such questions by concentrating attention on the looks and feels, so much as by asking: Am I awake or dreaming? Am I in a street or at a theatre? How did I get here? etc., i.e. by reference to routines.

I must add that I do not want to restrict 'feels' to what is felt in a tactual sense. I want to include also such objects as Hamlet was referring to when he said:

But I have that within which passeth show;
These but the trappings and the suits of woe.

But I should object to the use of the word 'within' here (see below, p. 268, where *atopical* relations are defined).

When once we have taken note of sensible objects we see that we have two relations to deal with which are quite foreign to the physical sciences. First, there is the relation between a sensible object and a physical object, or a person, when the former is said to be *of* the latter in veridical perception. This has already been mentioned in Part I, and I have called it the relation **OF**. Secondly, there is the relation **S** between person and sensible object when the former is aware of or is sensing or getting the latter. It is clear that the relation between a person and an object belonging to the converse domain of **OF**, when the former is said to be perceiving the latter, is definable as the relative product of **S** and **OF**.*

* See Note 1, p. 320.

What I have just said about the relation **S** gives a very inadequate characterization of it. I do not want to restrict it to cases of simple awareness or sensing, if, indeed, there is such a thing. I want it rather to represent the Boolean sum of a number of cognitive relations, just as I want to use 'sensible object' in a very wide sense. Perhaps I can indicate sufficiently clearly for my purpose what is intended if I quote the following passage from a recent paper by Professor Aubrey Lewis.* He writes:

> Perception was accounted for until fairly recently in terms of sensation and association, but now perceptions are viewed as organized mental structures selectively taken from the unstructured stimulus field. Perception is not isolated from affect and memory: as F. C. Bartlett put it, 'inextricably mingled with it are imaging, valuing and those beginnings of judging which are involved in the response to plan, order of arrangement and construction of presented material. It is directed by interest and by feeling, and may be dominated by certain crucial features of the objects and scenes dealt with.'

I assume that Professor Lewis's 'perceptions' are my sensible objects. Calling them 'mental' commits us to a particular *theory* about them.

If we consider relations **S** and **OF** a little we notice that they differ very much from the relations with which we are familiar in the physical sciences. Physical objects stand in spatio-temporal relations to one another; one can be before another in time, north of another on the earth's surface, and one can be inside another. But this is not the case with sensible objects. It is true that the sensing of one sensible object can occur before that of another in time, and that looks and feels can have quasi-spatial relations; but a sound cannot be north of or inside a look or a smell—sensible objects do not have insides—and can it be meaningful to ask where a sensible object was before it was sensed, or where it is after it has ceased to be sensed? We can say that sensible objects (or some of them) *appear in*, or are sensed in,

* Aubrey Lewis, 'Philosophy and psychiatry' in *Philosophy* (1949), vol. XXIV, p. 108.

places, but can we test statements which assert that they *are in* places?

All this is very puzzling and irritating from the point of view of the physical sciences. The early days of physics were largely occupied by efforts to banish mention of sensible objects from its theoretical discourse. My own attempts in Part II to banish 'characters' from theoretical genetics provide an example of this tendency. It is not at all surprising, therefore, if neurologists get into difficulties with sensible objects and sometimes treat them as if they were physical objects.

Names of sensible objects only appear in the zero-level theoretical statements of the physical sciences under the guise of so-called property names. Thus if a botanist says that some buttercups are yellow, I should interpret that, according to my nominalistic attitude, as translatable into 'Some buttercup *looks* are yellow'. And when I say that a certain sensible object *is* yellow, I am not using the 'is' of predication, but the 'is' of strict identity. I am saying that a certain sensible object is identical with one of the objects named by the shared name 'yellow' among English-speaking people. Now when neurologists speak of nervous impulses 'giving rise to' or 'producing' sensible objects (of the kind they usually call sensations) they have obviously gone beyond the bounds of the language of the physical sciences. They have therefore ceased to regard persons as purely physical objects.*

Many people appear to believe that because persons can be successfully dealt with under the abstract notion of body, i.e. as physical objects, for many purposes, that therefore they *are* physical objects in some absolute or metaphysical sense. But

---

* When I say that persons are not physical objects I am not claiming to be saying anything metaphysical about them, I am saying simply that they cannot be adequately described for *all* purposes (as we shall see) with the help only of the language of the physical sciences, as at present constituted. But of course if you *widen* the vocabulary of the physical sciences sufficiently, then they would (by definition) be physical objects. The notion of person, like that of physical object, is a hypothetical one. It differs from the hypothetical notions of natural science in not being deliberately invented. We find ourselves in possession of it as soon as we come to reflect about such matters.

I hold that we cannot say what anything belonging to the con-verse domain of **OF** *is* in any metaphysical sense. We can only *name* it, and with the help of this name and others formulate hypotheses about it which can be tested, but not verified in the literal sense of the word. The shared name 'physical object' can be usefully applied to persons, but there are many shared names which can be usefully applied *only* to persons. In the same way the shared name 'animal' can be usefully applied to persons, although there are some shared names which can be usefully applied to persons but not to other animals.

Leaving such questions aside for the moment and returning to other examples of peculiar relations, it is clear that the relation **S** between a person and a sensible object is also not a spatial relation. In order to express the distinction between these rather peculiar (but by no means unfamiliar) relations and the spatio-temporal relations of the physical sciences I call them *atopical* relations. I call a relation atopical if at least one of the terms is a sensible object.

To quote Whitehead once more: 'Space-perception accom-panies our sensations, perhaps all of them, certainly many; but it does not seem to be a necessary quality of things that they should all exist in one space or in any space.'*

One consequence of the atopical nature of the relation of sensible objects to persons and physical objects is that we cannot *do* anything to them in the same sense in which we can *do* some-thing to physical objects. To do something to a physical object usually means changing its spatial relations. Whence it follows that we cannot do anything to a sensible object in that sense. When I pick up a piece of white paper I do not pick up a white sensible object. I can no more pick up a look than I can pick up a sound or a smell. When I turn over a piece of white paper at which I am looking I do not see the back of the white sensible

---

* A. N. Whitehead, *Introduction to Mathematics* (1910), p. 244. The common sense view, which is taken over (perhaps too uncritically) into neurology seems to be that our life is passed in a big box called 'space', and that everything that *is* at all must *be in* some particular part of this box. (See also the remark about localization in the footnote on p. 288.)

object which I saw at first. I see a new sensible object which is
OF the back of the piece of paper. I suspect that this has something to do with the unpopularity of sensible objects in the
physical sciences.

Something more must now be said about persons. The two
criteria I shall employ for distinguishing persons are (i) belonging
to the domain of **S**, i.e. sensing or having other cognitive relations to sensible objects, and (ii) being able to communicate
with one another by means of statements constructed of shared
and unshared names together with formative signs. These criteria
(as I understand them) render the set of persons identical with,
or at least confined to, the set of human beings. I may be asked
why I thus exclude dogs and apes and other animals. Do they
not communicate with us and with each other? My reply is
that we do not know whether the language of these animals
satisfies the second criterion. Moreover, the difference between
communication between man and animal and between person
and person is so vast that we cannot satisfactorily confirm the
hypothesis that they sense sensible objects, however strongly
we may *believe* that they do. The language of persons is so rich
in vocabulary, and so complex in structure, that we can communicate with a degree of subtlety far surpassing anything that
is possible between persons and other animals. It is characteristic of persons that they have secrets and that they sometimes
communicate them—now and again inadvertently, as when we
speak of a person 'giving himself away'. Other animals, if they
have secrets, are not able or willing to communicate them to us.
Hence the expression 'dumb animals'.

With persons we must distinguish between 'being directly
aware *of*', which is contained in the relation **S**, and 'being
directly aware *that*', which appears to be a different relation.
I can not only be directly aware *of* a sensible object, but I can
also be directly aware *that* I am aware of it. I can also be directly
aware that I can remember the date of my birth; I can be
directly aware that I am angry, or pleased or frightened and so on.
This is what I have in mind when I say that persons have secrets.

We do not know whether dogs and apes can be 'directly aware *of*' anything, or whether they can be 'directly aware *that*'. At the same time this ignorance does not provide an excuse for cruelty to animals. If animals do not feel pain it is impossible to be cruel to them. But I have not said that they do not.

Returning after these explanations to our original theme, it will, I think, be clear that we have to deal not with two languages but with *four*: first, the language of the physical sciences which speaks exclusively of physical objects; second, the language of sensible objects. The statement that this yellow sensible object is more orange than that one would be an example of a statement belonging to this language. Third, we have the person language, to which such statements as 'Tom loves Mary', 'Tom is trying to remember his telephone number', belong. Fourth, the community language. By way of example I may quote the opening paragraph of Tolstoy's *Anna Karenina*: 'All happy families resemble one another. Each unhappy family is unhappy in its own way.' That is a possible zero-level statement in the theory of families or medical psychology. To this of course belong statements in the theory of government and of law. Most of the statements in our daily newspapers belong to person language or to community language or to both.

Now in a natural language like English all these languages are hopelessly muddled up. The first is the most easily sorted out, although its syntax and semantics are by no means so well known that it is impossible to talk nonsense in it without being found out. But with the others there is chaos. What is wanted for scientific purposes is a working out of rules for their construction and use, and especially rules for their meaningful combination. In the case of genetics I was able to offer an actual specimen of a carefully worked-out language in order to illustrate what I had to say about the language of that science. Unfortunately, in the present case I am not able to do this. I have not devoted sufficient time to the problem. Here is a completely untilled field calling for workers.

But when I say that what is wanted for scientific purposes is a working out of rules for the construction and use of these languages, I do not mean the general syntactical and semantical rules of these languages as such, but rules for their use in actual particular scientific *theories*. That is to say, if we are using one of these languages (or two or more of them in combination, as in fact some neurologists do), we should not take them quite naïvely from their embeddedness in natural language. We must deliberately build up the theory on the basis of explicitly stated rules governing the combination and use of the words we are proposing to admit into the theory.

In this connexion it is desirable to say something about the notion of the reducibility of one theory to another, about which so much has been written. Strictly speaking we can only fruitfully discuss such relations between theories when both have been axiomatized, but, outside mathematics, this condition is never satisfied. Hence the futility of much of the discussion about whether theory T_1 is reducible to theory T_2 'in principle'. Such questions cannot be settled by discussions of that kind but *only by actually carrying out the reduction*, and this is not done and cannot be done until the theories have been axiomatized.

It is also important to distinguish between *reducibility* of a theory T_1 to a theory T_2, and the *interpretability* of a theory T_1 in a theory T_2. I will deal with reducibility first.

We can say that a theory T_1 is *reducible* to a theory T_2, if and only if the following conditions are satisfied:

(1) All the primitive or undefined functors of T_2 are also functors of T_1, but T_1 contains some primitive functors which do not occur in T_2. T_1 is thus richer in content than T_2.

(2) For every primitive functor F of T_1 which does not occur in T_2 it is possible to construct a biconditional

$$A \equiv B, \tag{1}$$

such that 'A' consists of a matrix constructed with the help of F alone, and 'B' consists of matrices (combined by means of the operators on statements) which are constructed with the help of the primitive functors of T_2 but contain none belonging only to T_1.

(3) The biconditionals of kind (1) are theorems and tested statements of T_1.

(4) All the postulates of T_1 are either tested theorems of T_2 or they become tested theorems of T_2 after the elimination from them of all those undefined functors of T_1 which do not belong to T_2 by the application of the biconditionals of the kind (1).

By way of an example, suppose T_2 is a chemical theory containing the primitive functors 'F', 'G' and 'H', and suppose T_1 is a biochemical theory containing the same functors and in addition the biological undefined functor 'C' (for example, 'C' might denote the set of all cells). In order that T_1 should be reducible to T_2 it is necessary and sufficient that it should be possible to formulate a biconditional

$$x \in C \equiv (\ldots x, F, G, H, \ldots), \tag{2}$$

where the expression on the right-hand side consists of one or more matrices containing only such functors as 'F', 'G' and 'H', and this biconditional must further be a tested theorem of T_1 and, finally, all the postulates of T_1 must either be tested theorems of T_2 or become such when 'C' is eliminated in favour of 'F', 'G' and 'H' by the help of the biconditional (2).

Now it is at once obvious that, if T_2 is a theory in the physical language and T_1 a theory in the sensible-object or person-language, the above definition of reducibility is not applicable. In such cases the notion of interpretability is much more important.

We shall say that a theory T_1 is *interpretable in* a theory T_2, if and only if the following conditions are satisfied:

(1) For *every* undefined functor F of T_1 it is possible to construct a biconditional

$$A \equiv B, \tag{3}$$

such that 'A' consists of a matrix constructed with the help of F alone, and 'B' consists of one or more matrices (compounded by means of the operators on statements) constructed with the help of functors belonging only to T_2.

(2) Suppose that S is a postulate of T_1 and S' is the statement obtained from S by eliminating all the functors belonging to T_1,

which occur in it, in favour of functors belonging to T_2 by means of the biconditionals of the kind (3). If S' is a statement of T_2, i.e. derivable from the postulates of T_2, which has not yet been tested, it must be tested. If it survives testing, it then becomes an accepted statement of T_2. But it may happen that S' is not derivable from the postulates of T_2. In that case, if it survives testing, it must be added to the postulates of T_2 to form a new theory T_3.

(3) The above procedure must be carried out for *all* the primitive functors F and *all* the postulates S of T_1.

If these conditions are satisfied we should have, corresponding to every statement of T_1, an equivalent statement either in T_2 or in a theory T_3, differing from T_2 not in its primitive functors but only in having one or more additional postulates.

It is clear that in considering possible relations between a theory T_1 in person language and a theory T_2 in physical language only interpretability, not reducibility, is applicable.*

Returning now to our four languages, it is possible with their help to characterize certain doctrines. The doctrine that neurology and the study of behaviour should confine itself exclusively to the physical language is the doctrine of *behaviourism*. This I believe to be the most essential characteristic of behaviourism, not the doctrine that only what is called 'overt behaviour' is observable. I shall return to this question later.

The doctrine that all statements in natural science can and should be expressed in the sensible object language is known as *phenomenalism*. This has been proposed as a method of overcoming the body-mind dualism. It is a somewhat drastic method and one which is extremely difficult to carry out consistently, owing to the poverty of vocabulary in this language.† A theory is said to be *animistic* or *anthropomorphic* if it uses the person

---

* I am indebted to Professor A. Tarski for drawing my attention to this distinction and for help in formulating these definitions.

† This is a somewhat too brief and misleading characterization of phenomenalism. It might be more correct to say that this doctrine does not regard names belonging to physical language as names of objects of a totally different kind from sensible objects, but rather as a means of *classifying* the latter.

language, especially when this language is applied to objects other than persons. Even the community language has been used outside its own original sphere. The doctrine of the cell-state in biology is an example of this.

Before I deal with the central problem of mixed languages in relation to neurology I should like to say something more about the physical language in behaviour studies. I had the privilege at one time of working with Professor Clark Hull in the Institute of Human Relations at Yale, and I found the following method useful. I took, as my units, lives and time-stretches of lives. We have first to consider possible relations between two distinct time-stretches when they are both parts of the same life. To define these relations all we need are the notions of the *first moment* or *beginning*, $\mathbf{B}(x)$, of a time-stretch x, the *last moment* or *end*, $\mathbf{E}(x)$, of a time-stretch x, and the asymmetrical and transitive relation $\mathbf{T}$ of being *before in time*.

(1) The first relation I call *adjoining* ($\mathbf{A}$). I say that $x\mathbf{A}y$, if and only if $\mathbf{E}(x) = \mathbf{B}(y)$.

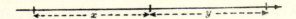

(2) The next relation is *disjunction*. I say that a stretch x is disjunct from a stretch y, if and only if there is a stretch z such that $x\mathbf{A}z$ and $z\mathbf{A}y$. This is equivalent to saying $x\mathbf{A}^2y$.

(3) I say that a time-stretch x is *contained initially* in a time-stretch y, if and only if $\mathbf{B}(x) = \mathbf{B}(y)$ and $\mathbf{E}(x)\,\mathbf{T}(\mathbf{E}(y))$. I write this $x\mathbf{Ci}y$.

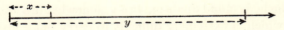

(4) I say that a time-stretch x is *contained terminally* in a time-stretch y, if and only if $\mathbf{E}(x) = \mathbf{E}(y)$ and $\mathbf{B}(y)\,\mathbf{T}(\mathbf{B}(x))$; $x\mathbf{Ct}y$.

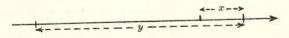

Only two more relations remain, both of which can be defined with the help of $\mathbf{Ci}$ and $\mathbf{Ct}$.

(5) The relation of being *contained medially* (**Cm**) can be defined as the relative product of **Ci** and **Ct**. That is to say, a time-stretch x is contained medially in a time-stretch y, if and only if there is a time-stretch z in which x is contained initially, and which is contained terminally in y.

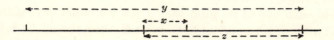

(6) The last relation, overlapping, can be defined as the relative product of the *converse* of **Ct** and **Ci**. That is to say, a time-stretch x overlaps a time-stretch y ($x\mathbf{O}y$), if and only if there is a time-stretch z which is contained terminally in x and initially in y.

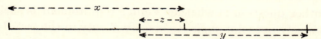

All these relations are asymmetrical. The first is intransitive and the last is neither transitive nor intransitive. For if we have $x\mathbf{O}y$ and $y\mathbf{O}z$, x may stand in **A** or $\mathbf{A}^2$ or **O** to z. All the remaining four relations are transitive. All these relations are mutually exclusive; if any one holds between two time-stretches not one of the others can also hold. On the other hand, if we take any two distinct time-stretches of the same life, one of these relations *must* hold between them.*

The composition functor for individual objects (as opposed to sets) is often useful in connexion with these relations. Thus if we have two time-stretches x and y such that $x\mathbf{A}y$, we have at once '$\mathbf{c}(\mathbf{A}, x, y)$' as a designation for the single time-stretch composed of x and y.

Now we proceed to consider the *classification* of time-stretches. Let us suppose that we are confining attention to animals all belonging to some one species, say domestic dogs. Let S be the set of all time-stretches of such lives which are in process of being stimulated in some specific way. For example, S might be

* See Note 2, p. 320.

the set of all time-stretches of such lives during which certain areas of skin are being flea-bitten or similarly irritated. In the same way let R be the set of all time-stretches of such lives during which the animal is exhibiting a certain characteristic response. For example, R might be the set of all time-stretches of lives during which the dog is scratching the above-mentioned areas of skin with one of its hind legs. Then we might say: if for all x and all y, if xAy and $x \epsilon S$, then $y \epsilon R$, then the set $\mathbf{C}(\mathbf{A}, S, R)$ is a *reflex*. In the case of the example mentioned, it would be what is called the *scratch reflex* in dogs. Of course we are not necessarily limited to the relation $\mathbf{A}$. We might more often have $\mathbf{O}$, or possibly $\mathbf{A}^2$. That would depend upon when we are to suppose that the stimulus stretch x ends. We could of course classify reflexes according to which relation is involved.

Another question is whether Venn's requirement is satisfied. It obviously does not *suffice* to specify S only in the way I have specified it. It must be supposed that members of S are *not* under the influence of anaesthetics or certain other drugs, that they have *not* had those afferent nerves cut which supply the area of skin in question and so on. Corresponding assumptions are presupposed regarding the time-stretch y. But there is still another important point concerning y. No reference has been made to its environment. Unless this is suitable, x will not be followed by a time-stretch which is a member of R. Some reference must therefore be included to a specific homogeneous set E of environments. We must consequently amend our definition of reflex as follows: We can say that the set $\mathbf{C}(\mathbf{A}, S, R)$ is a reflex with respect to the set E of environments if and only if, for all x and all y, if xAy and $x \epsilon S$ and $\mathbf{en}(y) \epsilon E$, then $y \epsilon R$.

We can now proceed to the *conditioned* reflex. This is a somewhat complicated notion. In this case, in order not to limit the definition to the relation $\mathbf{A}$, I shall use '$\mathbf{K}$' to denote the Boolean sum of $\mathbf{A}$, $\mathbf{A}^2$ and $\mathbf{O}$, thus $\mathbf{K} = \mathbf{A} \cup \mathbf{A}^2 \cup \mathbf{O}$.

By an *n-repeat* of a reflex X with time interval t^* will be meant a time-stretch of a life having n parts (n being a natural number

* See Note 3, p. 322.

greater than 1), each of which is a member of X and stands in **A**
to a time-stretch which is not a member of X and has a time-
length not exceeding t units of time, or stands in converse of
A to another time-stretch which is not a member of X and also
has a time-length not exceeding t units of time. In other words,
an n-repeat of X with time interval t is a string of n occurrences
of X in the same life separated by time intervals, each not
exceeding t units of time in length.

Now we can say that $Z = \mathbf{C}(\mathbf{K}, S'', R)$ is a conditioned reflex
established in the life x with respect to E and a time-length of
t' units if and only if there are distinct sets, S and S', of stimulus-
stretches of x and R is a homogeneous set of response stretches
such that $\mathbf{C}(\mathbf{K}, S \cap \bar{S}', R)$ is a reflex with respect to E ($\bar{S}'$ being
the complement of S'), S'' is a sub-set of S', all members of which
succeed an n-repeat of $\mathbf{C}(\mathbf{K}, S \cap S', R)$ with some time-interval t,
which is a reflex with respect to E, after a time-interval of length
not greater than t' units, and $\mathbf{C}(\mathbf{K}, S'', R)$ is a reflex with respect
to E. ($\mathbf{C}(\mathbf{K}, S \cap \bar{S}', R)$ is called the unconditioned reflex and
stretches belonging to $\mathbf{C}(\mathbf{K}, S \cap S', R)$ are called conditioning
processes.)

An alternative procedure would be to make explicit use of
a functor like **dlz** but without the restriction to zygotes and with
some other modifications made with a view to its use in
physiological contexts. We define '**dl** (x, y, z)' as an abbrevia
tion for '$x = \mathbf{B}(z)$ and $y = \mathbf{en}(z)$', z being a time-stretch of a life.
We define '**Dl** (X, Y, Z)' as an abbreviation for 'for all x, y, z,
if **dl** (x, y, z) and $x \in X$ and $y \in Y$, then $\mathbf{E}(z) \in Z$'.

Returning now to the general question of the exclusive use of
the physical language, there is no doubt that this has many
advantages. By this method we avoid all the perplexities and
confusions of mixing. The physical sciences contain many hypotheses which we can borrow and so save ourselves the trouble
of inventing new ones. And any hypothesis which will suggest
experiments will yield *some* results, even if not those expected
or hoped for. Their general methods and ways of thought are well
established and familiar. They hold out to us the lure of success,

since the physical sciences are by far the most successful. There seems to be no limit to the successful application of physical hypotheses except perhaps the limits of human ingenuity. Moreover, the physical method offers the lure of unity. If we use only the physical language there is no obstacle to our results becoming incorporated into the theoretical systems of the physical sciences.

On the other hand, exclusive adherence to the physical language is not without its disadvantages. It cannot cope with sensible objects. It carries with it the bifurcation of nature against which Whitehead protested in the first Tarner Lectures.* People who speak about nervous impulses causing or producing sensible objects, no less than those who speak about wishes and feelings causing or producing or directing nervous impulses (as perhaps Darwin did when he said: 'No doubt extreme joy by itself tends to act on the lacrymal glands'),† such people, I say, have ceased to talk physics or physical physiology. It is important to be clear about that. Causal laws in physics are not between physical objects and sensible objects, but between physical objects only.

Neither can the method, which uses the physical language exclusively, deal with persons, except by means of the abstract notion of body. This method undoubtedly suffices for many purposes. But, as we shall see, it has serious disadvantages in medicine and it involves ignoring almost all to which we as persons, but not as scientists, attach most importance. This leads many people to contradict in their lives what they say in their laboratories.

So much for some of the advantages and disadvantages of the exclusive use of the physical language. Anyone who wishes to play for safety may be recommended to follow the well-established grooves of the physical method. But people are not always content when they have found a good thing. They want to believe

---

* A. N. Whitehead, *The Concept of Nature* (1926), pp. 30, 185, 187.
† C. Darwin, *The Expression of the Emotions in Man and Animals*, Chapter VIII.

it is the *only* good thing. Consequently we find that many who follow this course do so because they honestly believe it to be the only possible one, or, at least, the only one which can be called scientific, because they *identify* science with physical science.

We saw, in our consideration of genetics, some instances of the curious but powerful tendency among biologists, when confronted with alternatives, to regard them as *mutually exclusive*; it has so often been 'heredity *or* environment', 'nucleus *or* cytoplasm', but *not both*. This tendency was the incentive to the writing of my book *Biological Principles* as well as its principal theme. Now we find the same tendency manifesting itself in connexion with the so-called rival points of view in psychology.

Psychologists seem to be particularly prone to discussions on the relative merits of what they call *concepts*. But it is not the concepts that matter but the *statements* in which they occur (cf. *The Parable of the Four Islands*, p. 177), and the mutual relations between these statements in theories. It is especially important to decide what statements are to be regarded as observation records by which other statements (above all, statements belonging to levels above zero level) are to be tested. Words belonging to theoretical levels need not all be 'intelligible' or 'picturable' (cf. Note 19, p. 72). If this were better understood there would be much less controversy over concepts, and words would not be dismissed merely on the ground that what they are supposed to name is 'subjective' or 'cannot be proved to exist', etc.

Now as I wish to do what I can to rectify the above tendencies and to encourage the outcasts who refuse to be bullied by the advocates of the *exclusive* attachment to physical methods, I propose to examine some of the arguments which have been used against other alternatives. Some of these arguments have recently been stated in Professor Hull's *Principles of Behaviour*.* Although I very much admire the ingenuity of some of Hull's hypotheses and his appreciation of the value of the axiomatic

---

* Clark L. Hull, *Principles of Behaviour* (1943).

method, yet I cannot agree with *all* that he says in the first two chapters of his book.

First, a word about a general belief which is not mentioned in Hull's book. If we speak the language of the body-mind dualism, we may say that the prejudice in favour of physicalism is partly supported by the belief that bodies are tangible and visible objects and minds are not. I am not using this language. I would only point out that this doctrine rests only on the naïve realism of everyday life and that physical objects and persons both belong to the converse domain of **OF**.* I have mentioned that all we can say about them can only be by way of hypotheses which are tested, but cannot be verified, by observing the sensible objects which stand in **OF** to them. I have already mentioned that 'observability' is not the point at issue, since behaviourists themselves have recourse to unobservable dispositions, stimulus-traces, etc. These are unobservable in the sense that there are no sensible objects standing in **OF** to them. What is aimed at is the exclusion of all but physical objects in order to remain within the physical language.

Hull expresses regret that what he calls the 'molar science of behaviour' cannot be derived from 'the subsidiary science of neuro-physiology'. He says: 'Nearly all serious students of behaviour like to believe that some day the major neurological laws will be known in a form adequate to constitute the foundation principles of a science of behaviour.' This does not directly raise the issue of physicalism, but I mention it because I believe it to be mistaken for two reasons. First, in building a theory we do not begin at the top of the pyramid and work down to the zero level. That is what we do when we axiomatize and already have the raw materials. We must first have generalizations of observation records *of behaviour* and *then* seek first-level explanatory hypotheses for groups of them. In the second place, the existing neuro-physiological laws are not laws about behaviour at all. They are, for the most part, laws concerning the interaction of parts in decerebrate animals or in animals which have

* See p. 28.

been deprived of all parts of the central nervous system above the spinal cord. It would be surprising if hypotheses of such an origin sufficed for the derivation of the laws of behaviour. This does not mean that they will not be helpful in providing hints for the required explanatory hypotheses of behaviour theory. Professor Konorski has pointed out that

...when undertaking the investigation of the function of the cerebral cortex, we should be prepared for the fact that this organ does possess certain specific properties distinguishing it from other parts of the nervous system, and that the language in which its activity has to be described needs to be enriched by certain new terms. But we cannot expect this language to be fundamentally different from that of the physiology of the spinal cord. And yet the situation at present is precisely that the two languages are quite different, and there is not even a dictionary to explain the one in terms of the other.*

(Professor Konorski owes his appreciation of the linguistic aspect of these problems to the fact that he attended the famous Polish School of Methodology, led by Leśniewski, Łukasiewicz, Kotarbiński and Tarski, which flourished in Warsaw before the late war).

I am glad to find that Professor E. C. Tolman also shares the view I am maintaining. He writes:

...But the thesis I am actually going to try to uphold here is the reverse and, at first sight, seemingly absurd one, to wit: that the facts and laws of psychology are, rather, in some part dependent on those of sociology and that the facts and laws of physiology are similarly in some part dependent upon those of psychology.†

This is to be expected in view of what I have said about the four languages. It means that, in specifying the environments of persons, words belonging to the community language must be used.

In theories relating to behaviour, and especially in those belonging to neuro-physiology, a large part in the construction

---

* J. Konorski, *Conditioned Reflexes and Neuron Organization* (1948), p. 5.

† E. C. Tolman, *Psychology Review* (1938), vol. XLV, pp. 228–41.

of hypotheses is played by micro-anatomical studies. This is an example of the tendency to seek hypotheses of the higher levels which are expressible with the help of the composition functor. But unless they have been checked by physiological experiment such hypotheses can be very misleading.

Hull objects that non-behaviouristic theories are guilty of what he calls anthropomorphic subjectivism. Now it seems to me that the doctrine of subjectivity has been greatly exaggerated. Statements in the person language at all events, such as 'Mary loves John', seem to me to be just as objective as statements involving both persons and physical objects, such as 'Mary is making a cake'. Both are hypotheses in the sense that we may be mistaken in both cases. But confirmation and falsification are also possible in both cases. Moreover, they *both* require the use of language *and* the belief, that *persons in general are not habitual liars*, for their confirmation. For, owing to the fact that **S** is a one-many relation (that at least seems to be the generally accepted view) even the so-called objective statements must in the long run owe their inter-subjectivity to communication.*

In order to exorcize the spectre of anthropomorphism, Hull recommends thinking 'in terms of the behaviour of sub-human organisms, such as chimpanzees, monkeys, dogs, cats and albino rats'. But this is not enough because, according to Hull, the infirm theorist 'begins thinking what he would do if he were a rat, a cat, etc.', and 'when that happens, all his knowledge of his own behaviour, born of years of self-observation, at once begins to function in place of the objectively stated general rules or principles which are the proper substance of science'. The only way of avoiding such lapses, Hull explains, is 'to regard from time to time, the behaving organism as a completely self-maintaining robot, constructed of materials as unlike ourselves as may be'.

From the point of view of the physical sciences, which of

---

* A relation R is said to be one-many if and only if whenever we have xRy and zRy, we must have $x = z$. Thus the relation of father to child is one-many: a child can have only one father.

course is Hull's point of view, this attitude is no doubt correct and indeed the only possible one. I am not criticizing it from that point of view at all. But from a wider point of view it certainly seems most extraordinary that, in order to study one thing you must think of something quite different—as unlike it as may be. This seems to involve a complete departure from the supposedly empirical attitude of science. We are frequently told that in science facts are not to be distorted and squeezed to fit into pre-determined theoretical moulds, but that the explanatory hypo-theses must be constructed to accommodate the facts. Here the reverse procedure seems to be advocated. It might be answered that no harm can result because the observations will disprove the theory if it is false and lead to its rejection. But there is nothing to compel us to reject a theory. We can always introduce new complications, if we are clever enough, which will restore the situation. The limit is not set only by the facts but by the limits of our capacity to invent and readjust hypotheses. That is why it is so important not to be content with only one type of hypo-thesis.

Then again, why must we reject knowledge born of years of self-observation which in fact we all use every day of our lives? Not because it is unscientific or cannot be made so, but because it cannot be expressed in the physical language, only in the person language. Here again we see that it is the desire to have a homogeneous physical language which is the crux of the matter.

Regarding the charge of anthropomorphism, I should agree that it would be most unscientific to say that water runs down hill because it loves the sea. But that is because I have no reason for regarding water as a person; it does not satisfy my criteria. But how can the same objection be brought against the state-ment that Mary bakes cakes for John because she loves him? It has not been made at all clear why it should be scientifically pernicious to apply person language when we are speaking of persons, or why it should be a scientific sin to be anthropomorphic when we are dealing with ἄνθρωπος himself.

Hull also raises the following objection against what I call person language. He says:

> Our usual thoughtless custom is to speak of cycles of behaviour by merely naming their outcome...and practically to ignore the various movements which brought this terminal state about.... The end result of each angling exploit, for example, may be in some sense the same; but the actual movements involved are perhaps never exactly the same on any two occasions: indeed neither the angler nor perhaps anyone else knows or could know in their ultimate detail exactly what movements were made. It is thus inevitable that for purposes of communication we designate behaviour sequences by their goals.

The difference here between the outlook of one who uses the physical language and one who uses the person language seems to be one of *interest*. It does not seem to be only a question of thoughtless custom or lack of knowledge. When we are describing acts of persons in person language we are usually not at all interested in the precise details of how they are performed. What is of primary interest in the one case is quite secondary in the other. This suggests that perhaps, in spite of superficial appearances, person-acts and behaviour are not quite the same things, and that psychologists and students of behaviour are not, after all, concerned with the same problem. But I must confess that I do not feel at all clear about this point.

There is of course a long history behind all this—a history of squabbles about method. I agree with Professor Arne Næss when he says, in his *Notes on the Foundation of Psychology as a Science,*

> What disturbs me is a disharmony between the vast production of programs and terminologies and the meagre production of painstaking empirical studies of limited problems.*

Let me repeat that I am not arguing against the adherence to the physical language as a method; it at least can claim to have

* Arne Næss, *Notes on the Foundation of Psychology as a Science*, Filosofiske Problemer, utgitt av Filosofisk Klubb, Oslo 1948, Nr. 9 (mimeographed in English).

produced 'painstaking studies of limited problems', although how far they can be called 'empirical', in view of what has just been said, is another matter. I am only arguing against its claims to be the *only* method, and the dangers which may arise if that claim is generally admitted. There have been repeated attempts to limit all scientific hypotheses to one type. About the middle of the last century Helmholtz wrote:

> Finally, therefore, we discover the problem of physical material science to be to refer natural phenomena back to unchanging elements, to attractive and repulsive forces whose intensity depends only upon distance. The solution of this problem is the condition of the complete comprehensibility of nature.
> And its vocation will be ended as soon as the reduction of natural phenomena to simple forces is complete and the proof given that this is the only reduction of which the phenomena are capable.*

In spite of the fact that this dogma has been abundantly falsified by the subsequent development of physics, it is still possible to find behaviourists writing in the same vein. Another example is furnished by the polemic conducted by Haeckel against His's attempt to found physiological embryology, on the ground that only evolutionary explanations were permissible in embryology.

It is a great misfortune that psychologists so often regard their hypotheses as mutually exclusive and as providing a basis for polemics rather than co-operation. It has not been shown that a psychological theory in person language is impossible, and in the next lecture an example of such a theory will be discussed.

* Quoted by Einstein and Infeld, *The Evolution of Physics* (1938).

LECTURE VII

§ 1. SOME LINGUISTIC DIFFICULTIES
IN NEUROLOGY

At the beginning of the last lecture I mentioned three methodological problems to which I suggested we might reasonably
hope to find answers. The first was: How do you know what
belongs to the language of neurology and what belongs to that
of psychology? The second was: Why must they not be mixed?
And the third: Assuming that there is no objection in principle
to their mixture, what are the rules governing the mixing?

I have explained my view that we have to deal, not with two,
but with four, languages; the physical language, the sensible-
object language, the person language and the community
language. I have pointed out that from the point of view of its
application to persons the physical language is exceedingly
abstract, in the sense that if used quite rigorously it must
necessarily omit a great deal that we believe about persons.
I have urged that no compelling reason has been brought forward against the mixing of these languages, but that rules
regulating their combination for scientific purposes have not
yet been worked out.

Our next task is to examine some specimens of the mixed
statements which occur in neurological writings and which
I mentioned at the beginning of the last lecture. Among the
commonest mistakes, as it seems to me, are: (i) treating sensible
objects as though they were physical objects, for example, by
identifying stimulus or neural impulse with sensible object;
(ii) identifying person with brain, i.e. putting a person into his
own head; and (iii) being too easily satisfied with metaphors, as
when neurologists speak of 'pictures' being 'projected on the
cortex' as though the brain were a kind of private cinema.

An example which illustrates most of these points is provided
by the following passage from a well-known work on pathology:

Paradoxical as it seems, pain cannot exist in the tissues; a pain in the foot is a disturbance of those nerve cells in the brain whose function it is to receive stimuli conveyed to them by the afferent nerves from that region...we must recognize two orders of tissues, irritation of which may set up the sensation of pain, but in the one this process is accurately localized, while in the other the sensation is localized by the brain as originating in some other area or areas.

Thus pains are treated as though they were physical objects and identified with nerve cells in certain states. But the process of localization is *not* a process of saying where the pain *is*. A pain, being a sensible object, can only be atopically related to other objects. Localization is a process of saying where the pain *appears in*. And this is performed by the person, not by the brain, because it is a characteristic of persons that their *parts are not persons*; although certain of their parts are capable of *becoming* persons, otherwise surgery and reproduction would be impossible.* The same point is curiously illustrated in the following passage where the writer speaks in one place of 'the female cerebral cortex' and in another of 'a woman'. It is from a letter in *The Lancet* in reply to a previous letter:

First, he [the author of the previous letter] asks why in women renal pain is not referred to the ovaries whereas in men it is referred to the testes. The answer is that the female cerebral cortex (where localization of pain actually takes place) has never really had the chance to determine the position of the gonads; ovaries do not normally suffer specific traumata, whereas testes often do by reason of their somatic isolation. Mr Brown need only ask a woman where her ovaries are, and the comparative indefiniteness of her answer will soon convince him that in this respect, even without pain, women cannot be compared with men.

This seems to me to be an extraordinary argument. Because testes protrude, in a sense, outside the body, male cerebral cortices know where they are and refer renal pain to them. Why they should do so is not stated. Ovaries, on the other hand, do not stick out, so female cerebral cortices are not so learned in

* See Note 4, p. 323.

anatomy and do not refer renal pain to them. But in order to examine them in this subject you must ask, not the female cerebral cortex, but the woman who possesses it.*

Difficulties of a different kind are illustrated by the following passage from a paper by a celebrated neurologist:

> Clearly, in any attempt to discover the realities underlying the phenomena experienced by the human mind it is a matter of the utmost importance to know something of the apparatus through which the effects of an external stimulus are conveyed to those parts of the brain which provide the physical basis for mental activity. On this will partly depend the answer to the question: how direct is the relation which a conscious sensation bears to the nature of the original stimulus?...Of great importance is the question whether impulses which arise in peripheral receptors are in any way modified in their passage to the cerebral cortex, for on this depends the accuracy with which the human mind can apprehend the exact nature of an external stimulus.

This seems to contain an epistemological mix-up. First, it seems to assume that persons sense neural impulses, not sensible objects. Secondly, it seems to assume that physiology is in an especially favoured position as compared with other sciences. It seems to say: In order to learn anything about the converse domain of **OF** you must first make a thorough study of brains. But as brains themselves belong to the converse domain of **OF** how are we ever to begin?†

We frequently read of *messages* travelling along nerve fibres and of *information* arriving at the cerebral cortex. We are told that *pictures* are projected on to the cortex in one place and get themselves *recognized* or *interpreted* in another. If neurology sticks to its own language it can only speak of volleys of nervous impulses reaching and leaving the cortex. Is anything really

---

* Lashley's experiments strongly suggest that neurologists in the past have been somewhat too naïve in their attitude towards all so-called localization problems. This is a region where common sense can hardly be expected to provide a very trustworthy guide. It calls for quite independent and original thinking. See *Symposia of the Society for Experimental Biology*, No. IV (1950), pp. 455–82.

† See Note 5, p. 324.

gained by borrowing words like 'message', 'information', 'picture', 'recognize', etc., from person language and sensible-object language?

Then there is frequent oscillation between 'the brain' and 'the mind'. On one page we may read that

From time to time this information may also be needed by the brain when it determines the next thing that the body should do.

and on the next be told that

The mind orders a particular movement, but leaves its execution to the lower levels of the nervous system.

If the brain determines the next thing that the body should do, why drag in the mind to give orders?

It is sometimes difficult to discover what exactly the non-behaviouristic neurologists are trying to do. One of their number has recently stated that

The final objective is to find out how the activity of the brain is related to that of the mind.

and adds that

if it is found that physical mechanisms cannot even explain all that happens in the brain, we shall have to decide when and where the mind intervenes.

I must confess that I find this very puzzling. How shall we know when physical mechanisms cannot explain all that happens in the brain? Will it not simply mean that, for the moment at least, we have come to an end of our ingenuity in inventing hypotheses? In any event, there will always be *something* happening in the brain which is not explained, because at any stage of neurological research there must be *some* hypotheses which are at the highest level in the theory as it stands at that stage, and these will not be explained until they cease to constitute the highest level. It will therefore be quite arbitrary when we decide that 'the mind intervenes'.*

* It is most important to notice that the phrase 'what goes on in the brain' does not, in neurological theory, belong to the level corresponding to that occupied by the phrase 'what goes on in the House of Commons' in sociological theory. We can discover something about the latter processes by paying

When neurologists use person language, but substitute 'the brain' for the name of the person, they are identifying that person with one of his own parts—putting him into his own head. If we do this, then it will be the brain that will decide when all that goes on in itself is to be explained by reference to itself or to a mind—a somewhat curious situation. Novelists frequently use 'brain' and 'mind' interchangeably. But the usages of natural language provide a somewhat erratic guide in such situations. We say 'Tom is still breathing', not 'Tom's lungs are still breathing'. But we say 'Tom's heart is still beating', not 'Tom is still beating'. Again, we say 'Tom is eating' not 'Tom's mouth is eating' or 'Tom's brain is eating'. We say 'Tom wants a poached egg' not 'Tom's brain wants a poached egg' or 'Tom's mind wants a poached egg'. Yet in all these cases Tom's brain is presumably involved in these processes.

If we substitute 'x's brain' for 'x' in some person statements, in which 'x' occurs as the name of a person, we sometimes get plain nonsense and sometimes plain falsehood. For example:

    (i)   Tom loves Mary

becomes   Tom's brain loves Mary's brain.

    (ii)   Mary is baking a cake for Tom

becomes

        Mary's brain is baking a cake for Tom's brain.

    (iii) When Tom swallows this he gets a taste of vinegar

becomes

    When Tom's brain swallows this it gets a taste of vinegar.

    (iv)   Tom gets a good view of Tom in this mirror

becomes

  Tom's brain gets a good view of Tom's brain in this mirror.

a visit to the Strangers' Gallery. But statements concerning what goes on in the brain will all be in the form of hypotheses, *invented by neurologists themselves* in order that statements may be derived from them which can be tested by observation records and which will not contain the phrase 'what goes on in the brain'.

This at least seems to be false. But some people might find nothing wrong with the next example.

(v)   Tom gets a fine view of the sea from this window

becomes

Tom's brain gets a fine view of the sea from this window.

In the absence of carefully formulated rules governing such substitutions we have no guide apart from personal preferences for deciding when their results are, in general, significant.

Sometimes these difficulties are recognized by neurologists but are dismissed as unimportant compared with the claims of brevity of expression, as in the following passage:

It will be only too evident that in this account a good many ill-defined and perhaps misleading terms have been used to describe what goes on in the nervous system. It is often considered improper to speak of a 'message' sent along the nerves when we are referring to the discharge of impulses, and to speak of their 'conveying information' to the brain. For those who think precisely this conjures up a disquieting figure of a little hobgoblin sitting up aloft in the cerebral hemispheres with a series of maps to look at. Both physiologists and philosophers have drawn attention to the fact that there is no such person. Indeed, Pavlov showed that a refusal to consider his existence may be a necessary condition for progress. He held that the physiologist is lost when he begins to use psychological terms and he managed to avoid them in describing his conditioned reflexes. This would be impossible in describing sensation, and if we are all aware of the dangers it will certainly save a good deal of circumlocution to keep those terms which mix up mechanical and mental similes. So let us continue to say that sights and sounds are of more interest to the brain than touches and pressures, for there is not much risk that it will lead us astray.

In the first place, is it even meaningful to say that sights are of *interest* to the brain? How can this eminent author be so confident that the use of such expressions will not lead us astray? Surely they commit us to putting the person into his own head, whether this is acknowledged or not, because the word 'interest' belongs to person language. Secondly, he has mentioned dangers but not specified them. Thirdly, what matters primarily in a scientific language is not what images it conjures up, nor in the first instance whether it enables us to avoid circumlocution, but *whether it has the right structure*. Until we have worked out the syntactical and semantical rules of a theory using mixed language we cannot know whether the latter is leading us astray.

Many such passages could be quoted, but these will suffice to show what a muddle we are in and how much neurology is in need of linguistic purgation. Here is a vast scope for the application of the results of the Boole-Frege movement. All that is lacking is a supply of trained workers able to carry out the task.

Now, with suitable precautions, there is no great difficulty in the use of mixed statements at the zero level in a theory, otherwise physiological psychology would be impossible. It is when we come to explanatory hypotheses that the serious difficulties begin. These difficulties are referred to by Whitehead, when he speaks of

the extreme difficulty of exhibiting the perceived redness and warmth of the fire in one system of relations with the agitated molecules of carbon and oxygen, with the radiant energy from them, and with the various functionings of the material body.*

There is also a passage in the *Monadology* of Leibniz which is interesting in this connexion:

We are moreover obliged to confess that *perception* and that which depends on it *cannot be explained mechanically*, that is to say by figures and motions. Suppose that there were a machine so constructed as to produce thought, feeling, and perception, we could imagine it increased in size while retaining the same proportions, so that one could enter as one might a mill. On going inside we should only see the parts impinging upon one another; we should not see anything which would explain perception.†

It is clear that the inventor of Leibniz's mill would only know whether he had succeeded if the mill were able to communicate

---

* A. N. Whitehead, *The Concept of Nature*, p. 32.
† Leibniz, *Monadology*, §17.

in the same sense and manner in which persons are able to communicate.

I think these quotations make it quite clear that the source of the difficulties referred to is the demand that an explanation must be not only an explanatory hypothesis in the sense used in Part I, but also an *intelligible* or picturable explanation in the sense there explained; and this is obviously ruled out in the present case. We cannot represent in the imagination an excited nerve cell, or system of nerve cells *and* the sensible objects which are in some way connected (in physiological theory) with their state of excitation. This is because **OF** is the only relation between sensible object and nerve cell with which we can be said to be familiar, and the relation in question is not the relation **OF**. But it is another atopical relation and there lies the difficulty. Now if every scientific explanation *must* be intelligible in the above sense this would constitute an insuperable barrier. But we have seen that this is very far from being the case; and even in the case of intelligible hypotheses it is not to their intelligibility that they owe their place in theories but to their *structure* and structure alone. This suggests a way out from our difficulties. It has not been shown that there is *any obstacle whatever*, apart from the limitations of human ingenuity and inventiveness, to constructing a theory which mixes physical language, sensible-object language and person language in its lower levels, *provided it is purely abstract in its higher levels*. In such a construction the composition functor could not be used exclusively because it involves the notion of spatial part.

The important questions which neurologists must ask themselves are (1) what are the most firmly established zero-level statements in neurology? and (2) what hypotheses can we invent which will have these zero-level statements among their consequences and will suggest further experiments? Both neurology and psychology are still in too primitive a state (judged by the number of theoretical levels in these sciences) to enable their mutual relations to be discussed profitably. Only when theory creation has progressed further will it be possible to construct them axiomatically and then to see how hypotheses involving mixed language could be introduced.

Whitehead, in his *Process and Reality* (p. 144), writes about physical physiology and psychological physiology. He says: 'Physical Physiology has, in the last century, established itself as a unified science; Psychological Physiology is still in the process of incubation.' Some readers may find what he says about psychological physiology helpful. But I must confess that I do not understand it.

§ 2. A DISCREPANCY BETWEEN THE TEACHING AND PRACTICE OF MEDICINE

I said at the beginning of the last lecture that there were two topics I wanted to discuss. I have now said all I can say at present about the first. The second problem was referred to as a discrepancy between the training of medical students and the practice of medicine. I hope what I have to say under this head will dispel any beliefs there may be that the problems with which I am attempting to deal are of only theoretical interest. We shall see something of their immense practical importance in medicine.

For the first two and a half years of his training a medical student learns about persons under a system of abstractions which treats them as purely physical objects. Even during the rest of his training—in the clinical period as it is called— although he will attend lectures on psychiatry, the physical point of view still vastly predominates, and it is left entirely to his own common sense, the pressure of social opinion and the sheer hard facts of the situation, to teach him that persons cannot always be regarded simply as physical objects. Only in recent years has the suggestion been made (but not carried out) that some psychological lectures should be given in the pre-clinical period, and only comparatively recently has there been talk about social medicine. But if we recognize that patients are persons, and that most persons are members of families, we shall wonder how the medical outlook could come to be so one-sided, and we shall see that in some degree all medicine must be, not only applied biology, but applied sociology, and especially that part of it which treats morbid conditions arising out of family relationships.

Some of the consequences of the body-mind dualism in medicine are startling and deplorable. Medical men make a distinction between organic and functional diseases. It is one of the prevailing canons of diagnosis that every effort must first be made to 'exclude the organic' (as it is called) before labelling the patient as 'functional' and handing him over to a psychiatrist.*

This procedure often has unfortunate consequences, which have recently been described as follows:

Many psychiatric cases are not recognized for what they are, or the recognition is unduly delayed to the great detriment of the patient; for a ruthless determination to rule out any possibility of physical disease beyond the least shadow of doubt before diagnosing a functional condition may ruin a patient permanently both in pocket and self-confidence....Little emphasis is laid and little direct instruction given on the importance of assessing a patient's happiness, work and social relationships, and it is implied that this can safely be left to his unaided common-sense....Fear of missing the organic also frequently leads to an incorrect emphasis on some minor physical abnormality. A thorough physical examination is rightly regarded as essential, but a reasonably thorough assessment of the mental and emotional aspect of all patients should equally be regarded as essential.†

The literature of psychological medicine abounds in examples of the consequences of the prevailing view. The authors just quoted describe the case of a girl who developed an abdominal pain and consulted a surgeon. He recommended an operation for appendicectomy which was accordingly performed. But after recovery and convalescence the girl again

* See Note 6, p. 325.
† D. Curran and E. Guttman, *Psychological Medicine* (1945).

complained of abdominal pain. This time she was advised to consult a surgeon with a view to treatment for adhesions resulting from the first operation. Fortunately, the second surgeon referred the girl to a psychiatrist from whose investigations it transpired that the girl's education had been such that she believed it to be possible to become pregnant by being kissed. The first abdominal pain had appeared after the experience of being kissed by an undergraduate during his vacation. After the recovery from the operation this girl was again kissed by the same undergraduate with a similar result. When the relevant facts about human reproduction had been explained to her the girl had no further trouble and when last heard of she was rowing in a women's eight.

This story, which might have had a less happy ending, doubtless contains many lessons for parents and undergraduates. But let me give another example. In this case a secretary in an office complained of dyspepsia. She was recommended to take a rest from work and to have her teeth removed. After she had recovered from this operation and taken a holiday she returned to work, whereupon the same symptoms returned. But this time, having no more teeth to be removed, she consulted a psychiatrist who discovered that she had fallen in love with her employer. The situation being such that marriage was impossible, and the girl having been virtuously brought up, she had been unable to acknowledge to herself that she was in love, and had expressed her feelings in a too whole-hearted devotion to her employer's business. She recovered when she found other employment.

Here, then, we have two examples of totally unnecessary surgery, involving the irrevocable loss of a harmless appendix and of a presumably good set of teeth, solely as a result of the prevailing doctrine that persons must be regarded first and foremost as physical objects.

I have said that the discovery that persons are not purely physical objects was very largely left to the common sense of the student and the sheer hard facts of the situation. That these sources of information do not suffice in all cases is illustrated from the following account in *The Lancet* of a lecture by a physician on the Seven Sins of Medicine.* Lest it should be supposed that there are no more than seven, the lecturer is careful to point out at the beginning that these are only the seven *worst* sins. Before I give extracts I should mention that the tools used in medicine fall into three sets: the tools of the surgeon, the tools of the physician, and the tools of the psychiatrist. The principal tool of the psychiatrist is the *language* by means of which he communicates with his patients as persons. But surgeons and physicians also have to deal with persons and they also use the psychiatrist's tool. That they do not always handle it with the skill and care of the psychiatrist and that they sometimes forget that words as well as knives can wound, will be clear from the following passages. The two sins which principally concern us are called cruelty and bad manners:

Cruelty [says the lecturer] is probably the most important and prevalent sin in the list I have chosen. Usually it is due to thoughtlessness and not deliberate. *Mental cruelty* is common and arises in three ways: (1) by saying too much; (2) by saying too little; and (3) by the patient being forgotten. By saying too much we often burden a patient with a load of anxiety which adds to the illness we are trying to relieve....Before telling a patient anything of his illness it is essential to consider whether it will help him or harm him....

By saying too little one can cause the fear of the unknown; the gaps may be filled in by the patient with alarming inventions and superstitions...in these cases reassurance is more important than medicine, and it is the doctor's duty to dig out these fears if possible.

Lastly, forgetting the patient. I refer to that kind of bedside teaching and discussion where the patient is treated as if he were unconscious, or discussed as if he already lay on the necropsy slab. It must be remembered that patients have ears, and that *sotto voce* murmurings about polysyllabic diseases strike needless terror into their hearts.

* Richard Asher, *The Lancet*, 27 August 1949, p. 359.

Physical Cruelty. . . . Do not wheel elaborate trolleys to a patient's bedside and start sticking needles in him until you have given him a word of reassurance and explanation.

Regarding the sin of bad manners the lecturer said:

If students do not learn good manners while they are learning medicine they will be at a great disadvantage in dealing with patients, nurses, and colleagues. . . . I once asked a student to examine the abdomen of a patient lying in an outpatient cubicle. He dashed into the cubicle where she lay, flung back the blanket, plumped his hand on her abdomen, shouted 'Gosh, what a beauty' (he was referring to the patient's enlarged spleen and not to her personal appearance), and dashed out again. Such behaviour must be condemned.

Is it not truly extraordinary that such admonitions should be necessary? And yet, is it not surely to be expected that a training which is almost exclusively physical should have such results? You will see now what I mean by a discrepancy between the teaching and the practice of medicine. In teaching, persons are regarded under the abstract notion of body. But when it comes to practice medical men are forced to amend this attitude. A doctor who consistently behaved towards his patients as if they were physical objects would very soon have no practice at all.

How has this state of affairs arisen? Historically speaking, the prevailing view presumably owes its origin to the Cartesian dualistic doctrine and the subsequent success and consequent prestige of the physical sciences. To the dualism we owe the doctrine that patients are tangible bodies with an intangible and unimportant appendage called a mind which is the exclusive concern of specialists. To the prestige of the physical sciences we owe the belief that nothing else is necessary or even possible. This prestige is now so enormous that it permeates and overpowers our thoughts as much as it overshadows our practical activities like a great mushroom-shaped cloud.

The physical sciences have won this enormous prestige by their spectacular achievements in the realm of technology, which are witnessed by everybody, so that the men who perform these miracles take the place of the magicians of older cultures

in the popular imagination. I use the word 'miracle' here in
the sense in which Bernard Shaw uses it when he makes the
Archbishop of Reims say: 'A miracle my friend is an event
which creates faith.'* Modern statesmen do not employ priests
to examine the livers of recently killed oxen before making
important decisions, they consult physicists, chemists and even
biologists. The difference in the attitude of governments to
scientists in the two world wars is a measure of the speed with
which the prestige of the physical sciences has increased in
recent years.

But the success of the physical sciences not only has this
effect on the popular imagination, it also has an overpowering
effect upon workers in other branches of science, who tend to
feel that unless they copy the methods and borrow the ideas of
the physical sciences they cannot be genuinely scientific. From
this it is to be expected that workers in the less developed
sciences will be discouraged from approaching their problems
in a really empirical spirit, in the way that must have been
followed by the pioneers of the physical sciences themselves,
who had no precedents to guide them. But before we succumb
to the assumption that the methodological principles and types
of hypotheses which are successful in the physical sciences are
all that we need, and that nothing new in that direction remains
to be discovered, it is, I think, important to remember that procedures which seem so obvious and even commonplace now have
only become so during a slow process extending over centuries.
It may well be that new methods remain to be devised and new
types of hypothesis to be invented, which are as alien to our
present ways of thinking as those once were to our predecessors,
which seem to us to-day so obvious and inevitable.†

* G. B. Shaw, *St Joan*, Scene ii: 'A miracle, my friend, is an event which
creates faith. That is the purpose and nature of miracles. They may seem very
wonderful to the people who witness them, and very simple to those who perform them. That does not matter: if they confirm or create faith they are true
miracles.'

† The scientific investigation of the so-called para-psychological phenomena
seems to have been carried so far forward that it is becoming increasingly
difficult to ignore them or to explain them away as the outcome of fraud, in

By way of example I would mention the exceedingly slow spread of the appreciation of the method of hypothesis and testing by experiment. It is very well illustrated by the story of scurvy. There are six important dates beginning with 1535 and ending with 1795, a period of 260 years. In 1535 the men of an expedition exploring those parts of America which lie westward of Newfoundland began to sicken during the long winter. They were rapidly cured by taking a decoction, made by the local women, of the bark and leaves of a certain tree. In August 1600 the crews of an expedition to the East Indies, consisting of four ships which had last touched land on 7 May, began to shows signs of scurvy, except those in one ship. The commander of this ship had brought with him bottles of lemon juice, three spoonfuls of which were given to each man every morning. One hundred and thirty-four years later, in 1734, Johannes Bachstrom published *Observationes circa Scorbutum*, in which the importance of fresh vegetables in the diet was clearly recognized. He coined the word 'antiscorbutic'. James Lind published his *Treatise on the Scurvy* in 1753. It contained an account of what appears to have been the first deliberate experiment in this field. On 20 May 1747 he had taken to sea twelve patients suffering from scurvy:

2 were given 1 quart of cider daily.

2 were given 25 drops of elixir vitriol 3 times daily.

2 were given 2 spoonfuls of vinegar 3 times daily.

2 were given a course of sea-water, half a pint daily.

2 were given 2 oranges and 1 lemon daily.

2 were given 'the bigness of a nutmeg 3 times a day of an electuary recommended by an hospital surgeon, made of garlic, mustard-seed, horse radish, balsam of Peru, and gum myrrh, using for common drink barley water boiled with tamarinds.'

Those who got the oranges recovered in six days, those with

---

order to preserve purely physical hypotheses in science. But even if such phenomena became widely recognized they would not in fact have the kind of metaphysical results which seem to be expected of them. Physicists would simply invent a new kind of energy (or something of that sort) with laws which the para-psychological phenomena would be said to exemplify.

the cider improved slowly, of the rest it is reported that they 'proved disappointing'. At last, in 1795, 42 years after the publication of James Lind's *Treatise*, the Admiralty decided to adopt lemon juice as the principal antiscorbutic. The consequences were spectacular. Whereas there had been 1754 cases of scurvy in the Royal Naval Hospital, Haslar, in 1760, in 1806 there was only one.*

I have offered this as an example of the slow spread of ideas, and of the way in which hypotheses and procedures which seem so obvious and commonplace to us to-day were by no means obvious when they were first introduced. You may say: Yes, but we have changed all that; you yourself have mentioned the speeding-up of this process between the two world wars. I reply: Admittedly, but that was all within the realm of the physical sciences. It is easy to follow the crowd along the well-worn paths. But perhaps it is not so in other fields. The slow spread of the Boole-Frege movement might itself be cited as a counter example. Things move very slowly in the world of education. But apart from this is there any serious obstacle to the introduction of some of the elementary ideas which have emerged from this movement into school teaching as a preparation for, if not as a substitute for, some of the mathematics that is now taught?

§3. A THEORY IN PERSON LANGUAGE

In order to support and illustrate my thesis that medical psychology is really a branch of sociology, especially the sociology of families, and also in support of my thesis that medical psychology needs no dualistic language in the ordinary sense of that phrase, I should like now to give a brief account of what I believe may prove to be an important hypothesis in this field. It is the hypothesis invented by Dr Ian Suttie and expounded with a wealth of illustration in his book, *The Origins of Love and*

* Data have been taken from J. C. Drummond and A. Wilbraham, *The Englishman's Food* (1940).

Hate,* which was published very shortly before his untimely death in 1935. I should in honesty explain that I am strongly biased in favour of this hypothesis. I first became acquainted with Suttie when he was serving as medical officer in the infantry regiment in which I was a subaltern, during the first world war, in Mesopotamia, as we then called it. We fought side by side in the Battle of the Shumran Bend which led to the retreat of the Turks from Kut-el-Amara. We marched together to Baghdad in the pursuit, we went sick together at the fall of that city, and we were evacuated together to the same base hospital. This was the beginning of an intimate friendship which lasted until his death. It was Suttie who first aroused my interest in methodology. His own interest in this subject is reflected in his book, which is in part a criticism of the Freudian doctrines, based on Suttie's own experience in psychiatric practice and his very wide reading. His methodological understanding led him to reject some of the more phantastic elements in Freud's teaching. I like especially Suttie's appeal to common sense.† Speaking of his hypotheses in the closing words of his book, he says: 'In fact it seems to me (in moments of enthusiasm) they reintroduce common sense into the science of psychology.'

Suttie begins by pointing out that when we make a *comparative* study of social life, the important fact emerges that 'social animals as a rule nurture their young, and conversely that nurtured animals tend to be more or less social. The social disposition seems to be a modified continuance of the infant's need for the nurtural parent's presence (even when the material need is outworn). Into it enter also nurtural or parental impulses, but there is no need to postulate a special social instinct.'

The child begins post-natal life in an ideal mutual love-relation with its mother. The mother gives to the child food,

---

* Published by Kegan Paul, London, 1935.

† Not because I regard common sense as a system of unchallengeable hypotheses, but because, in this particular field, it provides a valuable check on scientific hypotheses, the only important check we have at present for hypotheses in person language.

approbation, attention, interest. The child is helpless to give, in a material sense; it has only its pleasure and good will, and these it gives freely. This blissful symbiotic relationship, as Suttie calls it, must inevitably come to an end. It is interrupted by

  (i) the exigencies of life itself (advent of another child),

  (ii) the demands of culture (cleanliness-training),

  (iii) the demands of the community on the mother (e.g. the working mother must leave her babies).

Suttie's main contention is that, apart from genetic factors, the type of person that develops depends primarily upon the way in which this exclusive dependence on mother love is overcome.

It is part of Suttie's hypothesis that the baby not only starts life with a benevolent attitude but the need to give continues as a dominant motive throughout life and, like every other need, brings anxiety when it is frustrated. The need to give is as vital therefore as the need to get. The feeling that our gifts are not accepted is as intolerable as the feeling that others' gifts are no longer obtainable. Yet one or the other of these feelings may dominate an individual life. The process of psychotherapy is nothing but the overcoming of the barriers to loving and feeling oneself loved. Suttie was fond of quoting the saying of Ferenczi that the patient is cured by the love of the physician.

If the process of freeing the child from exclusive dependence on mother love—person-weaning as we might call it—is carried out gently and skilfully, the child develops interest in physical objects, and love relationships with other persons, during play, and so is gradually prepared for his place in the community. The mother's will and capacity to enforce this renunciation will vary directly (*a*) with the quality of her own character, and (*b*) with her own domestic status and dignity in the child's eyes, and inversely with (*c*) the importance of the child in her own emotional life, relative to other attachments and interests (i.e. her own dependency on the child).

What most commonly happens is that early in life the infant discovers that the benevolence of others is whimsical or conditional, and that its own gifts in turn are apt to be criticized and rejected. Love turns to anxiety, or to hate if frustration is severe. But this ambivalence of love and hate is intolerable, and the child will react in various ways which tend to preserve the love relationship or to provide substitutes for it.

(1) The child may take an aggressive attitude of fighting for its rights, leading perhaps to delinquency.*

(2) It may have recourse to surreptitious regressions or substitutes:

(i) it may regress to infancy in phantasy, which may lead to a complete turning away from social life, as in schizophrenia, or in lesser degree to utilization of illness; or

(ii) it may take the form of renunciation of the mother as bad and the adoption of the father as a substitute. If this does not lead to father-fixation in girls it may lead ultimately to a normal adoption of the whole social environment in lieu of the mother; or

(iii) security may be sought in power to exact services, leading perhaps to delinquency or to paranoia.

(3) Finally, the child may submit and avoid the pain of privation by repression. This is what Suttie calls the *taboo on tenderness*, the self-weaning from affection by a blindness to pathos of any kind. He regards this taboo as the leading feature of our own culture and the main reason for the substitution of the power technique for that of love. He says:

The view that tenderness is more or less an artifact and that asexual love is a myth of the idealists is fairly well established in our tradition and everyday life. The glorification of toughness is a revenge upon and a repudiation of the weaning mother, on the defensive principle of 'sour-grapes'.†

* See Note 7, p. 326.

† Anyone who has doubts about the glorification of toughness in our times need only pay a visit to a cinema or read about the treatment of political deviationists in the totalitarian countries.

But

what we call tender feeling and affection is based not on sexual desire, but upon the pre-oedipal emotional and fondling relationship with the mother and upon the instinctual need for companionship which is characteristic of all animals which pass through a phase of nurtural infancy.

In our culture in particular, says Suttie,

the brusqueness of the cleanliness-training, the frequent and prolonged separation of mother and infant, and the mother's own intolerance of tenderness (the result of her 'puritanical' upbringing) bring about a precipitate 'psychic parturition' [as Suttie calls it], attended by anxiety, acquisitiveness and aggressiveness which is reflected in our culture and economic customs and attitudes.

In this connexion it is perhaps worth recalling William James's division of philosophers into the tough-minded and the tender-minded, with their emphasis on the physical and personal aspects of experience respectively. And one may wonder whether the taboo on tenderness may not also be a factor in establishing the prevailing fashionableness of the physical sciences, even when we are dealing with persons. Suttie himself asks at the very beginning:

In our anxiety to avoid the intrusion of sentiment into our scientific formulations, have we not gone to the length of excluding it altogether from our field of observation?

He also remarks that

it is even rather absurd that some psychologists should idealize the formulations of physical science at a time when physicists themselves are not agreed as to the *kind* of formula which is desirable.

On account of the taboo on tenderness,

anything that tends to rearouse pathos and sentiment is resented, exactly as the prude resents an erotic suggestion and for the same reason. The taboo upon regressive longings extends to all manifestations of affection until we can neither offer nor tolerate overt affection. The hard puritanical character thus developed is intensely jealous and intolerant. We force our own children to grow up too quickly to allow them time to outgrow their childishness. We make them 'serious', preferring success to enjoyment—efficient competitors in the struggle for existence. But have we not mistaken a mere desertion or suppression of the open-mindedness of childhood for maturation and manhood, and regarded this negative quality— a defensive reaction—as good in itself?

I must omit any attempt to describe how Suttie finds support for his hypothesis in ethnology and comparative religion, as well as his interesting comparison of patriarchal and matriarchal cultures. Neither is it necessary to say anything about his criticism of Freud.*

It is clear that this theory is stated in the person language. It is a developmental and social theory in the sense that it attempts to derive statements concerning types of adult persons from general statements concerning the various possible results that may follow upon types of events in early life, namely, the types of person-weaning, as I have called it. But it does this at present only in a very general way. There is no attempt to establish anything like precise general laws. We cannot yet specify all the types of person-weaning in detail and correlate each exactly with a specific type of adult person.† Moreover, although mishandling of person-weaning has such serious effects in adult life, on account of what I have called the magnifying effect of development, because it occurs relatively early, yet this is not intended to mean that occurrences subsequent to this early period are not without permanent effect, otherwise psychotherapy would be impossible.

Supposing the types of adult person to be what in Part II were called phenotypes, we can use our **Dlz** functor in this

---

* I should be sorry if the above very brief account of Suttie's hypothesis were to give any reader the impression that Suttie regarded the factors to which he drew attention as of such importance as to justify neglect of all others, or that he believed that therapy based on his views would be a cure-all. Suttie was in no sense a fanatic or a one-sided man. He thought of his hypothesis as being quite capable of incorporation in the general Freudian outlook.

† It may well be that this will always be impossible from the nature of the case. It may be that in this field as in some others we must content ourselves with probability statements.

connexion in order to contrast the present problem with that in genetics. In the latter, as we saw, when we have a law of the form $Dlz(Z, E, P)$ the emphasis tends to be upon Z rather than on E, because the adult environmental range is usually contained in the P-environmental ranges. But in person development we have the converse situation. E is recognized as having an enormous variety of sub-sets, and Z tends to be ignored because, for one thing, we know very little about it, and, for another, it seems to be assumed that varieties of Z are unimportant for the types of P in which we are interested.

If I ask myself why I am biased in favour of this theory, I think the answer is because it is an optimistic theory, and I see no reason why a theory can only be truly scientific if it is pessimistic. Suttie's theory is optimistic because it offers some hope to mankind. It offers a procedure by which we might greatly diminish the population in our mental hospitals and the number of people needed to look after them.* It offers a receipt for producing happy families. Tolstoy's generalization finds a place in Suttie's theory. All happy families resemble one another, each unhappy family is unhappy in its own way, on account (among other reasons) of the variety of ways in which person-weaning may go wrong.

But what hope is there that Suttie's theory will be put to the test of experiment? Here there is less ground for optimism.† Will not the taboo on tenderness itself be an obstacle? We often read nowadays of the contrast between our knowledge of and control over the physical world and our lack of knowledge of and control over ourselves and our social institutions. But it is not *only* lack of knowledge; it is our unwillingness or inability to accept and to apply to ourselves the knowledge we already have about persons, which should be contrasted with the almost terrifying speed with which we not only learn, but accept and use, our knowledge of physical objects. Some

---

* I am assuming that people of the most diverse political and ethical opinions would agree that this is desirable.

† See Appendix C, p. 354.

consequences of Suttie's doctrines have been before the world, in the form of religious and moral teaching, for over 2000 years. But G. K. Chesterton's saying still seems to be applicable: that Christianity has not been tried and found wanting, but found difficult and not tried.* This is because toughness is self-perpetuating and salvation is therefore not to be reached in one generation. To eliminate the taboo on tenderness we must persuade people to provide their children with a social environment which will not drive them to seek this refuge. But the beating of children has had the approval of Christian pastors for centuries. Our tragedy is not so much lack of knowledge about how to change the world, as lack of ability to agree about the direction in which to change it, because the world desired by the tough is different from the world desired by the tender.

From the point of view of practical applications and the possible consequences of such applications, I think Suttie's theory compares very favourably with those which confine themselves to the physical language. I would like to add one or two further criticisms of the latter from this point of view.

First, there is what I will call the sincerity requirement. All persons, according to Suttie, have primarily a need for love. But this does not mean that they only want other people to behave towards them *as if* they loved them. They are not satisfied with that: they want people to *feel* love towards them. 'The best way', said Jeremy Bentham, 'to win men to you is to seem to love them; and the best way to seem to love them is to love them indeed.'† Now if a person x behaves towards a person y *as if* he loved him but does not in fact feel love for him, we say that x is behaving insincerely towards y; and y will sooner or later detect this, unless x is an unusually successful and persistent actor who is never caught off his guard. I am

---

* Suttie's hypothesis relieves us from the assumption that this is a result of some 'inherent wickedness' or 'original sin' in persons. What is the sense of exhorting a person to love his enemies if he has been so mishandled in early childhood that he is incapable of loving anybody? I have in mind here the ethical, not the theological, doctrines of Christianity.

† Quoted in J. Morley's *Life of Gladstone* (1903), vol. II, p. 60.

told that even quite young children are able to detect insincerity. Consequently there is nothing intrinsically private, subjective, unobservable or unscientific about the notion of love. There is therefore no reason why a theory of persons should not contain it. But for behaviourism the sincerity requirement cannot even be formulated, because it essentially involves person language. Incidentally, I may point out that in a properly formulated scientific theory the word 'love' would not enter as the name of a feeling, but as a shared name of each couple x, y such that x loves y.

Secondly, I ask whether it is good empiricism and good science to postpone the study of persons until you have completed a behaviour theory, founded on the study of white rats and robots, in the hope that you will then be able to deduce the statements descriptive of persons from the postulates at which you have arrived from your experiments on rats? The behaviourist programme is a long-term policy. We do not know whether it will ever be completed. It would surely be foolish to reject a theory which is expressed in the person language and refuse to try to extend and improve it simply on the ground that it cannot be translated into the physical language.

My third point is that Hull's theory, for example, contains one feature which would, as it stands, rule it out as a theory of human conduct. A fundamental part is played in this theory by the notion of *need*. But need, as Hull understands it, is defined purely in terms of survival. Now the notion of need in relation to persons is clearly very much wider than this.* Persons have supra-biological needs, and consequently the notion of need would require radical revision if Hull's theory is to have the wide scope he claims for it.

Finally, I come to the question whether it is possible to be impartial and to exclude all consideration of possible social consequences of our hypotheses when we are dealing with persons. We are told that the final test of a hypothesis is in successful applications, and, in connexion with psychological

* See Appendix C, p. 341.

hypotheses, there is always the possibility that people may change in the direction to which a particular hypothesis points. Thus if some people are told often enough that they are robots they may in time come to believe it, and even to become very good imitations of robots. If, on the other hand, they believe they have an urge to love one another and that they are the victims of a taboo on tenderness, then they may in time grow to love more and hate less. These two possibilities are likely to appeal to different people in different ways according to whether they belong to the tough or the tender. The first, for example, should appeal to advertising agents and to propaganda ministers in totalitarian states.

Such considerations raise the question how far the example of the physical sciences offers an altogether trustworthy model for a science of persons. We are told, for example, that the aim of the physical sciences is 'prediction and control'. But what if persons, except when they are ill, do not want to be predicted and resent being controlled? Who is to do the controlling? Suttie's theory does not exactly do this. It says to mothers: *if* you want a happy family of healthy children you must, among other things, be very careful and very gentle in their person-weaning.*

A purely physical theory of persons has no relish of salvation in it. It must necessarily lead to a de-personalization of our attitude towards persons—a process which again may recommend itself to the tough but not to the tender.† Suttie's hypothesis enables us to see why this should be so. Some years ago Lord Russell wrote:

Only the most abstract knowledge is required for practical manipulation of matter. But there is a grave danger when this habit of manipulation based upon mathematical laws is carried over into our dealings with human beings, since they, unlike the telephone wire, are capable of happiness and misery, desire and aversion. It would therefore be unfortunate if the habits of mind which are appropriate and right in dealing with material mechanisms were allowed to dominate the administrator's attempts at social constructiveness.‡

* See Note 8, p. 327.   † See Note 9, p. 327.   ‡ See Note 10, p. 328.

In constructing scientific hypotheses we disregard everything that is not immediately relevant to obtaining the result desired. We are concerned with the satisfaction of purely intellectual or practical (material) needs. When we come to apply scientific theories to persons, some of the factors from which abstraction has been made may, however, be relevant if the application is to be successful. Some persons have what are called emotional and spiritual needs, as well as intellectual and material ones. It therefore becomes necessary to see that there is no conflict or frustration when scientific hypotheses, in which no account is taken of such needs, are applied to persons. We have seen how this can happen, with unfortunate consequences, in the case of medicine, when its problems are approached from a purely physical point of view. This is a particular instance of what Whitehead has called 'the intolerant use of abstractions'.

Let us consider this question of applied behaviourism a little more closely. I must first describe two attitudes which, from time to time, we may adopt towards fellow-members of a community. Suppose O is some scientific observer who is observing some subject-matter S in which he is interested. He will not think of himself as part of S but as being *outside* it and able, in most cases, to interfere in it in order to set up experiments with a view to discovering the laws of S. He will also think of himself as being able to choose between possible alternative hypotheses regarding S and to direct his experimental procedure accordingly.

Now suppose we introduce a second observer O'. He may do either of two things: he may be primarily interested in S and regard O as well as himself as outside S and as a co-observer with himself. Or, he may be interested in the relation of O to S, and so he regards both O and S as parts of a wider system S'. But he will still regard himself as outside S' and as able to consider hypotheses about it and to investigate its laws. He will, however, deny this ability regarding S to O. He will not think of O as being able to choose regarding S but as subject to the laws of the system S'. And this will be so whether he formulates the laws of S' in the physical language or in the person language. This, however, presupposes that O is not aware that O' is regarding him in this way. If he does become aware of this he may willingly submit, like one sitting for his portrait, or he may resent the attitude of O' and become a spoil sport. I call each observer's attitude to his system the 'outside the system' attitude.

This same attitude may be adopted in other situations than those of scientific inquiry. Those of my friends who differ from me in their political opinions are clearly the victims of propaganda. But in *their* view I, who differ from them, am equally clearly the victim of propaganda. But as we live in a country in which more than one type of political propaganda is permitted, a further hypothesis is required to explain why one of us is the victim of one type of propaganda and the other the victim of another. This is provided by a developmental person hypothesis according to which my upbringing has predisposed me towards one type and theirs has predisposed them to another. These are explanations which are forced upon us because each of us takes the 'outside the system' attitude towards the other.

But there is another attitude, according to which each of us thinks of himself, not as a product of a type of upbringing and a type of propaganda, but as being able to consider each side on its merits and to decide that the view he has adopted is both a correct political theory and one which would lead to the kind of life which he regards as best for himself and his fellows. In the same way we may have two psychologists holding different theories. One may regard the other as hopelessly biased and the victim of various extraneous influences, but he does not regard himself in this way.*

There are thus two attitudes which we may take towards fellow-members in a community: we may take the attitude 'I am outside the system and you are inside it'; or we may take the co-operative attitude of allowing our fellow-members the same status that we assume for ourselves.

* See Note 11, p. 328.

Let us see now how these attitudes will appear in a community regulated in accordance with the principles of applied behaviourism. Referring to 'the oncoming youth, those now in training and those to be trained in the future', an American behaviourist writer has recently expressed the hope that

Perhaps they will have the satisfaction of creating a new and better world, one in which, among other things, there will be a really effective and universal moral education.

Why is it that the enthusiasts for the application of a new scientific theory to persons so often assume that the results will be beneficial, when they see around them instances of such applications, regarding the beneficial effects of which there is at least some room for differences of opinion? Is it not because they always take the 'I am outside the system and you are inside' attitude? Would everyone agree with this author's view of what would be a better world? If not, how would it be decided *which* version of a better world was to be realized in practice, and made the basis of a really effective and universal moral education? Would all sections of the population of the United States of America agree upon this? Surely this question has only to be asked, to be answered immediately in the negative, because the better world of the tough is different from the better world of the tender, and the better world of the rich is different from the better world of the poor.

Suppose we find ourselves confronted with two alternative, mutually exclusive, courses of action, A and B, between which we regard ourselves as being able to choose. After due deliberation of their possible consequences and a weighing of the pros and cons of each, we finally decide to follow one, say A. It may be that we are aware of *wanting* very strongly to follow B and that a special effort and vigilance are required in adhering to A. However, in a community which was the subject of applied behaviourism there would be no question of choice, except on the part of the Minister of Propaganda. He and his governmental colleagues would alone be outside the system. If *he* decided that actions of type B were to be forbidden, then it would be his business to see that the members of the community, by proper conditioning, maintained by suitable reinforcing states of affairs, always performed actions of type A, when the occasion arose. If the members of this community thought of themselves as exercising a choice between A and B, that would be a purely private affair not officially recognized in the system; and whether they felt any residual longings for B, or enjoyed the virtue of choosing A, would be equally irrelevant. Such possibilities could not even be formulated in the official language. Any aberrant individuals who *did* insist upon exercising choice, and were misguided enough to follow actions of type B, would (if we may judge by historical precedents) be dealt with by the technique of the midnight warning, the rubber truncheon and the concentration camp. This would be a really effective and universal moral education and, as far as I can see, the only kind of education that would be possible within a community governed on strictly physical lines.

Now all this presupposes that there is just *one* minister of propaganda, who keeps a strict rein on all sources of information and opinion and is supported by an efficient secret police who will report to him at once any murmurings of discontent among the population. Relax these conditions but a little, so as to admit at least two independent sources of information and alternative opinions, and at once the system breaks down —the possibility of choice presents itself together with discussion, deliberation and decision. Conditioning then becomes impossible, just as it would be impossible in a behaviour laboratory in which there were two professors, each independently using the same white rats. Professor A arrives in the morning and conditions the rats in one way, but as soon as his back is turned in comes Professor B and begins a separate set of experiments which completely frustrates Professor A's efforts.

Thus we have two possible worlds: one governed by a minister of propaganda who takes the 'outside the system' attitude towards the population, and one which allows alternatives, discussion and co-operation. We are therefore confronted with the problem of deciding which possibility will provide a better world. If we choose the first alternative—perhaps because we enjoy the exercise of power and entertain ministerial ambitions, or because we like being told what to do—then clearly in order to realize it we must, by hook or by crook, contrive to get an all-powerful minister of propaganda installed in his office at the earliest possible moment, in order to deal effectively with those who would choose the second alternative. This clearly requires the technique of the *coup d'état* and the revolution. Thus the doctrine of applied behaviourism would seem to be a direct incentive to revolution—a result which is all the more surprising in view of the popularity of behaviourism in the United States of America.*

Lord Russell has recently written:

It is hoped that by studying the psychology of belief those who control propaganda will in time be able to make anybody believe anything. Then the totalitarian state will become invincible.

But so long at least as more than one kind of propaganda is allowed in a community there is always the possibility of encouraging people to examine critically, and to resist, propaganda. I think well enough of my fellow-men to hope that such an attempt as Lord Russell describes would in the long run defeat its own ends. Should we not take the attitude of Hamlet in his rebuke to Guildenstern:

Why, look you now, how unworthy a thing you make of me! You would play upon me; you would seem to know my stops; you would pluck out the heart of my mystery; you would sound me from my lowest note to the top of my compass: and there is much music, excellent voice, in this little organ; yet cannot you make it speak. 'Sblood, do you think I am easier to be play'd on than a pipe? Call me what instrument you will, though you can fret me yet you cannot play upon me.

*   *   *   *

* See Note 12, p. 329.

In conclusion, let me summarize the main points which I have been trying to illustrate by these lectures. First, the need for a critical attitude towards language in science. I hope the many examples I have given will suffice to remove any doubts about this. In the first lecture I said that I would test the hypothesis that only five sentential connectives (as they are commonly called) are needed in science: 'not', 'and', 'or' (in the inclusive sense), 'if...then...', and '...if and only if...'. This hypothesis has been upheld. Next, emphasis was laid on the extensional point of view and the avoidance of abstract entities. This too has worked out quite well, except that it has not been possible at all places to avoid sets of sets and the quantification of dummy names representing sets (as opposed to individuals). In Appendix B I had to use undefined sets of sets, and it was not possible, therefore, to treat their signs as abbreviators. Moreover, in using relation signs as names of ordered couples we do not avoid abstract entities because ordered couples are such entities. This applies of course just as much to a natural language as to an artificial one. Moreover, I have made free use of natural and rational numbers without any attempt to bring them under the theory of shared and unshared names. But apart from these technical problems, with which biologists as such need not much concern themselves, I hope the many illustrations I have given of the usefulness of elementary set-theory will suffice to convince the reader of the desirability of cultivating it, since it enabled us in Part II to construct the combined algebra there explained, and to reach a generalization of elementary genetics and a classification of genetical systems.

Another point which I discussed in Part I and which has, I hope, been sufficiently illustrated in the remaining lectures, is the notion of *structure* in connexion with scientific theories. I stated how the consequence relation, upon which scientific theories are built, depends only on the structure of the statements involved, not on any *particular* meaning that may be given to the functors they contain. I have also explained the

notion of levels of theoretical statements, which emerge in the
course of methodological analysis. It is important that we
should try to be aware of the level at which we are working,
and it is always desirable to avoid formulating a statement in
terms belonging to level n if it can be satisfactorily formulated
(for the purpose in hand) in terms belonging to level $n-1$.
The establishment and preservation of the continuity of steps
between the levels is also important; the lack of this continuity
sometimes makes it difficult to connect biological with physical
and chemical statements. I have also emphasized in several
places the desirability of remembering Venn's requirement and
the constant factor principle.

Regarding epistemological problems, which have occupied
such a large part in many Tarner Lectures in the past, I have
tried to say as little as I could. So long as we remain within the
language of the physical sciences such problems do not seem
to be very pressing. It is when we consider the problems raised
in Part III that they become important. I have maintained
the hypothesis that there is an irreducible antithesis between
feeling or sensing (interpreted very widely) on the one hand,
and doing on the other. Persons have traffic with both the
domain and the converse domain of **OF**. With the domain
by way of sensing, with the converse domain by way of
doing.

Regarding the problems of Part III the important point
seems to be to keep alive the spirit of inquiry and not to allow
ourselves to be satisfied with traditional attitudes and traditional language in which so much of traditional belief is embedded. My principal aim has been to urge that we should try
to find a new starting point in a *pre-dualistic* language which
I have called person language. Words like 'psycho-somatic'
are only invented to heal a breach which need never have been
made. I have maintained that medicine has no need for a dualistic language (in the usual sense) and would be better without
one. If we use person language we can see that medicine is
involved in the sociology of family life and that the so-called

medical psychology deals with problems arising from the difficulties of living together under one roof of persons related by the parental or some derived relation. I have also drawn attention in Part III to some of the special difficulties which may present themselves when scientific hypotheses are applied to persons, and to the desirability of being prepared to meet and overcome such difficulties.

Regarding other problems raised in Part III, I hope I have made it clear that if you want to remain within the boundaries of the physical sciences you must rigorously confine yourself to the physical language. If you do not wish to confine yourself to the physical language, then you cannot remain within the boundaries of the physical sciences, but must face the task of inventing new hypotheses which can only be of the abstract kind expressed in a deliberately constructed language.

Throughout these lectures I have emphasized the importance of hypotheses in natural science and the impossibility of knowing whether a hypothesis is true. Science is not based only on observation and experiment. Like most other human activities it is based on the celebrated trio, faith, hope and charity: faith in the results, hope that this faith will continue to be justified in the future, and charity towards fellow-workers, especially those engaged in the less developed sciences.

I hope I have said enough to show that something useful is to be learnt from the Boole-Frege movement about the use of language in science. For, in spite of what has been said, the natural languages have taken us a long way, and some knowledge of the Boole-Frege movement can be of great help in showing us how to make the best use of them. However, as the sciences develop something more is required and, for some of the projects which I have suggested, a more technical knowledge will be necessary.

One other thing is necessary—patience! Important results will not be easy of attainment. We must be prepared for laborious and persistent toil, and this requires patience and still more patience.

He that would have a cake out of the wheat must needs tarry the grinding.

Have I not tarried?

Ay, the grinding; but you must tarry the bolting.

Have I not tarried?

Ay, the bolting; but you must tarry the leavening.

Still have I tarried.

Ay, to the leavening: but here's yet in the word 'hereafter' the kneading, the making of the cake, the heating of the oven, and the baking; nay, you must stay the cooling too, or you may chance to burn your lips.

Note 1 (p. 206). By the relative product of two two-termed relations P and Q, written $P \mid Q$, is meant the relation in which an object x stands to an object y when there is an object z such that x stands in P to z and z stands in Q to y. Thus uncle is the relative product of brother and parent, because if x is uncle of y there is a z such that x is brother of z and z is parent of y. The relative product of **S** and **OF** is the relation in which a person x stands to an object y when there is a sensible object z such that x stands in **S** to z and z is **OF** y. The square of a relation R (R^2) is a particular case of relative product, since it is the relative product of R with itself.

Note 2 (p. 275). The following is a derivation of the statement in the text that, if x and y are any time-stretches of one and the same life, then one stands to the other in one of the following relations: **A, A², O, Ci, Cm, Ct** or $x = y$. We shall denote the first moment of any time-stretch u by $\mathbf{B}(u)$ and the last moment by $\mathbf{E}(u)$. We shall write '$x\mathbf{T}y$' for 'x is before y in time'. The above statement will be derived from the following assumptions:

(i) The relation **T** with its field limited to the moments of any one life is connected, i.e. if u and v are any such moments we must have $u\mathbf{T}v$ or $u = v$ or $v\mathbf{T}u$.

(ii) For any time-stretch x, $\mathbf{B}(x)\,\mathbf{T}\,\mathbf{E}(x)$ and $\mathbf{B}(x) \neq \mathbf{E}(x)$.

(iii) If, for any moments u and v of the same life we have $u\mathbf{T}v$, then there is a time-stretch z which is part of that life and such that $u = \mathbf{B}(z)$ and $v = \mathbf{E}(z)$.

(iv) **T** is transitive, i.e. if for any time-stretches x, y and z we have $x\mathbf{T}y$ and $y\mathbf{T}z$, then we have $x\mathbf{T}z$.

(v) If for any time-stretches x and y we have $\mathbf{B}(x) = \mathbf{B}(y)$ and $\mathbf{E}(x) = \mathbf{E}(y)$, then $x = y$.

Derivation: From assumption (i) it follows that if x and y are any time-stretches of the same life we must have

A. $\mathbf{B}(x)\,\mathbf{T}\,\mathbf{B}(y)$,　or　B. $\mathbf{B}(x) = \mathbf{B}(y)$,　or　C. $\mathbf{B}(y)\,\mathbf{T}\,\mathbf{B}(x)$.

It also follows that with *each* of these three possibilities we also have three possibilities regarding the last moments of x and y,

I. $\mathbf{E}(x)\,\mathbf{T}\,\mathbf{E}(y)$, or II. $\mathbf{E}(x) = \mathbf{E}(y)$, or III. $\mathbf{E}(y)\,\mathbf{T}\,\mathbf{E}(x)$.

Thus we have in all nine combined possibilities:

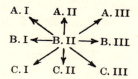

Opposites in this array, as indicated by arrows, will be found to be converses of one another, except in the case of B. II which has no opposite and corresponds to a symmetrical relation. In each of the nine possibilities, except A. I and C. III (its opposite), it is possible, with the help of assumptions (ii) and (iv), to deduce the relation of $\mathbf{B}(x)$ to $\mathbf{E}(y)$. But in the exceptional cases mentioned there are again three possibilities:

In the case of A. I we can have

A. I (i) $\mathbf{B}(y)\,\mathbf{T}\,\mathbf{E}(x)$, or A. I (ii) $\mathbf{B}(y) = \mathbf{E}(x)$,

or A. I (iii) $\mathbf{E}(x)\,\mathbf{T}\,\mathbf{B}(y)$.

And in the case of C. III we can have

C. III (i) $\mathbf{E}(y)\,\mathbf{T}\,\mathbf{B}(x)$, or C. III (ii) $\mathbf{E}(y) = \mathbf{B}(x)$,

or C. III (iii) $\mathbf{B}(x)\,\mathbf{T}\,\mathbf{E}(y)$.

In case A. I (i) since $\mathbf{B}(y)\,\mathbf{T}\,\mathbf{E}(x)$ there must be, by assumption (iii), a stretch z such that $\mathbf{B}(y) = \mathbf{B}(z)$ and $\mathbf{E}(x) = \mathbf{E}(z)$ so that $\mathbf{E}(z)\,\mathbf{T}\,\mathbf{E}(y)$, hence $z\mathbf{C}i y$, and since $\mathbf{B}(y) = \mathbf{B}(z)$ and $\mathbf{B}(x)\mathbf{T}\,\mathbf{B}(y)$, we have $\mathbf{B}(x)\,\mathbf{T}\,\mathbf{B}(z)$ and $\mathbf{E}(x) = \mathbf{E}(z)$, hence $z\mathbf{C}t x$ and hence by definition $x\mathbf{O}y$.

Similarly, in case C. III (iii) we have $y\mathbf{O}x$.

In case A. I (ii) we have $\mathbf{B}(y) = \mathbf{E}(x)$, hence by definition $x\mathbf{A}y$.

Similarly in case C. III (ii) we have $y\mathbf{A}x$.

In case A. I (iii) since we have $\mathbf{E}(x)\,\mathbf{T}\,\mathbf{B}(y)$, there must be, by assumption (iii), a stretch z such that $\mathbf{B}(z) = \mathbf{E}(x)$ and $\mathbf{E}(z) = \mathbf{B}(y)$, hence a stretch z such that $x\mathbf{A}z$ and $z\mathbf{A}y$, hence $x\mathbf{A}^2 y$.

Similarly, in case C. III (i) we have $y\mathbf{A}^2x$.

In case A. II we have $\mathbf{B}(x)\,\mathbf{T}\,\mathbf{B}(y)$ and $\mathbf{E}(x) = \mathbf{E}(y)$, hence $y\mathbf{Ct}x$.

In case C. II we have $\mathbf{B}(y)\,\mathbf{T}\,\mathbf{B}(x)$ and $\mathbf{E}(x) = \mathbf{E}(y)$, hence $x\mathbf{Ct}y$.

In case A. III we have $\mathbf{B}(x)\,\mathbf{T}\,\mathbf{B}(y)$ & $\mathbf{E}(y)\,\mathbf{T}\,\mathbf{E}(x)$. Hence, by assumptions (ii) and (iv), we have $\mathbf{B}(x)\,\mathbf{T}\,\mathbf{E}(y)$. And, by assumption (iii), we have a stretch z such that $\mathbf{B}(z) = \mathbf{B}(x)$ and $\mathbf{E}(z) = \mathbf{E}(y)$. But if $\mathbf{B}(x)\,\mathbf{T}\,\mathbf{E}(y)$ and $\mathbf{B}(x) = \mathbf{B}(z)$, we have $\mathbf{B}(z)\,\mathbf{T}\,\mathbf{E}(y)$ and since $\mathbf{E}(z) = \mathbf{E}(y)$, we have $y\mathbf{Ct}z$. And since $\mathbf{E}(y) = \mathbf{E}(z)$ and $\mathbf{E}(y)\,\mathbf{T}\,\mathbf{E}(x)$, we have $\mathbf{E}(z)\,\mathbf{T}\,\mathbf{E}(x)$ and since $\mathbf{B}(z) = \mathbf{B}(x)$, we have $z\mathbf{Ci}x$. So, since $y\mathbf{Ct}z$ and $z\mathbf{Ci}x$, we have $y\mathbf{Cm}x$. (Note that $\mathbf{Ct} \mid \mathbf{Ci} = \mathbf{Ci} \mid \mathbf{Ct}$, see Note 1, above.)

Similarly in case C. I we have $x\mathbf{Cm}y$.

In case B. I we have $\mathbf{B}(x) = \mathbf{B}(y)$ and $\mathbf{E}(x)\,\mathbf{T}\,\mathbf{E}(y)$, hence we have $x\mathbf{Ci}y$.

In case B. III we have $\mathbf{B}(x) = \mathbf{B}(y)$ and $\mathbf{E}(y)\,\mathbf{T}\,\mathbf{E}(x)$, hence by definition we have $y\mathbf{Ci}x$.

In case B. II, since we have $\mathbf{B}(x) = \mathbf{B}(y)$ and $\mathbf{E}(x) = \mathbf{E}(y)$, we have, by assumption (v), $x = y$.

Now the foregoing exhaust all possibilities and consequently we must have $x = y$, or x stands in one of the six relations $\mathbf{A}$, $\mathbf{A}^2$, $\mathbf{O}$, $\mathbf{Ci}$, $\mathbf{Cm}$ or $\mathbf{Ct}$, or its converse, to y. And this is the statement to be derived.

Note 3 (p. 276). Anyone who wishes to introduce a time-metric into a strictly formulated biological theory may find the following postulates useful. The phrase 'the time-length of x with respect to the unit y is equal to ξ' is taken as undefined. All the other expressions are used in the same sense in which they occur in my *Axiomatic Method in Biology*.

Definition: '$\mathbf{a}$' is first defined to denote the set of all objects x such that x has a first time-slice (or moment) and a last time-slice; and for every y, if y is a momentary object such that the first slice of x stands in $\mathbf{T}$ to y and y stands in $\mathbf{T}$ to the last slice of x, then there is a time-slice z of x such that y stands neither in $\mathbf{T}$ nor its converse to z.

Postulate 1: If x and u belong to **a**, and u is nct momentary, then the time-length of x with respect to the unit u is a positive real number equal to or greater than zero.

Postulate 2: If u is a member of **a** but not momentary, then the time-length of u with respect to u is equal to 1.

Postulate 3: If x, y and u are members of **a**, and u is not momentary, and the first time-slice of x stands neither in **T** nor its converse to the first time-slice of y, and the last slice of x stands neither in **T** nor its converse to the last slice of y, then the time-length of x with respect to u is identical with that of y with respect to u.

Postulate 4: If x, y and u are members of **a**, and u is not momentary, and the last time-slice of x stands neither in **T** nor its converse to the first time-slice of y, then the time-length of the sum of $[x, y]$ is identical with the sum of the time-length of x with respect to u and the time-length of y with respect to u.

Postulate 5: If x and u are members of **a**, and u is not momentary but x is momentary, and ξ is a real number, then there is a y such that x stands neither in **T** nor its converse to the first slice of y, and the time-length of y with respect to u is equal to ξ.

Postulate 6: If x, u and v belong to **a**, and u and v are not momentary, then the time-length of x with respect to v is identical with the time-length of x with respect to u multiplied by the time-length of u with respect to v.

(I am indebted to Professor Tarski for help in formulating these postulates.)

Note 4 (p. 287). When an organism is accidentally or surgically cut into two parts we have the following possibilities: (1) each part survives and becomes a whole; (2) only one part survives and becomes a whole, the other dies; (3) neither part survives. In the case of persons (as far as I know) only possibilities (2) and (3) are realized. When, in organisms, a part survives and becomes a whole this may happen *either* (i) in consequence of a regenerative process by which the lost part is restored, *or* (ii) without any such restoration. In the case of persons, usually only the second method is followed. A person can thus be a whole (in one sense) without being 'complete in space' (in another sense). In the surgical treatment of infantile hemiplegia the entire cerebral hemisphere of one side (excluding the hippocampus) is removed. After recovery from the operation the person is 'more whole' than before, but the missing cerebral hemisphere does not regenerate. (See the article by Sir Hugh Cairns and M. A. Davidson, *The Lancet*, 6 Sept. 1951, pp. 411–15.) Biologists in general do not seem to attach much importance to the notions of part and whole, but W. Bateson wrote: 'The discovery of a true delimitation of the properties and attributes of individuals, which distinguish them from parts, would constitute a great advance in biological theory' (*Mendel's Principles of Heredity*, 1909, p. 275). The fact that the parts of persons are not persons not only makes it ridiculous to identify person with brain, since this involves putting a person into each person's head, but has as a consequence the impossibility of using the notion of person in the composition functor in explanatory hypotheses concerning persons, at least in so far as this involves the notion of spatial part. There is nothing especially peculiar about the fact that the parts of persons are not persons. The parts of dogs are not dogs.

In connexion with the tendency to identify neural impulse with sensible object, I notice that the following question was set in an anatomy paper in a Second Examination for medical degrees: 'State what you know of the central fibre tracts by which sensations from the left lower limb reach the cerebral cortex.'

Note 5 (p. 288). Behind this passage there seems to lurk a belief about perception which may be stated somewhat as follows (it is stated in much the same form in Karl Pearson's *Grammar of Science*): 'The human mind' is a sort of homunculus, born and bred in a dark chamber which is locked from the outside. But in this chamber is installed a television set with which the human mind amuses himself in his waking hours. But not content with watching the pictures he is compelled to invent something he calls 'the world around us' (another name for which is 'the reality underlying' the picture on the screen), although why such a thing should occur to him in view of his situation is not explained. But having taken this step he tortures himself from time to time by wondering how closely this unattainable world resembles the pictures. In the passage quoted, however, he is allowed to know quite a lot about the works in the television set (how this is possible is again not stated), and he is urged to avail himself to the utmost of this information in the confident hope that it will provide a solution of the major problem.

The passage quoted certainly seems to suggest that physiology, especially neurological physiology, is in a privileged position among the sciences, and that the final assessment of the results of the other sciences must in some way require the seal of physiology's approval. As a statement of the scope and task of neurology this passage seems to be clearly erroneous.

This putting a person into another one's head in order to explain perception leads to an infinite regress, because in order to explain the internal person's perceptions we must put a person into *his* head and so on *ad infinitum*. This is another example of the 'outside the system' attitude (see above, p. 311). An observer O' observing another observer O observing a subject-matter S, puts S inside O's head together with a miniature observer o to observe it. But he does not put the system S', consisting of S and O into his *own* head. He regards S' as outside himself and as obeying laws independently of him.

Note 6 (p. 295). Surely it is high time that the sharp antithesis between organic and functional was abandoned. Also the Platonistic tendency to regard diseases as entities which patients 'have'. There are no such things as diseases—only sick persons. It would probably be correct to say that a person is never sick only in the organic way or only in the functional way, but always in some degree in both ways. The object of treatment is not to combat a disease but to restore health, and the object of diagnosis is not to label a disease but to discover the best way to restore health. These ends will be best achieved if both ways of being sick are always kept in mind. The organic-functional antithesis, like the tough-tender antithesis and most other antitheses, illustrate what Hempel and Oppenheim call *bipolare Ordnungsbegriffe*, see their *Der Typusbegriff im Lichte der neuen Logik* (1936).

Note 7 (p. 304). In an account given in *The Times*, 12 May 1950, of the report, commissioned by the Carnegie United Kingdom Trust and issued under the title of *Delinquency and Human Nature*, dealing with the work carried out over a period of four years by Mr D. H. Stott, it is stated that

While it was the reaction that developed when a boy has for several years been unable to establish a relationship of affection with a parent or parent-substitute that was mainly responsible for the juvenile housebreaker—the most overt type of delinquency—it was the reaction which was an inhibition of the instinctive urge, common to all mankind, to establish a relationship of fellow-feeling one with another which had in the long run the most serious social consequences. Dishonesty of a sly and deliberate character, laziness and bad workmanship, treachery towards one's fellows and in a few cases physical violence were seen as the outcome of years of starved affection. Beneath the wickedness was perceived a human being in distress. It was true of all the most withdrawn types that they found the lovelessness of their situation intolerable and struggled blindly to escape from it.

It was encouraging to observe from case history what mites of interest and sympathy seemed to suffice to avert breakdown or amend it. There was evidence in at least two cases that breakdown was delayed by the boys finding parent-substitutes in their school teachers.... The member of the staff of an approved school must train himself to have always the thought in his mind that the greater the hate the greater the need for love.

Mr Stott's report (which does not mention Suttie's hypothesis) is obtainable from the Carnegie United Kingdom Trust, Dunfermline, Fife. It contains abundant confirmation of Suttie's hypothesis as far as delinquency is concerned.

See also Bowlby, *Forty-four Juvenile Thieves; Their Characters and Home Life* (1946). (Forty-four juvenile thieves were compared with forty-four children who did not steal who had been referred to the Tavistock clinic. Eighteen of the thieves had parents or grandparents suffering from psychosis. Comparable figures are not available for the control group. Seventeen thieves had separation for six months or more from mothers or established foster-mothers before the age of five. Only two controls had similar separations. Of fourteen thieves classified as affectionless characters, twelve had such separations. Of the remaining thirty thieves only five had such separations.) I am indebted to Dr John Klauber for giving me this reference. See also the article 'Mental health and the mother' in *The Lancet*, 26 May 1951, p. 1165.

Note 8 (p. 310). Is it possible to be unbiased in the psychological and social sciences? In order that this should be possible we should have to provide a scientist who was entirely devoid of any ethical or political preferences and was completely indifferent to the fate of mankind. If such a robot cannot be found (and even the tough man who claims to be completely objective may be a victim of the taboo on tenderness) we must reconcile ourselves to the fact that most hypotheses in these sciences will be influenced by such preferences. Even the collection of data will be so influenced, because the type of hypothesis you have in mind when you collect your data, however rudimentary or tentative it may be, will have some influence on what is admitted as a datum or on what is selected. But this is not so deplorable as it may seem at first sight, so long as criticism and discussion are permissible in the community in which the theory is promulgated, because theories are judged by their logical consequences, not by their psychological antecedents. (This is further touched upon in Appendix C.)

Note 9 (p. 310). There are certain dangers attending the too early teaching of science in schools, especially for boys. First, it may seem to them too much like a continuation of play on the nursery floor, so that their interests become fixated at an adolescent stage. Second, science teaching in schools may be too much simplified and therefore may be presented too dogmatically. Unless he subsequently studies methodology a boy may never escape the effect of such early influences. The older classical type of education had the advantage that it dealt very largely with persons—grown-up persons. Boys therefore learnt about persons first, before becoming immersed in the fascinations of impersonal natural science. They were therefore less in danger of taking the de-personalized attitude towards human affairs referred to above. The older type of education also had the advantage of inculcating a deliberate, as contrasted with a purely intuitive, use of language.

Note 10 (p. 310). B. A. W. Russell's article, 'Relativity: Philosophical consequences', *Encyclopedia Britannica*, 13th ed., new vol. III, p. 332.

At present, if we want to learn about persons it is not to physical theories that we turn, but to medical psychology couched in the person language and to the works of the great epic and dramatic writers and those of the great novelists, all in the person language. The psycho-analysts have pointed out the astonishing psychological insight manifested in Shakespeare's *Hamlet*. We may recall also Mary Shelley's insight in placing the source of the hate and rage of the synthetic monster in her *Frankenstein* in his *inability to arouse love*. In literature of this kind we seem to have a place where science and art overlap. The investigation of the precise nature of this overlap would provide a fascinating topic for someone with the requisite understanding of both science and literature and a knowledge of the Boole-Frege technique of linguistic analysis.

Note 11 (p. 312). Thus Professor Hull writes as follows about opposition to his views:

There will be encountered vituperative opposition from those who cannot or will not think in terms of mathematics, from those who prefer to have their scientific pictures artistically out of focus, from those who are apprehensive of the ultimate exposure of certain personally cherished superstitions and magical practices, and from those who are associated with institutions whose vested interests may be fancied as endangered. *Principles of Behaviour*, p. 401.

NOTES TO PART III

But to me it seems that good *reasons* can be brought forward against regarding persons exclusively as purely physical objects, as we must do if we reject all theories which use any but the physical language. Let me summarize them as follows:

(i) In the theoretical or speculative sphere you are committed to using the abstract notion of body; you are therefore bound within the limits imposed by this method of abstraction and cannot deal with those aspects from which abstraction has been made.

(ii) In the practical sphere you make enemies, because persons resent being regarded as physical objects. Persons want to be loved, or at least respected, by other persons. Wider sociological consequences are described in the text.

(iii) In the special sphere of medical practice you risk being an unsuccessful doctor (a) because you will limit yourself to using only physical methods of diagnosis and treatment, and (b) because an attitude of resentment (see (ii)) between patient and doctor is not favourable to the patient's return to health.

There is another puzzle connected with this problem. With one voice we are told that the purpose of science is to enable us to control our environment; with another we are told that we must confine ourselves to constructing hypotheses about the behaviour of persons which depict them as robots entirely controlled by their environments. As Professor Broad has remarked, 'however convenient this may be in practice, it is intolerable in theory to anyone with a tidy mind who has become aware of the facts'. See C. D. Broad, 'Some methods of speculative philosophy', *The Aristotelian Society, Suppl.* vol. XXI, p. 10.

Note 12 (p. 315). Countries like the U.S.A. and the U.S.S.R. which have successfully completed one revolution are understandably reluctant to embark upon another. None the less incitements to revolution have not been wanting in the United States. By way of example I may mention Jefferson's remarks on Shay's Rebellion: 'God forbid that we should ever be twenty years without such a rebellion.... What country can preserve its liberties, if its rulers are not warned, from time to time, that the people preserve the spirit of resistance.... ? ' 'Let them take arms. What signify a few lives lost? The tree of Liberty must be refreshed from time to time with the blood of patriots and tyrants.'

A similar sentiment is expressed less bloodthirstily by Henry W. Nevinson in his *Essays on Freedom*:

For freedom, we know, is a thing that we have to conquer afresh for ourselves, every day, like love; and we are always losing freedom, just as we are always losing love, because, after each victory, we think we can now settle down and enjoy it without further struggle. ...The battle of freedom is never done, and the field never quiet. (Quoted in H. Laski's *A Grammar of Politics*, 1925.)

I note that Professor Norbert Wiener is aware of the sociological aspect of the problems discussed in the text; see the Introduction and Chapter VIII of his *Cybernetics; or Control and Communication in the Animal and the Machine*, New York, 1948. The following warning by Arne Næss is also relevant in this connexion:

The growing importance of psychological popularizations, especially the tremendously influential vague and propagandistic statements referred to as principles of 'modern education', makes it a major task for our universities to instruct our students about the difference between research reports and working hypotheses based on research, and between such statements and popularizations. The lack of critical (neither dogmatic nor sceptical) attitude towards popularizations may cause misunderstandings with immense consequences for education, morals, mental hygiene and our *mores* in general. This seems to me to furnish the most important practical argument for increased methodological clearness and explicitness in psychological research and in psychological publications of all kinds. (*Notes on the Foundation of Psychology as a Science*, Filosofiske Problemer, utgitt av Filosofisk Klubb, Nr. 9, 1948, Oslo, p. 48.)

APPENDIX C

NATURAL SCIENCE AND HUMAN AFFAIRS

What, art thou mad? art thou mad? is not the
truth the truth?   *Henry IV, Part I*, ii, iv.

In this appendix I wish to add something more about the relations between natural science and other human activities, in
order to explain why arguments about possible sociological
consequences of applied behaviourism were introduced into
Lecture VII. This takes us out of the field of methodology;
but it is still a topic belonging to the philosophy of science and
is not therefore beyond the scope of a Tarner Lecturer's task.
If anyone is scandalized by the introduction of such topics into
a book of this kind all I can say in explanation and excuse is
that I believe that scientific speculations should sometimes be
brought out of the specialized atmosphere of the laboratory and
workshop and confronted with the actualities of human life
in general.

In order to clarify this problem it is necessary to introduce
certain historical considerations and to say something about
what I shall call the *rationalist tradition*.* Pythagoras and
Plato were responsible for initiating the doctrine that men were
endowed with what was called reason and sense and that the
former was vastly superior to the latter. What could be discovered by sense was transitory and particular, whilst the
revelations of reason were eternal and universal. This doctrine
flourished right through the Middle Ages into the Renaissance

---

* In modern times the word 'rationalism' has been used in a special sense
for an anti-authoritarian, anti-religious movement. See, for example, J. B.
Bury's *A History of Freedom of Thought*. I am using the word in its traditional
philosophical sense of rationalism as opposed to empiricism. Consequently,
rejection of rationalism does not mean acceptance of irrationalism but of
empiricism.

and still persists in modern times. Thus we find Charles Darwin writing: 'Of all the faculties of the human mind, it will, I presume, be admitted that Reason stands at the summit.' During the Middle Ages rationalists were largely occupied with the search for proofs of the existence of God. It was believed that it was possible, by the exercise of reason, to discover certain very general statements from which it was possible to deduce the existence of the Deity.

For centuries, in fact from the time of Pythagoras, mathematics (especially geometry) seemed to support the rationalist tradition. But that was because Euclidean geometry was the only geometry that had been studied; and Kant was able to use this as a support for his doctrine of synthetic (as opposed to analytic) judgements *a priori*. With the invention of non-Euclidean geometries, and with the still more recent discovery that mathematical statements are analytic, this buttress of rationalism collapsed.

During the Renaissance, and even earlier, this doctrine had been challenged by the rival doctrine of empiricism, which assigned a much more important role to the senses. The conflict between rationalism and empiricism is well illustrated by the debates among early embryologists about preformation and epigenesis. According to the preformationists, development was simply a process of enlargement of a complicated structure which was already fully formed in the egg. The rationalist attitude is exemplified by the saying of Haller in a book called *Elementa Physiologiae* (1765–6), admitting that as far as observation goes the chick when it first appears is a small shapeless worm with a huge hernia arising from its intestine, but without signs of beak, limbs, viscera, or even heart. But, says he, 'We must not conclude that these parts did not exist before, but that they were so transparent that their outlines could not be recognized'. He says, further, that 'It would thus appear that the young chick arises gradually by various stages, and so passes into the adult animal. Nevertheless epigenesis is totally impossible! The foetus can never have been without a heart, since in the heart resides the principles of all life and movement, and the heart in its turn cannot exist without arteries and veins.'*

Another writer, Charles Bonnet, in a work published about the same time (1762), held that if development should seem to be accomplished by epigenesis then 'our senses deceive us. A mask of falsehood obscures the whole face of nature. Development is a complete illusion, or what appears to arise only emerges from a state of invisibility to one of visibility'; and he declared that 'The hypothesis of emboîtement is one of the most striking victories of the understanding over the senses'. Again, although Gesner, writing in 1735, denied that the homunculus had been seen in the sperm and pointed out that Leeuwenhoek never found anything more than a head and a tail, he nevertheless maintained that '*reason* compels us to believe that an entire man in miniature is enclosed in the little spermatic worm'. The empiricist attitude on the other hand is exemplified by the saying of Swammerdam that 'we must not surmise or invent, but *discover*, what Nature does'. We thus have one set of writers rejecting what is observed or seeking to explain it away on the ground that it is contrary to some statement which is supposed to be guaranteed by reason, and another set maintaining the view that the business of science is to discover, not to surmise or invent. What is the modern attitude towards this problem?

The modern attitude, or at least the modern attitude which I share, holds that the empiricists were wrong in saying that we must not surmise or invent; indeed, the invention of hypotheses is part of the business of science. But it differs from the rationalists in the way in which it regards these hypotheses. It does not regard them as revelations of metaphysical truths, by something called reason, which are to be adhered to at all costs and in the face of contradictory observation. It regards them as tentative guides to the business of observation itself,

* For an account of this controversy, see F. J. Cole, *Early Theories of Sexual Generation* (1930).

which are to be rejected when the results of that observation are not in harmony with them.

This attitude is traceable to the work of David Hume, who showed that there was no rational justification, as it was called, for scientific induction. That is to say, there is no principle by which such a procedure can be shown to be valid which is not itself equally in need of justification. All that reason can do, if I may continue in the traditional idiom, is to tell you when one statement *follows from* another, so that *if* you accept the latter you cannot, without inconsistency, reject the former. But it does not tell you *whether* to accept the second statement, and it does not tell you to avoid inconsistency. We try to avoid inconsistency because any other procedure gets us into hopeless muddles, and we accept certain theoretical statements, not because we can find a rational justification for them, but because they provide a guide to that kind of manual activity which is so characteristic of experimental science.* Successful manual activity begets faith as nothing else does. Macbeth rejected the dagger he saw before him because when he tried to clutch it, it was not 'sensible to feeling as to sight'. It was not therefore the kind of dagger that could be used for killing the unfortunate Duncan.

The precise role of explanatory hypotheses in natural science is as follows; they not only provide a means of grouping the statements of science into an ordered and consequently manageable system by means of the relation of logical consequence, but, just because they always say more than is warranted by observation, they also suggest new ways in which to direct the business of experiment. They provide a guide to the manual activity without which it would be blind. Every new explanatory hypothesis, if it is a good one, sets going new experiments, and so long as a hypothesis does this it continues

---

* It is easy for philosophers to overemphasize the intellectual aspect of natural science, and to forget to what a great extent success in it depends upon manual dexterity. It is for this reason that it is possible to attain eminence in science without paying any attention to the theoretical topics which have been discussed in this book.

to be accepted. If the new observations contradict it, it is either rejected or modified or supplemented until prediction and observation are once more in agreement. Thus the justification of such theoretical statements is not a rational but a pragmatic one.

In addition to the test of success in the laboratory there is the further test of success in the realm of technological application—the building of ships, bridges, aeroplanes, etc. So long as these activities are successful science does not trouble itself about the rational justification of its procedure. That is why science has not been troubled by Hume's destructive criticism.

Whitehead expressed the situation very well when, referring to the tests through which a scientific theory must pass, he wrote: 'Only one question is asked: Has the doctrine a precise application to a variety of particular circumstances so as to determine the exact phenomena which should then be observed? In the comparative absence of these applications beauty, generality, or even truth, will not save a doctrine from neglect in scientific thought.'*

We can in fact go further and say that the question of truth does not arise at all as far as theoretical statements of science are concerned, because a theory can continue to be useful even after it has ceased to be regarded as true. Thus Newtonian mechanics is still applicable in those spheres for which it was first invented, in spite of the fact that it has now been superseded as a universal theory in physics. Science is not pursued for the sake of discovering the truth of theories, but theories are set up to promote the continuation of scientific research.

The belief that it is possible to discover whether scientific theoretical statements are true is perhaps partly owing to the persistence of the erroneous supposition that it is possible to infer a statement 'A' from the two statements 'If A then B' and 'B'. But from the two statements, 'If Venus is visible then the night is cloudless' and 'the night is cloudless', I cannot infer the statement, 'Venus is visible'.†

---

* *The Principle of Relativity* (1922), p. 3.
† See p. 71, Note 17, quotation from Lord Russell.

Not only is it unnecessary that all the statements in a scientific theory should be true or known to be true, but it is unnecessary that all the functors in it should 'have meaning' or that we should know what they mean. It has already been explained that a scientific theory does its work by virtue of its structure. So long as it has the requisite structure, and so long as at *some* level its statements speak about objects which have sensible objects which are **OF** them, that is all that we can ask of it. If we persist in asking more we raise questions to which it does not seem to be possible for us to find answers.

Science in modern times is supposed to be thoroughly empirical, but the rationalist tradition still persists in the sense that many general theoretical statements appear to be strongly adhered to *in advance* of empirical investigation. We saw examples of this in the discussion of the role of purely physical theories in psychology.

Another manifestation of the same tendency is seen in the old controversy about the 'reduction' of the biological sciences to physics and chemistry. If all that is being asserted is that the techniques and hypotheses of physics and chemistry are *applicable* to biological objects, then there would be no occasion for controversy, since every day brings fresh and brilliant confirmation of this statement. We remain within the province of methodology. But people are not content to remain within the safe confines of methodology. Most people are natural metaphysicians, and it is an easy passage for them from the unassailable methodological doctrine, that physics and chemistry are applicable to biological objects, to the metaphysical doctrine, that living organisms are 'nothing but' physical systems. This might be harmless enough if it did not have methodological repercussions. But it does have such repercussions. It engenders a feeling of inferiority in biologists. It makes them feel that they are wasting their time unless they too become biophysicists or biochemists. It thus retards the search for explanatory hypotheses on the biological levels, just as a purely behaviouristic approach to psychology retards and discourages the search for other hypotheses in that science.* Owing to the comparative lateness of its birth, and the slowness of its development, biology is in the somewhat unfortunate position of a youngest child in a family of brilliantly successful elder brothers. Its own independent development may be stifled by the powerful example of its older brethren.

In more general terms we may say that the persistence of the rationalist tradition tends to make people believe that a successful system of hypotheses, just because it is successful, *must* be metaphysically or absolutely true and therefore excludes *all other* hypotheses and consequently discourages the search for them and so prejudices future discovery. But if we recognize that the scientific method is such that we can never know when a theoretical statement is *true*,† but only when it is *successful*, and if, mindful of the history of science, we recognize that the success of one hypothesis never excludes the possibility of other equally successful, or even more successful, ones, then nothing is lost and much may be gained in the future. But the attraction of a successful system of hypotheses is so strong, its power to generate belief so great and the difficulties of inventing new hypotheses and new methods of approach so enormous, that it is small wonder if young men who have their living to earn follow the tide that leads on to fortune.

There is one more point to be mentioned in connexion with the doctrine of the reducibility of biology to physics and chemistry: people who hold the doctrine do not in fact believe it. If they did they would not spend laborious hours experimenting in their laboratories; instead, they would spend

* If you adhere absolutely and dogmatically, in the rationalist tradition, to *any* system of hypotheses (not excluding the hypotheses of everyday life which are enshrined in common sense), you are bound to find that your observations are in agreement with it, because you will be driven to devise methods of explaining away *every* contradictory observation, and thus to exclude the possibility of challenging the system of hypotheses, just as the eighteenth-century preformationists were driven to explaining away what they observed through their microscopes.

† I use the word 'true' in Tarski's sense, i.e. in accordance with the correspondence theory of truth; see 'Der Wahrheitsbegriff in den formalisierten Sprachen', *Studia Philosophica*, Leopoli, **1935**.

equally laborious hours in their studies with paper and pencil reducing biology to chemistry and physics, because, as I pointed out on p. 271, reducibility is a purely paper and pencil affair. If you want to reduce biology to physics and chemistry, you must construct bi-conditionals which are in effect definitions of biological functors with the help of those belonging only to physics and chemistry; you must then add these to the postulates of physics and chemistry and work out their consequences. Then and only then will it be time to go into your laboratories to discover whether these consequences are upheld there. From the fact that people do *not* do this, I venture the guess that they confuse *reducibility* of biology to physics and chemistry, with *applicability* of physics and chemistry to biological objects. The truth of the latter is open to everybody to see, the truth of the former no one knows because we do not know whether anyone will have the wit enough to construct the required bi-conditionals, and we do not know what the postulates of physics and chemistry will be in the future if and when the required bi-conditionals have been constructed.

The modern Russian writers have not only completely repudiated the rationalist tradition, they have gone to the opposite extreme of complete *technological* pragmatism. They believe that all human activities are to be subordinated to the establishment of what is called the classless society. By this is meant (at least theoretically) a society in which the working class is the ruling class.* Consequently, scientific theories are to be judged, not by the customary intellectual criteria, but by whether or not they tend to promote or hinder the coming of this classless society. They believe that genetical theories which

---

* The reader who wonders why one class is singled out and exalted in this way should know that early in the nineteenth century the Goddess of History revealed to her high priest in her London (Bloomsbury) temple that she was stricken with remorse when she saw the rough deal which the working class had hitherto received at her hands, and that a resolution to correct this error had been recorded in her book of destiny. As is usually the case, not all philosophers agree about the authenticity of this revelation (see K. Popper, 'The poverty of historicism', I, II and III, *Economica* (1944–5), XI, pp. 86–103, 119–37 and XII, pp. 69–89). Some have even alluded to the service of this goddess as *the opium of the philosophers*.

have their origin in the hypotheses of Mendel and of Morgan
are not helpful in increasing agricultural production. But increased agricultural production is necessary for the establishment of the classless society. Therefore genetical theories which
spring from the hypotheses of Mendel and Morgan are to be
repudiated and research in these directions is to be discouraged.

In opposing these doctrines the anti-rationalism of the modern
Russian writers displays itself in another way. They do not
hesitate to use any means which they believe will promote
the ends they wish to achieve, so that *all* argument becomes
propaganda argument. Whether the arguments brought forward are logically irrelevant is of no consequence. Thus the
fact that Mendel was a Roman Catholic is logically irrelevant
to the truth or falsehood of his hypotheses, but this is no obstacle
to its use as a stick with which to belabour Mendel's theory.
As I have already pointed out, scientific theories in pure science
are *not* judged by their antecedents, historical, psychological or
logical, but by the success of their logical *consequences* in
agreeing with observations.* Even applied science is not judged
by its antecedents, but by the success of its *technological* consequences. Now the Russian subordination of everything to
technological considerations, that is to say, to success in promoting the advent of the classless society, has the result of
obliterating the distinction between pure and applied science,
because it does not leave room for recognition of any difference
in the criteria by which they are judged. This is no doubt
justifiable enough as an emergency measure and as a short-
term policy. But in the long run it must mean killing the
goose that lays the golden eggs.

Moreover, not only do the Russian biologists (or at least the
officially recognized ones) thus subordinate pure science to
applied science, but they believe that other scientists do the

* For this reason a critic of a particular scientific hypothesis cannot be
answered simply by saying that he is biased or that some psychological factor
has influenced his opinions. To answer him we must show that his critical
statements are false, either because they are contradicted by accepted observation records or because they are internally inconsistent.

same. Consequently the apparent rationalism of the latter seems in their eyes to be sheer hypocrisy. Thus it is easy for the Russian biologists to point to some of the eugenical writings of followers of Mendel and Morgan as evidence of their class bias. In doing this they may well be right. But this is logically irrelevant to the truth or falsehood of those theories in pure science. A theory may be well confirmed as judged by the criteria of pure science, even though we may not like its possible technological applications. In Lecture VII, I have myself drawn attention to certain possible consequences of applied behaviourism. But I do not regard the fact that many people dislike these consequences as an argument against behaviourism as a doctrine of pure science. In the same way the fact that the consequences of applying atomic fission may be unpleasant is logically irrelevant to the truth or falsehood of theoretical physics.*

But although the Russian writers repudiate the rationalist tradition in their attitude to science, their attitude to political theory exhibits some of the worst features of that tradition. This appears to be a result of the influence of German philosophy, especially that of Hegel.†

By contrast, British statesmen frequently repudiate the rationalist tradition in politics, although they sometimes express themselves in a rather odd way. Mr Attlee, for example, is reported to have said, in a speech on 9 May 1949, that

> Without the spirit of tolerance, our parliamentary system, which was not logical, would not work.... We had rather a horror of being too logical, and of tying ourselves to rigid formulae to be applied regardless of circumstance. We did not mind if something we did was illogical provided it worked. There were so many things which if worked out to their logical conclusion would result in disaster.

It seems clear that what is here repudiated is not logic in its technical sense but the rationalist tradition in practical politics.

---

* See the article by N. I. Nuzhdin in *Nature*, 1950, vol. CLXV, p. 704.

† See K. Popper, *The Open Society and its Enemies* (1945), especially vol. II, chap. 12.

The rationalist tradition is responsible for many, if not all, of the doctrinal quarrels which separate men into hostile groups by diverting attention from the practical maxims upon which they might agree, to a vain search for untestable abstract principles which are supposed to be necessary to provide such maxims with a so-called rational basis.

The mention of success in connexion with science reminds us that human beings engage in pursuits other than science, and that success in these other pursuits may have quite different and possibly conflicting criteria. Thus persons engage in business, in aesthetic and in religious activities. They are also all involved in the difficult art of living together in communities. Moreover, in all these activities we find, no less than in science, that *language* is involved. Without language these activities would be solitary, not social ones. Language objectifies and makes inter-personal what would otherwise remain secret and personal, because, associated with each of these and other activities, there are certain sentences, not necessarily general statements, but at least verbal formulations which have the appearance of statements and for which, accordingly, *rational justification* in each case is demanded and sought.

Now I wish to contend that the search for a rational justification is even more mistaken in these cases than it is in relation to the theoretical statements of science. I wish to contend that, in these activities also, the criterion is not a rational one but success, although what constitutes success is different in each case. These activities have for their goal the satisfaction of certain needs. We can divide the needs of persons into two groups, the biological needs and the supra-biological or social needs. Under biological needs I would place: air, co-ordination, food, information, movement, protection, removal of waste, sex, and water. Under supra-biological needs I would place, among others: adornment (which includes architecture, sculpture, painting, ceramics and jewellery), co-ordination, dancing, drama, information (including science), literature, love (which the tough do not distinguish from sex), movement, music, religion, removal of waste, power, protection, and sport.

You will notice that I have included the need for power, that is to say, power over other persons, among the supra-biological needs. But according to Suttie's hypothesis this would not be a primary need but a secondary one, in the sense that it is a manifestation of a frustrated need for love.

One important difference between the two kinds of need, namely, the biological and the supra-biological, is that whereas all persons share the former they do not by any means all share the same supra-biological needs. Thus a person may have a strong need for sport and dancing, but none at all for literature or religion.

Satisfaction of needs may be passive or active. A clarinet player in an orchestra may be providing music for others and enjoying it at the same time. A member of the audience will be enjoying it but not making it. The first will have active, the second passive enjoyment. In the same way a scientist may enjoy performing his experiments and recording and thinking about his results. His is active satisfaction. A person who studies his theories will have passive satisfaction. But a man who makes clarinets will have neither active nor passive satisfaction of musical needs. For although he will be providing for the satisfaction of musical needs of others he is not making music nor need he have musical needs of his own at all.

It will be noticed that some needs have been mentioned under both biological and social (or supra-biological) headings. But although the same word occurs in both places it will not have the same meaning in each. Consider what I have called co-ordination, for example. If we disregard the social activities of a person, co-ordination is a private affair of his own physiological processes, about which he, as a person, may know nothing, and with which he does not interfere. But on the social level every person (except the professional criminal) has active satisfaction of the need for co-ordination, from the private citizen to the government official. The professional criminal has only passive satisfaction. Under co-ordination I include the art of living together harmoniously under one roof, that is to say, co-ordination within the family.

Co-ordination requires communication between persons, and this is achieved either by making things with the hands or by making sounds with the voice or other instrument. It is in this way that personal experiences become shared and the satisfaction of needs becomes a social activity. The principal, but not the only, device for this purpose is *language* either in the form of marks on paper or in the form of spoken words. But language has three principal uses: the conveyance of information, calculation (i.e. the working out of the consequences of hypotheses) and the expression of feelings and attitudes. The employment of language in science exemplifies the first two uses; its employment in relation to conduct, religion, literature, etc., exemplifies chiefly the third use, although the three uses are not always neatly separated and confined to any of these activities. Let us speak of the first two uses of language as the *propositional* uses and the third as the *non-propositional* use. In both kinds we construct *sentences*, but in the first these are *statements*, in the second they are not.

We have seen that among statements it is possible to distinguish between those which can be known to be true and those which cannot. If I say 'Your house is on fire', you can go home and discover whether I am pulling your leg, or telling the melancholy truth. But if I say, 'All kettles boil when placed on a lighted gas-ring', it is impossible for you to discover whether this statement is true. It is no good going home and trying the experiment. However many times you try, this will still leave millions of inaccessible kettles untested. We believe this statement, not because we know it to be true, but because we have found it to be a useful guide to action in the past and we hope and trust it will continue to be so in the future. We might formulate it in the form of an instruction in the manner of a cookery book: If you want to boil a kettle try putting it on a lighted gas-ring. But in this form the statement would not be so useful for purposes of calculation, because the theory of calculation with such formulations has not yet been very well worked out.

For the non-propositional use of language the notions of truth and falsehood do not apply, at least not in the same senses of these words. Consequently 'belief' must also have a different meaning.

Now it is desirable to have a name for all these systems of sentences which cannot be known to be true but which are helpful in promoting the satisfaction of needs. I propose to call them *acceptances*—not in the sense of acts of accepting, but in the sense of formulations, towards which some persons take an accepting attitude. I wish to use this name in an entirely neutral way, as expressing neither approval nor disapproval. I want to treat acceptances—other people's as well as my own—as worthy of every respect, even when I do not subscribe to them myself. This wide term will thus cover the theoretical statements of science and all the non-propositional systems of sentences. We have economic and political acceptances, those connected with aesthetic and religious needs, and ethical and racial acceptances. All are judged by their success in their several spheres, although the criteria of success will differ very much in different spheres. Just because they are sentences we are prone to fall into the error of supposing that they must all be judged by *intellectual* criteria. As H. Granville-Barker said: 'Let us humbly own how hard it is not to write nonsense about art, which seems ever pleading to be enjoyed and not written about at all.'*

All these acceptances, by virtue of their verbal formulations, help to strengthen and give form and direction to the activities with which they are connected. Thus the political and economic acceptances of Marxism serve to stiffen the communist movement. The Nazi movement was similarly buttressed by racial and nationalistic acceptances. The various traditional religious acceptances support religious activities. The art of

* H. Granville-Barker, *Prefaces to Shakespeare*, First Series (1949), p. x.

living together rests on ethical acceptances, and so on. In each case success in promoting the activity in question is the criterion by which the acceptance in question is to be judged, not its truth or so-called rational justification.

Now it is clear that, if acceptances are to be judged by their success or failure in promoting the needs they serve, it will obviously be absurd to expect an acceptance which is satisfactory from the point of view of one need to be successful with regard to a totally different one. But this does not seem to be at all well recognized at the present day. Owing to its enormous success in satisfying our need for information and its technological applications which satisfy other needs, a great many people sincerely believe that all we require is more and more science in order to solve *all* our problems. Consequently great sums of money are now available for promoting scientific research, compared with former ages when such money would have been devoted to the arts and religion.

But if this happens it must mean that other needs will be relatively neglected and communities correspondingly impoverished, although it can be justly claimed that many scientific inventions have made the means for the satisfaction of such needs more easily available to larger numbers of people. Nevertheless it is much easier to earn enough to support life as a physicist, a chemist or an entomologist than as a poet or a painter.

There are three important points to be noted about acceptances: first, that they generate intense belief; secondly, that they are not shared by everybody; and thirdly, that they are frequently adhered to dogmatically and intolerantly.

People differ enormously in their needs and some have a passion for persuading or compelling others to have the same needs as themselves. This, coupled with the belief generated by acceptances, leads to the intolerant adherence to them. The divergence of needs is in its turn at least in part related to the divergence between the two main types of person mentioned in Lecture VII, the tough and the tender.

Among the philosophers of modern times, Nietzsche is the apostle of toughness and Lord Russell a representative of the tender. In the chapter on Nietzsche in his *History of Western Philosophy* Lord Russell relates an imaginary conversation in heaven between Buddha and Nietzsche. In the course of this he writes (p. 800):

Buddha, who in the courts of Heaven has learnt all history since his death, and has mastered science with delight in the knowledge, and sorrow at the use to which men have put it, replies with calm urbanity: 'You are mistaken, Professor Nietzsche, in thinking my ideal a purely negative one. True it includes a negative element, the absence of suffering; but it has quite as much that is positive as is to be found in your doctrine.... I too, have my heroes: my successor Jesus, because he told men to love their enemies; the men who discovered how to master the forces of nature and secure food with less labour; the medical men who have shown how to diminish disease; the poets and artists and musicians who have caught glimpses of the Divine beatitude. Love and knowledge and delight in beauty are not negations; they are enough to fill the lives of the greatest men who have ever lived.

So much for Buddha. Lord Russell then continues:

For my part, I agree with Buddha as I have imagined him. But I do not know how to prove that he is right by any argument such as can be used in a mathematical or a scientific question. I dislike Nietzsche because he likes the contemplation of pain, because he erects conceit into a duty, because the men whom he admires are conquerors, whose glory is cleverness in causing men to die. But I think the ultimate argument against his philosophy, as against any unpleasant but internally consistent ethic, lies not in an appeal to facts, but in an appeal to the emotions. Nietzsche despises universal love; I feel it the motive power to all that I desire as regards the world. His followers have had their innings, but we may hope that it is coming rapidly to an end.*

---

* The word 'innings' which occurs in this passage may greatly puzzle the foreign reader because it concerns a game called cricket which satisfies the sporting needs of a great many Englishmen during the summer months, but is quite unknown in many countries. This game is played between two sides or teams of eleven men each. The play consists in a member of one team violently propelling (technically 'bowling') a hard ball in the direction of a

The persistence of the rationalist tradition is well illustrated by Lord Russell's remark that he does not know how to prove that Buddha is right. If we understand the status of ethical acceptances we can see that they are the sort of things that cannot be 'proved to be right'. Neither can we speak of an 'appeal to the emotions' as an 'ultimate argument' against Nietzsche's philosophy. I am not objecting to the appeal, I am only objecting to the confusion of acceptances involved in calling it an argument. Nietzsche's own doctrine rests on such an appeal.

In illustration of what I have said about the desirability of trying to understand the mutual relations of acceptances of different kinds, let me say something about the impact of scientific acceptances upon some of the others. By way of example we can take the debate about evolution between biologists and geologists on one side and the leaders of the Church on the other, during the last century. The curious feature of this debate was that both sides approached it entirely from the standpoint of the rationalist tradition. Both sides appear to have agreed to treat the Book of Genesis, not as an expression of certain religious acceptances to be judged by their success or failure from that point of view, but as a text-book of geology. From the standpoint of the Church this was a fatal attitude to take, because it was easy for the men of science to show how inadequate it was as a text-book of geology. As a religious acceptance belonging to a primitive society existing at a time

member of the other team, who attempts to hit it with a flattened wooden club (called a bat). The player who wields this club (known as the batsman) is said to be 'having his innings'. The duration of this innings depends upon what happens to the ball after it leaves the hand of the bowler. At the termination of his innings the batsman is replaced by another member of the same team, until each of the eleven men has 'had his innings'. Then the team as a whole may be said to have 'had its innings'. There seems to be a slight inconsistency in Lord Russell's metaphorical use of this expression, because if the followers of Nietzsche have *had* their innings there would be no need to *hope* that it is coming rapidly to an end, it would already have *reached* its end. But Lord Russell may have had in mind the fact that in the game of cricket *each* team usually has *two* innings, and the followers of Nietzsche may only have had their *first* innings, and it is the second which Lord Russell hopes is coming rapidly to an end.

when the different uses of language had not been sorted out, it would have been much more easily defended and the recognition that it was an acceptance of this kind and not a scientific one would have revealed the fact that there was really no point of contact, that the whole controversy was not an intellectual one, but a conflict of need. It was also, in part, a struggle between a vested interest and one striving to become vested.

An intellectual acceptance cannot strictly conflict with a non-intellectual one and, since they relate to different needs, one cannot take the place of another. For example, with the decline in the older forms of religion we should expect a religious vacuum to develop, and this appears to have happened. And if this is so we should expect other forms of enthusiasm to arise to fill the vacuum. And this seems to be what has happened recently in Germany and Russia. National socialism filled the religious vacuum for many young men in Germany during the brief reign of Hitler, and Marxism is filling the religious vacuum for many young people in Russia and many other places. The religious element in these movements is seen in the conviction which they inspire, the desire for certainty which they satisfy, and in the way each has provided the figure of an all-wise father in the shape of a leader who knows what is good for those who put their trust in him, who will show them the path to a better world, will reward them when they obey his commandments and punish them when they deviate from the way they should go. It is partly because of a religious element in these movements, not merely through the promise of material reward, that people feel urged to join them. For the same reason it is useless for opponents of such acceptances to take a purely negative attitude towards them. Only some other positive movement which will arouse corresponding enthusiasm can successfully compete with them.

Now let me try to explain why scientific acceptances cannot take the place of ethical ones, in spite of the fact that many people have tried to build ethical acceptances on scientific ones. The purpose of scientific acceptances is, I have said, to sustain and direct observation and experiment in the satisfaction of intellectual needs and also to have technological applications in the satisfaction of other needs. *If* you want to build a power station certain scientific acceptances will offer you the only available guidance in setting about the satisfying of this need, but they cannot tell you *whether* a power station *should* be built. In deciding whether to build a power station many other considerations enter which are not scientific: such questions as whether the building will spoil the view and other amenities of the district, whether injustice will be done to the inhabitants if such a building is erected, how much compensation should be paid, and so on. In other words, there will be a conflict of needs which have to be reconciled or co-ordinated; and, in connexion with this conflict ethical acceptances will be relevant, because they are concerned with what *ought* to be done, not, like scientific acceptances, with *how* they are to be done.

Hume contested the rationalist tradition in ethics. 'Nothing is more usual in philosophy', he wrote, 'and even in common life, than to talk of the combat of passion and reason, to give the preference to reason, and assert that men are only so far virtuous as they conform themselves to its dictates.' He then continues:

Reason is the discovery of truth or falsehood. Truth or falsehood consists in an agreement or disagreement either to the *real* relations of ideas, or to *real* existence and matter of fact. Whatever therefore is not susceptible of this agreement or disagreement, is incapable of being true or false and can never be an object of reason. Now it is evident our passions, volitions and actions, are not susceptible of any such agreement or disagreement; being original facts and realities, complete in themselves, and implying no reference to other passions, volitions and actions. It is impossible they can be pronounced either true or false, and be either contrary or conformable to reason.

This argument, he continues,

proves *directly*, that actions do not derive their merit from a conformity to reason, nor their blame from a contrariety to it.

Finally, he says:

Nor does this reasoning only prove that morality consists not in any relations that are the objects of science; but if examined, will prove with equal certainty, that it consists not in any *matter of fact*, which can be discovered by the understanding....But can there be any difficulty in proving that vice and virtue are not matters of fact, whose existence we can infer by reason? Take any action allowed to be vicious...examine it in all lights, and see if you can find that matter of fact, or real existence, which you call *vice*...you find only certain passions, motives, volitions and thoughts....The vice entirely escapes you, so long as you consider the object. You never can find it, till you turn your reflection into your own breast, and find a sentiment of disapprobation, which arises in you, towards that action. Here is a matter of fact; but it is the object of feeling, not of reason. It lies in yourself, not in the object. So that when you pronounce any action or character to be vicious, you mean nothing, but that from the constitution of your nature you have a feeling or sentiment of blame from the contemplation of it.*

Now some men of science have supposed that it is possible to find a so-called rational basis for ethical doctrines within science itself, for example, in the theory of evolution. But in view of what Hume says about the role of 'the constitution of our nature', in deciding ethical attitudes, and in view of the tough-tender antithesis, it is not surprising to find that different people have believed that they could extract ethical doctrines of quite opposite tendencies from the theory of evolution.†

The involvement of this theory in ethical discussions is perhaps traceable to the use of the word 'progress' in this connexion. But this word may be used in at least two quite distinct senses. When we read on a notice board outside a lecture

* David Hume, *A Treatise of Human Nature*, Book III, Part I (Everyman edition). In thus quoting Hume I do not wish to suggest that his is the only possible ethical theory.

† The reader who is interested in ethical questions should not fail to consult C. L. Stevenson's *Ethics and Language* which unfortunately did not come to my hands until after this book was written, although it was published in 1944. In it the reader will find a thorough and detailed discussion of the complicated relations between the propositional and the non-propositional elements in ethical acceptances.

theatre: 'Lecture in progress', all we know (or are intended to believe) is that someone is lecturing inside—that something is happening. That is one sense of 'progress'. But more often when we use this word we not only mean that something is happening, but also that later stages of the process are in some sense *better* than earlier ones, in the sense, namely, that someone desires and approves of them more than the earlier stages. Thus when a physician tells his patient's wife that her husband is making progress he means that the state of the patient to-day is nearer one of health than it was yesterday. As it is his professional business to restore persons to health, from his point of view the patient is making progress in the second sense of the word. And in announcing this to his wife the physician assumes that she loves her husband and also desires his restoration to health. But suppose that the patient's heir has long lost all tender feelings for his father, that he has recently become a parliamentary candidate and, having been engaged in shady financial transactions, is anxious to inherit his father's wealth in order to be able to cover up the consequences before the election. Then from the heir's point of view the patient will *not* have been making progress.

But in this example of the second sense of 'progress', although an element of evaluation is involved, it is not *ethical* evaluation. Neither the physician nor the wife are supposing that the patient's recovery is an instance of *moral* betterment.

Now in connexion with evolution we can certainly use the word 'progress' in the *first* sense because something is happening. But if we say that in evolution there is progress in the *second* sense, then we are giving utterance to a statement which can form no part of biology and hence cannot belong to the theory of evolution itself. For the desires of biologists and their sentiments of approval form no part either of the subject-matter of biology or of its statements.

When we speak of the members of one species being *better* adapted to their environment than those of another, although the word 'better' occurs, this does not at all mean that any element of evaluation is involved, unless we suppose that the organisms concerned *desire* to be better adapted or that *someone* desires that they should be. But in biology no such assumptions are made, except perhaps in some Lamarckian doctrines which form no part of present-day biology. Consequently this use of the word 'better' has nothing whatever to do with moral progress. It is surely as nonsensical to say that man is morally better than a tape-worm as it would be to say that he is morally better than one of the square roots of 2. The attempt to base ethical acceptances on evolution is therefore a misuse of the rationalist tradition, and the author of such acceptances would be doing no more than giving expression to his own ethical predilections.

For different people, having (to repeat Hume's words) a 'different sentiment of blame from the contemplation of' the same mode of conduct according to the different constitution of their natures, will adopt different ethical acceptances. But owing to the persistence of the rationalist tradition and the objectifying effect of acceptances, they will fail to see the purely personal factors which have entered into their choice. Certain eugenical enthusiasts, for example, have from time to time advocated certain measures for what they call the betterment of the human race, while at the same time failing to see that there are many conflicting views about what would constitute betterment. For the betterment of the tough is quite different from the betterment of the tender, and the betterment of the rich is different again from the betterment of the poor. Such a procedure would therefore involve some people in paying a price for a change which they would not regard as betterment.

Another question in connexion with which there is conflict between the satisfaction of scientific needs and the claims of certain ethical acceptances is that of vivisection. Some scientific men appear to believe that there should be no restriction on vivisection, others hold that this type of experiment is only justified if it clearly and closely relates to the relief of human suffering. This is a difficult question and is related to the question of pure science versus applied science. Some scientific puritans appear to believe that the only science which is justified is that which promotes industrial or agricultural production and that all scientific research should be co-ordinated and planned with that end in view. The difficulty about this is that it is quite impossible to predict what applications may subsequently be found for a piece of pure science which is carried out primarily for the satisfaction of intellectual needs. The history of science shows abundantly that seemingly remote investigations, in pure mathematics for example, may ultimately have important technological applications which were not at all anticipated. Now if we admit the principle that vivisection is justified if it helps to relieve human suffering, then it is clear that the foregoing argument can be used to justify unrestricted vivisection.

But it is in connexion with technological applications that the scientific activity comes most strikingly into conflict with different attitudes towards the art of living together which are expressed in different ethical acceptances. Those who regard speed as part of the good life will welcome the advent of the internal combustion engine, in spite of the number of people who are killed annually on the roads or by bombing during successive world wars. Conflicts of this kind even raise doubts about the invocation of successful technological applications as part of the pragmatic justification of scientific acceptances. This will, however, depend upon the ethical type from the standpoint of which a particular technological application is judged. What is approved by the tough may be condemned by the tender.

But people of all ethical types have now had it vividly brought home to them that perhaps after all applied science is not an unmixed blessing. This is of course not so much a conflict of acceptances as a conflict of needs. Technological applications which satisfy some needs may make the satisfaction of others impossible. The invention of weapons of destruction of the most devastating kind threatens to make the satisfaction of *all* needs impossible, unless we adopt the Freudian acceptance that death is itself a need.

The passage from Lord Russell about Nietzsche which I have quoted ended with the words 'His followers have had their innings, but we may hope that it is coming rapidly to an end'. I must confess that I find it very difficult to share this optimism. Although the tough-tender antithesis by no means corresponds with geographical, political or racial boundaries, in this country we have slowly learnt to be less tough and to achieve social co-ordination by consent, rather than by coercion. We have long ago abolished the slave trade, duelling, public executions, arbitrary arrest, and other horrors. In spite of protests from some quarters we are trying to abolish the flogging of children and adults. From the standpoint of the tender these are steps in the direction of increasing civilization, but in the eyes of the tough they are merely manifestations of weakness and degeneracy. In some other countries, however, during the first half of the present century, there seems to have been a return to, or an increase in, the appeal to force and violence. History is very largely a dismal record of the consequences of the intolerant adherence to acceptances, and of the effort to impose them by force upon whole populations. Countless millions of people have been tortured or butchered in this process. In former days these persecutions were connected with religious acceptances, to-day they are used to enforce racial, nationalistic and political ones. If some reports are to be believed there is even persecution connected with scientific acceptances. The history of the Inquisition of the Roman Church is interesting in this connexion. It did not begin until early in the thirteenth century and was not finally abolished in Spain until the nineteenth. During all those centuries sects were constantly springing up, or persisting secretly, under the inspiration of men who were prepared to risk death or imprisonment for the right to live by acceptances of their own choosing. The story of the Inquisition thus illustrates the failure to impose acceptances upon people by coercion. Unhappily, applied science has placed in the hands of modern governments much more powerful instruments for this purpose than were available to the officers of the Inquisition.

Now the kind of society we achieve will depend in part on the kind of psychological, sociological and ethical acceptances we adopt. The kind of acceptances we adopt will depend upon the type of person we are, and the type of person we are will, according to Suttie, depend in part on the type of mother we have had. From the sociological point of view Suttie's doctrine is thus in the tradition of Robert Owen who proclaimed, to the deaf ears of his generation:

It must be evident to those who have been in the practice of observing children with attention, that much of good and evil is taught or acquired by the child at a very early period of its life; that much of temper or disposition is correctly or incorrectly formed before he attains his second year; and that many durable impressions are made at the termination of the first twelve or even six months of his existence.*

Suttie's great merit was to specify in detail some of the factors upon which in early infancy the development of the principal types of character depend.

Thus it is not *primarily* in economic conditions that the sources of wars and crimes are to be sought. The wars and peaces, the crimes and great social advances of the future are being secretly and unwittingly prepared in the millions of cradles and nurseries of the mansions, suburban villas and country cottages of the present day.

In the political oppositions to which I have alluded we have the tough and the tender in stark conflict—a conflict which may not be resolvable by compromise. Mankind seems to have devised but two ways of resolving such conflicts—the ballot and the bullet. If their opponents refuse to adopt the first alternative the tender are driven to use the very means which is most repugnant to them. It is to the refusal to acknowledge

A New View of Society (1813), third essay.

this most unpalatable situation that the failure of such institutions as the League of Nations has been traced.*

To repeat what was said in Lecture VII, our tragedy is not so much lack of knowledge of *how* to change the world, as lack of ability to agree about the direction in which to change it, and the means to be employed, owing to the existence of opposed psychological types. Suttie's doctrine offers perhaps one small gleam of hope. According to this the lust for power and the impulses towards violence are manifestations of the frustration of the need for love. Normality, then, is on the side of the tender. Were it otherwise it would be difficult to understand how, in this harsh world, the tender have survived at all. There is therefore some hope that, with the better education of mothers and the improvement of personal relations within families (provided the tough do not meanwhile, with the help of applied science, render the earth uninhabitable through radioactivity), toughness will ultimately become rarer. Only then will it be possible for the State to wither away. Perhaps it is in this sense that some day the meek will inherit the earth:

Though I speak with the tongues of men and of angels, and have not charity, I am become as sounding brass, or a tinkling cymbal.

And though I have the gift of prophecy, and understand all mysteries, and all knowledge; and though I have all faith, so that I could remove mountains, and have not charity, I am nothing.

* See Hans J. Morgenthau, *Scientific Man vs. Power Politics* (1947), p. 59.

POSTSCRIPT

(*see* p. 182)

After reading Professor Hogben's reassuring statement (quoted on p. 182) that 'genetical science has outgrown the false antithesis between heredity and environment' it is very discouraging to find the following passage in a paper by an eminent geneticist, written 20 years later (1951): 'One hears frequently that the organism is the product of heredity and environment. I cannot agree with this. Environment can affect the organism only within the limits set by its hereditary constitution. Beyond these limits there is no reaction or no organism. Thus, after all, it is heredity that makes the organism. This idea, a basic one, I think, is expressed best in Woltereck's definition of the genotype as a norm of reaction.'

This passage illustrates only too well many of the points which have been discussed in Part II—the use of abstract substantives like 'heredity', of metaphors like that of 'making' organisms, and the strange but not uncommon use of 'definition'. So long as geneticists continue to be satisfied with language of this kind in serious scientific discourse the false antithesis will not be outgrown. The author quoted omits to mention that its hereditary constitution can affect the organism only within the limits set by its environment. (The best genes in the world will do little in strong sulphuric acid, so again there is 'no organism'.) The use of a functor of degree three would prevent such omissions and reveal the falsity of the antithesis.

INDEX OF NAMES OF PERSONS

SUBJECT INDEX